OXFORD MEDICAL PUBLICATIONS

The Neuropathology of Schizophrenia

The Neuropathology of Schizophrenia

Progress and Interpretation

Edited by
Paul J. Harrison
University Department of Psychiatry, University of Oxford, Oxford, UK

And

Gareth W. Roberts
Opine Consultancy, Cambridge, UK

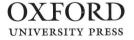

OXFORD
UNIVERSITY PRESS

OXFORD

UNIVERSITY PRESS

Oxford University Press, Great Clarendon Street, Oxford OX2 6DP

Oxford University Press is a department of the University of Oxford.

It furthers the University's objective of excellence in research, scholarship,
and education by publishing worldwide in
Oxford New York
Athens Auckland Bangkok Bogota Buenos Aires Calcutta
Cape Town Chennai Dar es Salaam Delhi Florence Hong Kong Istanbul
Karachi Kuala Lumpur Madrid Melbourne Mexico City Mumbai
Nairobi Paris São Paulo Singapore Taipei Tokyo Toronto Warsaw

with associated companies in Berlin Ibadan

Oxford is a registered trade mark of Oxford University Press
in the UK and in certain other countries

Published in the United States
by Oxford University Press Inc., New York

A catalogue record for this title is available from the British Library

Library of Congress Cataloging in Publication Data
The neuropathology of schizophrenia/edited by Paul J. Harrison and Gareth W. Roberts.
(Oxford medical publications)
Includes bibliographical references and index.
1. Schizophrenia–Pathophysiology. 2. Schizophrenia–Etiology. I. Harrison, P. J. (Paul
J.), 1960– II. Roberts, Gareth W. III. Series.
[DNLM: 1. Schizophrenia–physiopathology. 2. Brain–physiopathology. 3. Nervous
System–physiopathology. 4. Schizophrenia–etiology. WM 203 N49367 2000]
RC514.N446 2000   616.89¢8207–dc21   00-038497

1 3 5 7 9 10 8 6 4 2

ISBN 0 19 262907 7

Typeset by
Florence Production Ltd, Stoodleigh, Devon
Printed in Great Britain
on acid-free paper by
Biddles Ltd, Guildford & King's Lynn

Foreword

Janice Stevens

At the first International Congress of Neuropathology held in Turin, Italy in 1952, leading neuropathologists from the Americas, Europe, and Asia presented reports on the anatomical and histological pathology of schizophrenia. Using conventional techniques, and relying on their clinical experience rather than the now requisite blind comparison with controls, many of these investigators described a variety of abnormalities deemed pathological in the brains of patients with schizophrenia. Most of these findings have since been challenged, failed replication, were considered unrelated to the illness, or have been forgotten. With a few important exceptions, neuropathologists turned their attention to other, more data-rich areas such as the dementias, demyelinating disorders and neuromuscular disorders. For the next 25 years, neuropathological progress was primarily neurochemical, with the crucial discovery of the phenothiazines, and the emergence of the dopamine hypothesis.

The attention of psychiatrists to neuropathology in a structural sense was renewed by the study of Johnstone and colleagues (*Lancet* 1976, **ii**; 924–6), who reported enlarged ventricles in 15/17 (including four lobotomized) institutionalized, chronically ill patients with schizophrenia, compared to controls matched for age and pre-morbid socioeconomic status. This study was the first to use computed tomography to demonstrate ventricular enlargement, although its occurrence in a subgroup of patients had been described much earlier in the century both at autopsy and by pneumoencephalography. After the Johnstone *et al.* study, numerous confirmatory brain imaging results followed, brain banks were established, regional and international meetings were organized, and psychiatric journals – which had generally been devoted to psychological and behavioral aspects of the disorder – again included neurological and pathological studies of schizophrenia.

This unique volume chronicles and adds to the progress that has been made in unravelling the mystery of the neuropathology of schizophrenia by many of the leading investigators over the last 20 years. The progress has been driven by several advances. In contrast to the early reports, cases are now much more rigorously diagnosed using standard clinical criteria. Age and gender matched controls are included, and investigators are blind to diagnosis during examination and analysis of the material. New methods of anatomical and functional brain imaging, immunohistochemistry and molecular biology have made possible observations into entirely new parameters of neuropathology. Use of these techniques has produced a rich galaxy of recent findings.

The contributions in this book make it clear that significant strides have been made both in ruling in and ruling out potential features of the neuropathology of schizophrenia. However, they also show that in many areas, controversy over the data or their interpretation continue.

Three such themes are worth briefly highlighting here. The first concerns the question of pathological heterogeneity and the relationship of the clinical syndrome to the underlying structural substrate(s). The increasing number and variety of anatomical, histological and molecular findings reported in the brains from individuals diagnosed with schizophrenia suggests that the syndrome, like epilepsy or mental retardation, may be a final result of many different deviations, or an accumulation of such disturbances. If schizophrenia is a disorder of heterogeneous origin, obtaining consistent and significant results after pooling and averaging results from increasing numbers of cases will be difficult. The important pathological alterations reviewed in this volume occur in subgroups of patients and rarely if ever provide a clear distinction of cases from controls. To disaggregate the pathological endophenotype in search of significant factors, including genotype, study of statistical outliers for a given measure (who often account for the averaged differences) could lead to a new, biologically based classification of the syndrome. In support of this approach, similar disaggregation helped the identification of genetic anomalies in other complex neurological disorders previously deemed idiopathic, such as the epilepsies and muscular dystrophies. The pathological, but not pathognomonic, changes described in the elegant studies presented in these chapters should be invaluable springboards for segregating patients into cohorts who share similar deviations, and thus allow investigators to search more effectively for the causes of schizophrenia.

The second controversy concerns the location of the pathological changes. The focus of recent imaging and histological studies has largely been upon the cerebral cortex and hippocampus, yet there are reasons not to neglect other structures. For example, the most frequent gross pathologies in schizophrenia are enlargement of the third ventricle and lateral ventricles, both of which generally signify loss of sub-cortical tissue, most often thalamus, basal ganglia, or the pathways to and from these structures. Proponents of cortical pathology must also deal with the fact that the electroencephalogram, a sensitive record of cortical electrical activity, is considered normal in most individuals with schizophrenia, suggesting that the principal pathology may not be in the cortex in a majority of cases.

The final issue is one of the timing of pathology. The fact that skull and head size are normal in over 90% of individuals with schizophrenia, and that skull size depends on brain size, means that the cortical atrophy and reduced brain volume reported in the disorder must have occurred after brain growth ceases at around 6 years of age. This casts doubt on currently popular theories that schizophrenia is due to a pre- or peri-natal neurodevelopmental disturbance, a doubt amplified by the fact that in most if not all developmental neurological disorders, symptoms are manifest in infancy or childhood, whereas a majority of individuals with schizophrenia are considered normal prior to the onset of symptoms in late adolescence or adulthood.

These controversies are a sign of an active but difficult research field which has come a long way since the 1952 Congress, but which still has far to go. Rigour and ingenuity, as well as a willingness to cast out cherished ideas and shibboleths when necessary, will be needed for progress to continue. This volume is a comprehensive and critical overview of the neuropathology of schizophrenia as currently understood. It is also a timely one, as we pass the centenary of Kraepelin's delineation of the syndrome and his initial attempts to discover its pathological basis.

Contents

List of contributors

Mayada Akil, Clinical Brain Disorders Branch, Intramural Research Program, National Institute of Mental Health, Bethesda, MD 20892, USA

Nancy C. Andreasen, Mental Health Clinical Research Center, University of Iowa Hospitals and Clinics, Iowa City, Iowa 52242, USA

Steven E. Arnold, Center for Neurobiology and Behavior, University of Pennsylvania, 142 Clinical Research Building, 415 Curie Boulevard, Philadelphia, PA 19104, USA

Francine M. Benes, Laboratory for Structural Neuroscience, McLean Hospital, 115 Mill St, Belmont, MA 02178, USA and Program in Neuroscience and Department of Psychiatry, Harvard Medical School, Boston MA 02115, USA

Siew E. Chua, Department of Psychiatry, University of Hong Kong, Queen Mary Hospital, Pokfulam Road, Hong Kong

Margaret M. Esiri, University Department of Neuropathology (Clinical Neurology), Radcliffe Infirmary, Oxford OX2 6HE, UK

Peter Falkai, Department of Psychiatry, University of Bonn Medical Centre, Bonn, Germany

Albert M. Galaburda, Departments of Psychiatry and Neurology, Beth Israel Deaconess Medical Center and Harvard Medical School, Boston MA 02115, USA

Paul J. Harrison, Neurosciences Building, University Department of Psychiatry, Warneford Hospital, Oxford OX3 7JX, UK

Dorothy P. Holinger, Departments of Psychiatry and Neurology, Beth Israel Deaconess Medical Center and Harvard Medical School, Boston MA 02115, USA

Richard Hopkins, School of Psychiatry and Behavioural Sciences, University of Manchester, Manchester M20 8LR, UK

William G. Honer, Department of Psychiatry, University of British Columbia, Jack Bell Research Center, 2660 Oak Street, Vancouver, V6H 3Z6 Canada

Joel E. Kleinman, Clinical Brain Disorders Branch, National Institute of Mental Health, Bethesda MD 20892, USA

David A. Lewis, Departments of Psychiatry and Neuroscience, University of Pittsburgh, Pittsburgh, PA 15213, USA

Shôn Lewis, School of Psychiatry and Behavioural Sciences, University of Manchester, Manchester M20 8LR, UK

Barbara K. Lipska, Clinical Brain Disorders Branch, Intramural Research Program, National Institute of Mental Health, NIH, Bethesda MD 20892, USA

Peter J. McKenna, Fulbourn Hospital, Cambridge CB1 5EF, UK

R. Carl A. Pearson, Department of Biomedical Sciences, Sheffield University, Sheffield S10 2TN, UK

Jack Price, Institute of Psychiatry, London SE5 8AF, UK

Gareth W. Roberts, Opine Consultancy, The Grange, Church Street, Great Shelford, Cambridge CB2 5EL, UK

Susan K. Schultz, Department of Psychiatry, University of Iowa Hospitals and Clinics, Iowa City, Iowa 52242, USA

Janice R. Stevens, Department of Neurology and Psychiatry, Oregon Health Sciences University, Portland, Oregon 97201, USA

Daniel R. Weinberger, Clinical Brain Disorders Branch, Intramural Research Program, National Institute of Mental Health, NIH, Bethesda MD 20892, USA

Clint Young, Department of Psychiatry, University of British Columbia, Vancouver, V6H 3Z6 Canada

Introduction

Paul J. Harrison and Gareth W. Roberts

Few subjects have generated as much sustained controversy in the field of medicine as the neuropathology of schizophrenia—the Holy Grail of biological psychiatry. At times it has been considered a misguided or meaningless question to ask, reflecting contemporary opinions as to the nature of the relationship between mind and brain, distress, and disease. At the other extreme, eminent psychiatrists and neuropathologists throughout the twentieth century had described putative histological explanations for schizophrenia. Neither of these polarised views can be sustained, the nihilists falling into the dualist trap, and the empiricists finding that the results were not repeatable or were artefactual.

The failure to make unequivocal breakthroughs culminated with the infamous dictum that schizophrenia is the 'graveyard of neuropathologists' (Plum, 1972). The metaphor captured both the dearth of results and, by that time, the dearth of research activity. However, soon afterwards, another cycle of interest in the subject began, reflected in influential discussion papers concerning the anatomical basis of schizophrenia (Stevens, 1973; Torrey and Peterson, 1974) and the seminal report of Johnstone and colleagues (Johnstone *et al.*, 1976). It is the latter paper which really forms the starting point for this book, since it prefaced an ongoing generation of structural imaging studies which have shown with ever greater reliability and accuracy that there *is* a neuropathology of schizophrenia, at least at the macroscopic level. This realization in turn formed the prelude to, and stimulus for, contemporary microscopic studies of schizophrenia. Thus the book starts with a detailed review of the imaging literature, by Hopkins and Lewis (Chapter 1). The next four chapters cover the histological studies which have attempted to find the tissue correlates of the imaging alterations. Most of the work has concentrated on the hippocampus and cerebral cortex, covered by Arnold (Chapter 2) and Benes (Chapter 3), respectively. Honer, Young, and Falkai review the evidence for synaptic and dendritic pathology (Chapter 4), an area of current interest. Chapters 2 to 4 show how, over the past 15 years, attention has turned to the cortical cytoarchitecture—the morphology, arrangement, and connectivity of neurons—in schizophrenia. This has arisen partly because of the failure to find consistent evidence for gliosis (Chapter 5), and hence the implication that the disorder is developmental not degenerative. Another research theme is cerebral lateralisation, and in Chapter 6 Holinger, Galaburda, and Harrison review the neuropathological evidence for altered brain asymmetry in schizophrenia.

In different ways, the remaining chapters all focus primarily on the interpretation of the neuropathology of schizophrenia, something which has proven almost as controversial as the data themselves. Schultz and Andreasen discuss how neuropathology and pathophysiology in schizophrenia may be related, as illustrated by comparisons of the functional and structural imaging results (Chapter 7). The neurodevelopmental model of schizophrenia has become the most influential view of the nature of the disorder, so Akil and Weinberger review the hypothesis in terms of how it has affected, and has been affected by, the neuropathological findings (Chapter 8). Because the hypothesis needs to be informed by advances in developmental neurobiology, in Chapter 9 Price and Roberts cover the principles of brain development and the genes involved. Following on from this, Lewis describes the organisation of the cortical circuitry, linking its developmental origins to the ways in which it may be affected in schizophrenia. Broadening the perspective, in Chapter 11, Esiri and Pearson discuss how other neuropathological disorders, and the results of experimental lesions, can help refine interpretation of the findings in schizophrenia. Animal models provide another approach to neuropathology, and Lipska and Weinberger discuss the strengths and weaknesses of relevant models in Chapter 12.

The final three chapters discuss the limitations and difficulties of the field. Chua and McKenna (Chapter 13) provide an alternative view of the imaging and histological studies of schizophrenia, giving a valuable, sceptical critique and demonstrating that experimental and interpretational rigour remain essential if mistakes of the past are not to be repeated. The key methodological issues are reviewed by Harrison and Kleinman in Chapter 14, with discussion in Chapter 15 by Harrison of the specific problem of confounding by antipsychotic medication and other treatments.

We hope that the book provides a balanced, comprehensive, and up-to-date overview of the neuropathology of schizophrenia, a field now large enough to benefit from such a volume, yet one where the rate of progress is not so fast that it will become rapidly obsolete. Though the book documents clearly where the neuropathology of schizophrenia has got to, we can only speculate as to its future course. There are grounds for optimism that amongst the myriad of positive findings are a few which are genuine histological and molecular correlates of schizophrenia. With appropriately designed and powered studies this crucial stage of separating the wheat from the chaff should be completed in the next few years. As the cardinal changes emerge (and the broader understanding of brain development and disease progresses in parallel), the neuropathology of schizophrenia can be linked more clearly both to the clinical phenotype and to the key pathogenic and aetiological factors. The difficulty of this task should not be underestimated—research into the dementias shows just how complex the relationships between these facets of a disease can be. Nevertheless, at least the field no longer has to worry that there is no demonstrable pathology, and it can concentrate instead on maximising the speed and clarity with which it is revealed.

We thank all the authors for their contributions, Margaret Cousin for secretarial assistance, Sharon Eastwood for the index, and OUP for their patience.

August 2000
P.J.H.
G.W.R.

References to the Introduction

Johnstone EC, Crow TJ, Frith CD, Husband J, Kreel L (1976) Cerebral ventricular size and cognitive impairment in chronic schizophrenia. *Lancet* **ii**, 924–926.

Plum F (1972) Prospects for research on schizophrenia. Neuropathological findings. *Neuroscience Research Program Bulletin* **10**, 384–388.

Stevens JR (1973) An anatomy of schizophrenia? *Archives of General Psychiatry* **29**,177–189.

Torrey EF, Peterson MR (1974) Schizophrenia and the limbic system. *Lancet* **ii**, 942–946.

1 Structural Imaging Findings and Macroscopic Pathology

Richard Hopkins and Shôn Lewis

From its inception as dementia praecox over a hundred years ago, schizophrenia was considered to be a disorder of the brain (Kraepelin, 1896). There were numerous early attempts to isolate the presumed macroscopic and microscopic pathology (e.g. Alzheimer, 1897; Southard, 1915), mainly inspired by concurrent successes in the neuropathology of general paralysis of the insane. However, research was unable consistently to replicate findings, considerably hindered as it was by a lack of operationalised diagnostic criteria, problems with the selection of brains for analysis, postmortem artefacts, and inadequate controls (see Chapter 14). The diagnostic non-specificity of findings, and the absence of an overall hypothesis also hampered the development of a consensus view. Even Kraepelin, whilst remaining optimistic that a neuropathological basis for schizophrenia would

Table 1.1 Macroscopic postmortem findings in schizophrenia[1]

Parameter	Alteration in schizophrenia	Positive reports	Negative reports
General			
Brain weight	Decreased	Brown et al, 1986[2] Pakkenberg, 1987 Bruton et al, 1990[3]	Bogerts et al, 1990b Heckers et al, 1991 Arnold et al, 1995a Zaidel et al, 1997 Highley et al, 1999a
Cortical size	Decreased	Pakkenberg, 1987	Heckers et al, 1991
Brain length	Decreased	Bruton et al, 1990	
Ventricular size	Increased	Brown et al, 1986[2] Pakkenberg, 1987 Crow et al, 1989 Bruton et al, 1990	
Temporal lobe			
Overall size	Decreased	Highley et al, 1999c	Brown et al, 1986[2]
Hippocampal formation	Decreased	Bogerts et al, 1985 Falkai & Bogerts, 1986 Jeste & Lohr, 1989 Bogerts et al, 1990b	Heckers et al, 1990 Altshuler et al, 1990
Parahippocampal gyrus/entorhinal cortex	Decreased	Bogerts et al, 1985 Falkai et al, 1988 Altshuler et al, 1990	Brown et al, 1986[2]
Amygdala	Decreased	Bogerts et al, 1985	Heckers et al, 1990 Pakkenburg, 1990
Superior temporal gyrus	Decreased	Vogeley et al, 1998 Highley et al, 1999c	
Sulcogyral patterns	Abnormal	Jakob & Beckmann, 1986 Highley et al, 1998	Bruton et al, 1990
Other Areas			
Globus pallidus		Bogerts et al, 1985	Bogerts et al, 1990a Pakkenburg, 1990 Heckers et al, 1991
Caudate putamen	Increase	Heckers et al, 1991	Bogerts et al, 1985 Brown et al, 1986[2]
Nucleus accumbens	Decreased	Pakkenberg, 1990	Bogerts et al, 1985 Bogerts et al, 1990b
Corpus callosum	Abnormal size or thickness	Rosenthal & Bigelow, 1972 Bigelow et al, 1983	Brown et al, 1986[2] Highley et al, 1999a
Thalamus	Unchanged	Bogerts et al, 1985	
Mediodorsal thalamus	Decreased	Pakkenberg, 1990	
Periventricular grey matter	Thinned	Lesch & Bogerts, 1984	
Substantia nigra (lateral)	Decreased volume	Bogerts et al, 1983	
Locus coeruleus	Unchanged	Lohr & Jeste, 1988	
Anterior commissure	Unchanged	Highley et al, 1999b	

[1]For clarity, the table does not indicate studies which found interactions with gender or hemisphere. (See text, and Chapter 6.)
[2]Compared to affective disorder controls.
[3]Fixed but not fresh brain weights differed between groups.

eventually be identified, became sceptical of the 'brain mythologists' (Kraepelin, 1919). With the emergence of the psychoanalytic movement, particularly in the United States, and vocal disagreements between neuropathologists about the interpretation of findings, the focus moved from brain to mind. The nadir was reached in the 1970s, with the dismissal or disregard of essentially all extant neuropathological findings (Corsellis, 1976) and coining of the (in)famous quote that schizophrenia is the 'graveyard of neuropathologists' (Plum, 1972).

Subsequently, there has been a renaissance of interest in the subject, driven by *in vivo* brain imaging, initially with CT and more recently MRI. This chapter reviews the evidence for macroscopic alterations in brain structure in schizophrenia. Though the main focus is on imaging, macroscopic postmortem findings are mentioned, and are summarised in Table 1.1. Together the findings have provided a rationale and impetus to the new generation of microscopic and molecular neuropathological investigations covered in later chapters.

In vivo brain imaging in schizophrenia

Computed tomography

Johnstone *et al.* (1976) carried out the landmark CT study, reporting ventricular dilatation in a group of patients with chronic schizophrenia. There had been over 30 pneumoencephalography (PEG) studies during the preceding 40 years which in some cases had also shown gross ventricular enlargement and cortical atrophy. PEG was however a difficult and potentially dangerous procedure, and subject to the same diagnostic and other methodological limitations mentioned above. In their review, Weinberger *et al.* (1983) identified only six PEG studies worthy of mention; all but one reported some degree of ventricular enlargement in schizophrenia. In contrast to PEG, CT provided axial images of the brain which were much quicker, safer, and more comfortable to obtain. These factors, coupled with the introduction of operationalised criteria for schizophrenia during the 1970s, were crucial advances.

Despite its importance, the then state of neuropathological research in schizophrenia was such that the Johnstone *et al.* (1976) report was treated with initial scepticism. However, whilst it was 3 years before the next report of CT abnormalities in schizophrenia (Weinberger *et al.*, 1979) by 1990 there had been over 50 studies (Lewis, 1990). These generally confirmed a small but significant enlargement of the ventricular system in schizophrenia, primarily in the lateral and third ventricles. Problems in the selection of normal control scans may have over-estimated the degree of dilatation in earlier studies (van Horn and McManus, 1992) but, nevertheless, a significant ventricular enlargement remained a robust finding in systematic reviews (Raz and Raz, 1990; van Horn and McManus, 1992). The meta-analysis of Raz and Raz (1990) reported that lateral ventricular size was increased in schizophrenia with a medium average effect size (Cohen's d) of 0.70, representing a 43 per cent non-overlap between the patient and control distributions. There was a similar effect size for third ventricular enlargement ($d = 0.66$). There is also CT-derived evidence of an increased size of cortical sulcal spaces in schizophrenia suggestive of underlying cortical atrophy (Lewis, 1990), although there has been less consistency in how sulcal CSF spaces are measured, making systematic reviews more difficult. Despite this, Raz and Raz (1990) were able to calculate a significant average effect size for cortical sulcal CSF enlargement in schizophrenia, albeit of a lesser degree to that found for the ventricular system, with $d = 0.35$.

These cortical and subcortical CSF space abnormalities are clearly quantitative rather than qualitative. There has been no consistent evidence of bimodality in their distribution to suggest pathognomonic differences in patients or even a subgroup of patients (Harvey *et al.*, 1990; Daniel *et al.*, 1991). The hypothesis of Crow (1980) that there are two types of schizophrenia, type II being characterised by negative symptoms, poor treatment response, poor outcome, and structural brain abnormalities, generated much research but in the end received little experimental support. Other relationships between CSF space enlargements and aetiological, demographic, or illness-related factors have also proven inconsistent in the CT literature, although associations between ventricular enlargement, neuropsychological impairments, and negative symptoms have been reported (Lewis, 1990).

Magnetic resonance imaging

MRI is a safe, non-invasive technique for imaging the brain in any plane with a much enhanced resolution over CT, improved multiplanar imaging, and good grey–white matter differentiation. Modern scanning systems are able to obtain whole brain images within short time periods, particularly if equipped with echoplanar imaging. Unlike CT, the thickness of individual slices can be of the same order as the size of the pixels within each slice. Such isomorphic voxels (three-dimensional (3D) pixels) with a resolution of about 1 mm^3 reduce partial volume artefacts, which occur when large voxels contain significant proportions of two or more tissue types, and which were a significant source of measurement error in the CT and early MRI studies. With advances in image post-processing techniques, it is now possible to measure reliably the volumes of both cortical and subcortical structures in a semi-automated way. Most recently MRI has allowed high resolution 3D renderings of the brain to be constructed, with more accurate identification of anatomical landmarks, and allowing for *in vivo* 3D shape analysis (e.g. of cortical gyrification; see below). Because of the many advantages of MRI, CT is in most respects now a redundant research tool. Nevertheless, MRI studies of schizophrenia have their own methodological problems, which are summarised in the final section together with suggestions as to how they may be combatted.

Brain morphology in schizophrenia

Ventricular and sulcal abnormalities

Initial MRI studies attempted to replicate the CT findings by focusing on the sizes of the CSF spaces. They have generally confirmed that the ventricular system is enlarged in schizophrenia (Table 1.2). Most consistently reported are enlargements of the lateral ventricles, by a median of 28 per cent (range –30 to 92 per cent). Laterality and gender interactions with schizophrenia have been inconsistently reported (Table 1.2; see also Chapters 6 and 7). Examination of subdivisions of the lateral ventricles has also been limited, although the temporal horns appear to be most consistently affected. MRI studies show that the third ventricle is also enlarged in schizophrenia, with a median volume increase of 30 per cent. Third ventricular enlargement is of particular interest as adjacent structures, particularly the thalamus, may be a site of pathology (see below). No sex effects on third ventricular enlargement in schizophrenia have been found (Lauriello *et al.*, 1997; Pearlson *et al.*, 1997). Fourth ventricle enlargement was particularly difficult to measure with CT due to bony artefact in the posterior fossa. MRI has been used to image this ventricle in a handful of studies, with a median enlargement of 8 per cent. Its significance, both statistically and functionally, remains unclear.

Recent advances in morphometric analysis allow shape differences in the ventricular system to be examined. Buckley *et al.* (1999) failed to find any significant differences in women with schizophrenia, but in the male patient groups there was a significant shape difference in the region of the foramen of Monro and proximal temporal horns bilaterally, which appeared to be due to a dorsal shifting of identified temporal horn landmarks.

Cortical CSF spaces have also been found to be enlarged in schizophrenia (Table 1.2). The increases appear greater in the frontal (13 per cent), temporal (17 per cent), and parietal (20 per cent) areas compared with the occipital area (6 per cent). This apparent regional difference may be an artefact of the smaller number of studies which have examined regional, and in particular posterior volumes, as the overall cortical CSF increase is of the order of 11 per cent. Alternatively, it may reflect unequal underlying cortical tissue loss (Pearlson *et al.*, 1996). No gender effect on cortical CSF spaces has been reported, either globally or regionally. (Gender differences, and gender by hemisphere interactions do exist with regard to the Sylvian fissure; Chapter 6.) Significant lateralization effects for frontal cortical CSF have been reported in three of five studies, with right > left sulcal enlargement (Marsh *et al.*, 1997, 1999; Zipursky *et al.*, 1997); for temporal lobe cortical CSF, one of four studies found a similar asymmetry (Marsh *et al.*, 1999).

There is no apparent correlation between the volumes of cortical and ventricular CSF spaces, which has led some authors to suggest different mechanisms underlying their enlargement.

Intracranial and cerebral size

A number of studies have suggested reductions in head size, intracranial volume, and brain size in schizophrenia. Again this literature is at first sight inconclusive, with the majority of published studies reporting non-significant differences (Table 1.3). Nevertheless the majority of negative studies (89 per cent) show a difference in the direction of a reduction in the schizophrenic subjects, with a median decrease in brain size of 3 per cent. Nine studies have tested for hemisphere and seven for gender effects in schizophrenia, with no significant results.

Ward *et al.* (1996) carried out a meta-analysis of all the available postmortem, CT and MRI studies. Summarising all studies of adequate quality, they showed that in schizophrenia there is a highly significant reduction in brain size and to a lesser extent intracranial

Table 1.2 Intracranial CSF space volumes in schizophrenia*

Structure	Adjusted[a]	Decreased in schizophrenia — All trend (p > 0.05) except w (p < 0.05)	Increased in schizophrenia — Trend (> p0.05)	Increased in schizophrenia — Significant (p ≤ 0.05)	Summary of findings
Total CSF	Yes			Zipursky et al, 1998a Zipursky et al, 1997 Nopoulos et al, 1997a Nopoulos et al, 1995b Andreasen et al,1994b	*%difference[b]*
	No	Shenton et al, 1992 Gur et al, 1991[F]	Pearlson et al 1997 Gur et al, 1994 Harvey et al, 1993[F] Pearlson et al, 1993[I] Gur et al, 1991[M] Jernigan et al, 1991	Harvey et al, 1993[M]	*Median* Total: 12% Ventricular: 20% *Range* Total:–4 to 35% Ventricular:–26 to 70%
Ventricular CSF	Yes		Nopoulos et al, 1997a[F] Zipursky et al, 1997 Corey-Bloom et al, 1995 Gur et al, 1994[M]	Cannon et al, 1998 Zipursky et al, 1998a Nopoulos et al, 1997a[M] Rapoport et al, 1997[m] Corey-Bloom et al, 1995[I] Andreasen et al, 1994b Gur et al, 1994[F] Jernigan et al, 1991	*Sex × diagnosis[c]* Total:14% (7), M > F Ventricular: 17% (6), M > F
	No	Shenton et al, 1991	Gur et al, 1994[M] Woods et al, 1991	Rapoport et al, 1997[m] Gur et al, 1994[F] Degreef et al, 1992a Degreef et al, 1991	*Side × diagnosis[d]* Total: 0% (1) Ventricular: 0% (1)

Table 1.2 continued

Structure	Adjusted[a]	Decreased in schizophrenia	Increased in schizophrenia		Summary of findings
			Trend (p > 0.05)	Significant (p ≤ 0.05)	% difference[b]
Lateral Ventricles (LV)	Yes	Harvey et al, 1993[Mp]	Lawrie et al, 1999[n] Marsh et al, 1999[p] Roy et al, 1998 Woodruff et al, 1997b Rossi et al, 1994 Harvey et al, 1993[FRp] Pearlson et al, 1993[l] Shenton et al, 1992	Marsh et al, 1999[q] Sharma et al, 1998 Whitworth et al, 1998[no] Barr et al, 1997 Frazier et al, 1996[m] Lim et al, 1996b Flaum et al, 1995 Zipursky et al, 1994[e] Harvey et al, 1993[FLp] Dauphinais et al, 1990 Suddath et al, 1989 Kelsoe et al, 1988	*Median* LV: 28% TH: 28% *Range* LV: −30 to 92% TH: 10 to 133% *Sex × diagnosis[c]* LV: 13% (8), F > M 25% (8), M > F TH: 0% (3)
	No	Shenton et al, 1991	Roy et al, 1998 Frazier et al, 1996[m] Andreasen et al, 1994b[F] Rossi et al, 1994b Andreasen et al, 1990[F] Kelsoe et al, 1988	Barr et al, 1997 Lauriello et al, 1997 Lim et al, 1996a Lim et al, 1996b Lim et al, 1996c Woods et al, 1996 Nopoulos et al, 1995b Andreasen et al, 1994b[M] Gur et al, 1994 Degreef et al, 1992a O'Callagham et al, 1992 DeLisi et al, 1991a Andreasen et al, 1990[M] Dauphinais et al, 1990	*Side × diagnosis[d]* LV: 8% (12), L > R TH: 14% (7), L > R

Note on "Decreased in schizophrenia" column header: All trend (p > 0.05) except [w] (p < 0.05)

Table 1.2 continued

Structure	Adjusted[a]	Decreased in schizophrenia — All trend (p > 0.05) except w (p < 0.05)	Increased in schizophrenia — Trend (p > 0.05)	Increased in schizophrenia — Significant (p ≤ 0.05)	Summary of findings
Temporal Horn (TH)	Yes		Marsh et al, 1999[p] Woodruff et al, 1997b Flaum et al, 1995	Marsh et al, 1999[q] Roy et al, 1998	%difference[b]
	No		Pearlson et al, 1997	Roy et al, 1998 Barr et al, 1997 Degreef et al, 1992a	
Third Ventricle (3V)	Yes	Shenton et al, 1992	Roy et al, 1998	Marsh et al, 1999[pq] Lawrie et al, 1999[n] Woodruff et al, 1997b Laim et al, 1996c Flaum et al, 1995	*Median* 3V: 30% 4V: 8%
	No		Roy et al, 1998 DeLisi et al, 1991a Andreasen et al, 1990 Bogerts et al, 1990a Dauphinais et al, 1990	Pearlson et al, 1997 Lauriello et al, 1997 Lim et al, 1996a Lim et al, 1996c Marsh et al, 1994 Rossi et al, 1994b Pearlson et al, 1993[l] Degreef et al, 1992a Schwartzkopf et al, 1991 Barta et al, 1990	*Range* 3V: -5 to 73% 4V: -12 to 13% Sex × diagnosis[c] 3V: 0% (2) 4V: 0% (1)
Fourth Ventricle (4V)	Yes	Shenton et al, 1992	Lawrie et al, 1999[n] Woodruff et al, 1997b Jacobsen et al, 1997[am]	Aylward et al, 1994	
	No		Degreef et al, 1992a	Aylward et al, 1994	

Table 1.2 continued

Structure	Adjusted[a]	Decreased in schizophrenia All trend (p > 0.05) except w (p < 0.05)	Increased in schizophrenia Trend (p > 0.05)	Significant (p ≤ 0.05)	Summary of findings
Cortical CSF	Yes	Shenton et al, 1992 Shenton et al, 1991	Zipursky et al, 1998a Woodruff et al, 1997b Woods et al, 1996 Corey-Bloom et al, 1995 Gur et al, 1994	Cannon et al, 1998 Sullivan et al, 1998 Nopoulos et al, 1997a Nopoulos et al, 1995b Lim et al, 1996a Harvey et al, 1993 Jernigan et al, 1991	% difference[b] Median Total: 11% Frontal: 13% Temporal: 17% Parietal: 20% Occipital: 6%
	No	Gur et al, 1991[F]	Lauriello et al, 1997 Lim et al, 1996c Schlaepfer et al, 1994 Gur et al, 1994 Shenton et al, 1991	Woods et al, 1996 Lim et al, 1996a Gur et al, 1991[M]	Range Total:-7 to 27% Frontal:- 23% to 38% Temporal: 5 to 100% Parietal: 14–27% Occipital: 0–16%
Frontal CSF	Yes	Marsh et al, 1999[Lpfw] Marsh et al, 1999[Rpf] Marsh et al, 1999[qf] Marsh et al, 1997	Zipursky et al, 1997[Lg] Zipursky et al, 1997[h]	Cannon et al, 1998 Sullivan et al, 1998[gh] Zipursky et al, 1997[Rg] Woodruff et al, 1997b Turetsky et al, 1995 Andreasen et al, 1994b	Sex × diagnosis[c] Total: 0% (7) Frontal: 0% (3) Temporal: 0% (4) Parietal: 0% (2) Occipital: 0% (3)
	No		Woods et al, 1991		

Table 1.2 *continued*

Structure	Adjusted[a]	Decreased in schizophrenia — All trend (p > 0.05) except [w] (p < 0.05)	Increased in schizophrenia — Trend (p > 0.05)	Increased in schizophrenia — Significant (p ≤ 0.05)	Summary of findings
Temporal CSF	Yes		Marsh et al, 1999[L,p]; Zipursky et al, 1997[i,j]	Marsh et al, 1999[R,p]; Marsh et al, 1999[q]; Cannon et al, 1998; Sullivan et al, 1998[i,j]; Turetsky et al, 1995; Andreasen et al, 1994b	*Side × diagnosis*[d] Total: 0% (1) Frontal: 60% (5), R > L Temporal: 25% (4), R > L Parietal: (0) Occipital: 0% (1)
	No			Woods et al, 1991	
Parietal CSF	Yes			Sullivan et al, 1998; Andreasen et al, 1994b; Zipursky et al, 1997	
Occipital CSF	Yes	Zipursky et al, 1997[k]	Cannon et al, 1998[k]; Sullivan et al, 1998[k]	Andreasen et al, 1994b	

*Many of the studies include some subjects with schizophreniform or schizoaffective disorder.

[L]left; [R]right; [M]male; [F]female.

[a]Adjusted, i.e. whether controlled for height, head size, intracranial volume, or other relevant structure, by ratio, regression, or covariation. [b]% volume difference in schizophrenia; [c]% of studies finding a significant interaction (total number of studies); [d]% of studies finding a significant interaction (total number of studies); [e]body of lateral ventricles; [f]frontoparietal; [g]prefrontal; [h]frontal; [i]frontotemporal; [j]temporoparietal; [k]parieto-occipital; [L]Late-onset schizophrenia; [m]Child-onset schizophrenia; [n]first-episode patients; [o]chronically ill patients; [p]acutely psychotic patients; [q]chronic, severely ill patients.

Table 1.3 Intracranial and brain size in schizophrenia[*]

Structure	Decreased in schizophrenia		Increased in schizophrenia	Summary of findings
	Significant ($p < 0.05$)	Trend ($p > 0.05$)	Significant ($p \leq 0.05$)	
Intracranial size	Gur et al, 1998b[M] Gur et al, 1994	Gur et al, 1998b[F] Hirayasu et al, 1998[h] Keshavan et al, 1998 Lauriello et al, 1997 Lim et al, 1996c[h] Woods et al, 1996 Menon et al, 1995a Flaum et al, 1995 Buchanan et al, 1993 Harvey et al, 1993	Zipursky et al, 1997 McCarley et al, 1993 Shenton et al, 1992 Zipursky et al, 1992 Shenton et al, 1991	% difference[b] *Median* – 1% *Range* –6 to 4% Sex × diagnosis[c] 0% (3) Side× diagnosis[d] 0% (2)
Brain size	Tibbo et al, 1998 Whitworth et al, 1998[i] Woods et al, 1996 Jacobsen et al, 1997b[e] Andreasen et al, 1994b Gur et al, 1994 Harvey et al, 1993 Zipursky et al, 1992 Degreef et al, 1991	Hazlett et al, 1999 Velakoulis et al, 1999[hi] Buchanan et al, 1998 Gur et al, 1998b Sharma et al, 1998 Whitworth et al, 1998[h] Barta et al, 1997 Pearlson et al, 1997 Woodruff et al, 1997b	Lawrie et al, 1999[h] Roy et al, 1998 Shenton et al, 1991	% difference *Median* –3% *Range* –10 to 5% Sex × diagnosis[c] 0% (9)

Table 1.3 continued

Structure	Decreased in schizophrenia		Increased in schizophrenia	Summary of findings
	Significant ($p < 0.05$)	Trend ($p > 0.05$)	Significant ($p \leq 0.05$)	
		Cowell et al, 1996		Side $\times$ diagnosis[d]
		Kulynych et al, 1996		0% (7)
		Flaum et al, 1995		
		Nopoulos et al, 1995b		
		Bilder et al, 1994		
		Rossi et al, 1994		
		Schlaepfer et al, 1994		
		Kawasaki et al, 1993		
		Breier et al, 1992		
		DeLisi et al, 1991a		
		Woods et al, 1991		
		Barta et al, 1990		
		Dauphinais et al, 1990		
		Kelsoe et al, 1988		

*Many of the studies include some subjects with schizophreniform or schizoaffective disorder.

[a] No significance level given; [b] % volume difference in schizophrenia; % of studies finding a significant interaction (total number of studies); [d] % of studies finding a significant interaction (total number of studies); [e] Child-onset schizophrenia; [h] first-episode patients; [i] chronic patients; [M] male; [F] female.

size (including cortical CSF) irrespective of whether this was measured as an area or a volume. Extracranial size was unaffected. The effect size for brain size was small (–0.31, 95 per cent confidence intervals [CI] CI–0.41 to –0.20, $p < 0.0001$) and, in accord with Table 1.3, only seven of the 27 studies cited reported a significant finding. The smaller median decrease in intracranial size of 1 per cent (Table 1.3) is also in accord with Ward *et al.* (1996). Only four of 18 studies cited by them found a significant reduction in intracranial size and their reported effect size for this difference is very small with the upper 95 per cent CI approaching zero (effect size –0.16, 95 per cent CI –0.29 to –0.04, $p < 0.01$). Interestingly Ward *et al.* (1996) found that the average effect size was related to the plane of measure used in individual studies, indicating that the reduction in intracranial volume is primarily in the mediolateral direction. In broad agreement with the above findings, the systematic review of MRI studies by Lawrie and Abukmeil (1998) concluded that there is a 3 per cent reduction of brain volume (and a 40 per cent enlargement of the lateral ventricles) in schizophrenia.

Brain size is dependent on many demographic factors, such as age, sex, ethnic origin, and parental social class, which complicates its study in schizophrenia. How these factors exert their effects and interact is still poorly understood, though IQ may be one mediating variable (Andreasen *et al.*, 1993). Harvey *et al.* (1994) reported that intracranial volume in healthy subjects was dependent upon height ($p = 0.0001$) but, even after controlling for this, it was related independently to sex, ethnicity, and IQ. They did not find a significant correlation with age, although age has been shown to correlate inversely with brain volume in other studies. Likewise, Jones *et al.* (1994) demonstrated that ventricular volumes were related not only to intracranial volume, but also independently to age, sex, social class, and ethnicity. Both Harvey *et al.* (1994) and Flaum *et al.* (1994) reported that whilst there was a significant correlation between intracranial size and IQ, and brain size and IQ, in their normal subjects no such correlation was evident in their schizophrenic and male schizophrenic groups, respectively. Handedness may be another relevant variable to consider, given its relationship to temporal lobe structural asymmetries (Chapter 6). Most of the studies reported in this chapter have attempted to control for the main demographic variables, usually by group rather than case matching, although where this has been insufficient (e.g. Harvey *et al.*, 1994, sex; Zipursky *et al.*, 1997, age) the variables have been included in their multivariate analyses. It is also important to bear in mind that there is a danger of over-controlling for what may be disease-related variables, such as handedness (Shan-Ming *et al.*, 1985) and IQ.

Global versus regional changes

Reduced brain size may reflect uniform or localised pathology. This issue has been addressed in several ways, for example in terms of cortical versus subcortical structures, regional differences within the cerebral cortex, and grey versus white matter involvement. There has also been increasing interest in the occurrence of specific abnormalities (e.g. cavum septum pellucidum (see below).

Before considering the anatomical localisation of macroscopic brain changes in detail, it is worth considering how and whether regional measurements are normalised to overall brain volume. Intracranial or cranial size is the usual measure of choice for adjustment of raw regional volumes, although both height and ipsilateral lobar volumes have also been used. Such adjustment is carried out for two reasons. First, to attempt to control for any differences in stature between the two study groups. Secondly, to determine whether group differences in regional measures are simply a consequence of an overall reduction in brain volume, or whether they are localised disease effects. Controlling for whole brain volume is, however, not without its critics. Arndt *et al.* (1991) reported that controlling for head size decreased the reliability of brain measures compared with the analysis of raw volumes. Mathalon *et al.* (1993), whilst accepting this reduction in reliability, found that controlling for brain volume increased the criterion validity of the measure, better discriminating between patient and control groups. Although proportional scores such as the ventricle : brain ratio have traditionally been preferred, and have some validity, controlling for total brain volume in multivariate analyses has become more popular and is potentially a more accurate method (Arndt *et al.*, 1991). The method used is clearly important but a detailed analysis is beyond the scope of this chapter. Therefore the tables, excluding Table 1.3, simply list studies which have either controlled or not controlled for gross brain/body measures.

Grey versus white matter volume reductions

There have now been a number of MRI studies which have found significant global reductions, of the order of 4 per cent, in the volume of the cortical grey matter in schizophrenia, without concomitant white matter volume reductions (Table 1.4). This finding, also reported postmortem by Pakkenberg (1987), is most apparent when total brain volume has been controlled for, suggesting that the grey matter loss is of particular importance in the pathogenesis of schizophrenia. Its functional significance was highlighted by Zipursky *et al.* (1998*b*) who found that grey but not white matter or CSF volumes were significantly reduced in a subgroup of first-episode patients who required higher doses of neuroleptics. Schlaepfer *et al.* (1994) reported significant reductions in grey matter volume occurring primarily in areas of heteromodal association cortex (dorsolateral prefrontal cortex, inferior parietal lobule, and Wernicke's area), leading to the hypothesis that schizophrenia is a specific disorder of this kind of association cortex (Pearlson *et al.*, 1996). Sullivan *et al.* (1998) also found regionally specific deficits in grey matter volume in schizophrenia with greater decreases in prefrontal and anterior superior temporal areas than in posterior regions. This is in accord with median reductions of the order of 7 per cent in frontal and temporal areas compared with 4 per cent globally, and also with the regional cortical CSF findings discussed previously. There is no gender effect on grey matter volumes in schizophrenia, with only one of eight studies (Schlaepfer *et al.*, 1994) reporting a greater reduction in female subjects. Equally no consistent hemisphere effect has been reported, with only one of four studies (Marsh *et al.*, 1999) reporting an excess volume reduction in the right hemisphere. It has not yet been clarified whether the grey matter volume reduction is due to a reduction in thickness of the cortex (as suggested by some postmortem studies; e.g. Brown *et al.*, 1986; Pakkenberg, 1987; Selemon *et al.*, 1995), a reduction in cortical surface area, or both.

The median reduction of white matter in schizophrenia is 2 per cent globally and 0 per cent in frontal and temporal regions (Table 1.4). Despite its preserved volume, white matter may be affected in other ways, which can be studied with new imaging techniques. For example, diffusion tensor imaging has shown some promise in identifying *in vivo* decreases in corticocortical connections in schizophrenia (Lim *et al.*, 1999). It is too soon to draw any firm conclusions from this research, though it may well help in the future to clarify discrepancies in the literature on the callosal abnormalities discussed below.

The frontal lobe

The frontal lobe is an obvious area of interest in schizophrenia given the symptomatic, neuropsychological, and functional evidence implicating this area (Liddle and Morris, 1991; Morrison-Stewart *et al.*, 1992; Morice and Delahunty, 1996). Andreasen *et al.* (1986) first reported a reduction in frontal lobe volume in schizophrenia when controlling for brain size. This study did not control for the subjects' IQ and a further study, using the same probands and an IQ-matched control group, failed to find a similar effect (Andreasen *et al.*, 1990). As mentioned above, however, controlling for IQ, even premorbid IQ, is undesirable given its likely relationship to the schizophrenia disease process. Instead, controlling for predicted IQ can be approximated by using parental years of education or parental socioeconomic class as a proxy. Using these more appropriate variables, subsequent studies have shown some reduction in frontal lobe volumes, the median reduction being ~5 per cent (Table 1.5). However controlling for total cranial/cerebral size does not greatly improve the distribution of significant studies and therefore it is likely that the observed frontal lobe volume reduction is primarily associated with the generalised reduction in cortical size in schizophrenia. No gender-specific effects have been reported in the seven relevant studies. Fifteen of 18 studies investigating laterality have been non-significant; Marsh *et al.* (1997) reported a greater reduction on the right and Bilder *et al.* (1994) reported the same for premotor cortex but a reversed effect in the prefrontal cortex (Chapter 6).

Advances in identifying subregions of the frontal lobes on the basis of replicable cortical sulci on 3D-rendered images will help clarify whether any frontal lobe volume reductions are generalised or localise to specific gyri. Using this method, Buchanan *et al.* (1998) found a 13 per cent decrease of inferior prefrontal grey matter compared with an average of 5 per cent in other frontal regions.

The temporal lobe

Abnormalities in the shape and size of the temporal lobe in schizophrenia were observed in postmortem brains over 80 years ago (Southard, 1915) and in some more recent studies (Table 1.1). The importance of the temporal lobes, particularly the left, in epilepsy-related psychoses (Chapter 11) was highlighted by Flor-Henry (1969). Recent neuropsychological and functional imaging studies have also implicated this area in schizophrenia (Chapter 7).

Volumetric MRI studies report an overall ~4 per cent reduction in the sizes of the temporal lobes in schizophrenia, which is not disproportionate to the reported global cortical volume reduction (Table 1.5). Only two of 10 studies found a significant interaction of

Table 1.4 Grey and white matter volumes in schizophrenia*

Structure	Adjusted[a]	Decreased in schizophrenia Significant (p < 0.05)	Trend (p > 0.05)	Increased in schizophrenia Trend (p > 0.05)	Summary of findings
Total grey matter (GM)	Yes	Marsh et al, 1999[rs] Cannon et al, 1998 Zipursky et al, 1998a Zipursky et al, 1997 Lim et al, 1996a[n] Woods et al, 1996 Schlaepfer et al, 1994[e] Harvey et al, 1993	Sharma et al, 1998 Schlaepfer et al, 1994[f] Schlaepfer et al, 1994	McCarley et al, 1993	*% Difference[b]* *Median* GM: −4% WM: −2% *Range* GM: −12 to 2% WM: −8 to 10%
	No	Lauriello et al, 1997 Lim et al, 1996a[n] Lim et al, 1996c Woods et al, 1996 Schlaepfer et al, 1994[e] Woods et al, 1991	Pearlson et al, 1997 Rossi et al, 1994 Barta et al, 1997 Schlaepfer et al, 1994[f] Schlaepfer et al, 1994 Harvey et al, 1993		*Sex × diagnosis[c]* GM: 12% (8), F > M WM: 0% (5) *Side × diagnosis[d]* GM: 25%(4),R > L WM: 0%(3)
Total white matter (WM)	Yes	Cannon et al, 1998	Marsh et al, 1999[rs] Zipursky et al, 1998a Woods et al, 1996 Harvey et al, 1993	Zipursky et al, 1997 Lim et al, 1996a[n] McCarley et al, 1993	
	No		Pearlson et al, 1997 Lim et al, 1996c Woods et al, 1996 Woods et al, 1991	Lauriello et al, 1997 Lim et al, 1996a[n] McCarley et al, 1993	
Frontal Lobe GM	Yes	Marsh et al, 1999[irs] Cannon et al, 1998 Sullivan et al, 1999[jk] Zipursky et al, 1997[jk]	Baaré et al, 1999[j] Bryant et al, 1999 Wible et al, 1995[j]	Corey-Bloom et al, 1995[ho] Buchanan et al, 1993[ll]	*% difference[b]* *Median* GM: −7% WM: −3% *Range* GM: −13 to 2% WM: −17 to 12% *Sex × diagnosis[c]* GM: 0% (3) WM: 0% (4)
	No	Woods et al, 1991	Baaré et al, 1999[j] Corey-Bloom et al, 1995[go] Wible et al, 1995[j] Buchanan et al, 1993[jm] Breier et al, 1992[j] Suddath et al, 1989[j]		

Table 1.4 continued

Structure	Adjusted[a]	Decreased in schizophrenia Significant (p < 0.05)	Trend (p > 0.05)	Increased in schizophrenia Trend (p > 0.05)	Summary of findings
Frontal lobe WM	Yes	Bryant et al, 1999[j]	Baaré et al, 1999[j] Marsh et al, 1999[irs] Cannon et al, 1998 Sullivan et al, 1998[ik]	Zipursky et al, 1997[jk] Wible et al, 1995[j]	Side × diagnosis[d] GM: 12% (8), R > L WM: 0% (8)
	No	Breier et al, 1992[j]	Baaré et al, 1999[j] Buchanan et al, 1993[jlm] Woods et al, 1991	Wible et al, 1995[j] Suddath et al, 1989	
Temporal lobe GM	Yes	Marsh et al, 1992[rs] Cannon et al, 1998 Sullivan et al, 1998[pq] Zipursky et al, 1997[p] Harvey et al, 1993[R]	Sharma et al, 1998 Zipursky et al, 1997[t] Harvey et al, 1993[L]		% difference[b] Median GM: −7% WM: 0% Range GM: −19 to 0% WM: −10 to 6%
	No	Suddath et al, 1989	Woods et al, 1991		
Temporal lobe WM	Yes	Harvey et al, 1993[R]	Marsh et al, 1999[rs] Sullivan et al, 1998[q] Harvey et al, 1993[L]	Cannon et al, 1998 Sullivan et al, 1998[p] Zipursky et al, 1997[pq]	Sex × diagnosis[c] GM: 0% (3) WM: 0% (3)
	No		Suddath et al, 1989	Woods et al, 1991	Side × diagnosis[d] GM: 0% (4) WM: 0% (4)

*Many of the studies include some subjects with schizophreniform or schizoaffective disorder.
[L]Left; [R]right; [M]male; [F]female.
[a]Adjusted, i.e. whether controlled for height, head size, intracranial volume, or other relevant structure, by ratio, regression, or covariation; [b]% volume difference in schizophrenia; [c]% of studies finding a significant interaction (total number of studies); [d]% of studies finding a significant interaction (total number of studies); [e]heteromodal association cortex; [f]non-heteromodal association cortex; [g]dorsal frontal lobe; [h]medial frontal lobe; [i]frontoparietal reference area; [j]prefrontal lobe; [k]frontal lobe; [l]deficit syndrome cases; [m]non-deficit syndrome cases; [n]child-onset schizophrenia; [o]late-onset cases; [p]anterior superior temporal; [q]posterior superior temporal; [r]acute psychotic patients; [s]chronic severe patients.

Table 1.5 Frontal and temporal lobe regional brain volumes in schizophrenia*

Structure	Adjusted[a]	Decreased in schizophrenia — Significant (p ≤ 0.05)	Decreased in schizophrenia — Trend (p > 0.05)	Increased in schizophrenia — All trend (p > 0.05) except [w](p ≤ 0.05)	Summary of findings
Frontal lobe	Yes	Bryant et al, 1999[e] Marsh et al, 1997 Woodruff et al, 1997b[Rg] Nopoulos et al, 1995b Andreasen et al, 1994b Buchanan et al, 1993[l] Nopoulos et al, 1997a	Lawrie et al, 1999[en] Buchanan et al, 1998[e] Woodruff et al, 1997b Woodruff et al, 1997b[Lgh] Cowell et al, 1996 Frazier et al, 1996[m] Wible et al, 1995 Bilder et al, 1994[Ref] Bilder et al, 1994[Lf] Buchanan et al, 1993[k] Kelsoe et al, 1988[e]	Woodruff et al, 1997b[Rh] Bilder et al, 1994[Le]	% difference[b] Median −5% Range −10 to 14% Sex × diagnosis[c] 0% (7) Side × diagnosis[d] 6% (18), L > R 11% (18), R > L
	No	Buchanan et al, 1998[e] Frazier et al, 1996[m] Breier et al, 1992[e] Woods et al, 1991	Woods et al, 1996[g] Woods et al, 1996 Bilder et al, 1994[Ref] Bilder et al, 1994[Lf] DeLisi et al, 1991a Kelsoe et al, 1988[e] Suddath et al, 1989	Woods et al, 1996[i] Woods et al, 1996[jw] Bilder et al, 1994[Le]	
Temporal lobe	Yes	Bryant et al, 1999[ML] Marsh et al, 1997 Woodruff et al, 1997b[L] Harvey et al, 1993[R] Bogerts et al, 1990a[MR] Nopoulos et al, 1997a	Bryant et al, 1999[MR] Havermans et al, 1999[x] Altshuler et al, 1998 Roy et al, 1998 Woodruff et al, 1997b[R] Cowell et al, 1996 Jacobsen et al, 1996[m+]	Bryant et al, 1999[F] Havermans et al, 1999[w] Lawrie et al, 1999[n] Sharma et al, 1998 Swayze et al, 1992 Bogerts et al, 1990a[F]	% difference[b] Median −4% Range −14 to 4% Sex × diagnosis[c] 20% (10), M > F

Table 1.5 continued

Structure	Adjusted[a]	Decreased in schizophrenia		Increased in schizophrenia	Summary of findings
		Significant (p ≤ 0.05)	Trend (p > 0.05)	All trend (p > 0.05) except[w] (p ≤ 0.05)	
			Flaum et al, 1995 Nopoulos et al, 1995b Andreasen et al, 1994b Bilder et al, 1994 Harvey et al, 1993[L] Bogerts et al, 1990a[ML] Kelsoe et al, 1988		Side × diagnosis[d] 31% (13), R > L
	No	Barta et al, 1990[R] Dauphinais et al, 1990	Roy et al, 1998 Pearlson et al, 1997 Jacobsen et al, 1996[m] Bilder et al, 1994 Raine et al, 1992 Woods et al, 1991 Barta et al, 1990[L] DeLisi et al, 1991a Suddath et al, 1989 Kelsoe et al, 1988		
Amygdala–hippocampal complex	Yes	Bryant et al, 1999 Lawrie et al, 1999[n] Whitworth et al, 1998[no] McCarley et al, 1993[L]	McCarley et al, 1993[R] Hoff et al, 1992 Kelsoe et al, 1988		% difference[b] Median −8%
	No	Lawrie et al, 1999[Ln] Buchanan et al, 1993[kl] Breier et al, 1992 Shenton et al, 1992 Bogerts et al, 1990a[Mu] Dauphinais et al, 1990[Rr] Suddath et al, 1989	Lawrie et al, 1999[Rn] Jacobsen et al, 1996[m] Bogerts et al, 1993 DeLisi et al, 1991a Dauphinais et al, 1990[Lr] Kelsoe et al, 1988	Bogerts et al, 1990a[Fu] Swayze et al, 1992	Range −21 to 0% Sex × diagnosis[c] 33% (3), M > F Side × diagnosis[d] 14% (7), R > L

Table 1.5 continued

Structure	Adjusted[a]	Decreased in schizophrenia Significant ($p \leq 0.05$)	Trend ($p > 0.05$)	Increased in schizophrenia All trend ($p > 0.05$) except [w]($p \leq 0.05$)	Summary of findings
Amygdala	Yes	Breier et al, 1992 Shenton et al, 1992[LV]	Altshuler et al, 1998 Hirayasu et al, 1998 Whitworth et al. 1998[nv] Whitworth et al. 1998[ov] Jacobsen et al, 1996[m] Hoff et al, 1992 Shenton et al, 1992[Rv]	Havermans et al, 1999[vwx]	% difference[b] *Median* −8% *Range* −21 to 10%
	No	Pearlson et al, 1997[R] Rossi et al, 1994[L] Breier et al, 1992 Barta et al, 1990[L]	Jacobsen et al, 1996[m] Pearlson et al, 1997[ML] Rossi et al, 1994[F] Bogerts et al, 1993[R] Barta et al, 1990[R] Bogerts et al, 1990a[R]	Pearlson et al, 1997[FL] Bogerts et al, 1993[L] Bogerts et al, 1990a[L]	*Sex × diagnosis*[c] 50% (2), M > F *Side × diagnosis*[d] 11% (9), R > L 11% (9), L > R
Hippocampus	Yes	Velakoulis et al, 1999[o] Velakoulis et al, 1999[Ln] Altshuler et al, 1998 Hirayasu et al, 1998[L] Whitworth et al, 1998[nq] Whitworth et al, 1998[Roq] Woodruff et al, 1997b[L] Fukuzako et al, 1996 Flaum et al, 1995 Breier et al, 1992	Velakoulis et al, 1999[Rn] Csernansky et al, 1998 Hirayasu et al, 1998[R] Whitworth et al, 1998[Loq] Woodruff et al, 1997b[R] Jacobsen et al, 1996[m] Rossi et al, 1994[q] Hoff et al, 1992 Shenton et al, 1992[l]	Marsh et al, 1999[uv]	% difference[b] *Median* −8% *Range* −20 to 10% *Sex × diagnosis*[c] 25% (4), M > F *Side × diagnosis*[d] 14% (14), R > L 14% (14), L > R

Table 1.5 continued

Structure	Adjusted[a]	Decreased in schizophrenia Significant (p ≤ 0.05)	Trend (p > 0.05)	Increased in schizophrenia All trend (p > 0.05) except[w](p ≤ 0.05)	Summary of findings
	No	Barr et al, 1997[L] Fukuzako et al, 1996 Bogerts et al, 1993 Breier et al, 1992 Bogerts et al, 1990a[MR]	Csernansky et al, 1998 Barr et al, 1997[R] Jacobsen et al, 1996[Rm] Pearlson et al, 1997 Swayze et al, 1992 Bogerts et al, 1990a[ML]	Jacobsen et al, 1996[Lm] Bogerts et al, 1990a[F]	
Superior temporal gyrus (STG) (total)	Yes Marsh et al, 1997	Bryant et al, 1999 Flaum et al, 1995 McCarley et al, 1993[L] Shenton et al, 1992[L]	Havermans et al, 1999[x] Woodruff et al, 1997b McCarley et al, 1993[R] Shenton et al, 1992[R]	Havermans et al, 1999[w] Roy et al, 1998 Jacobsen et al, 1996[mW] Zipursky et al, 1994	% difference[b] Median Total:-5% Ant: -8% Post: -8%
	No	Barta et al, 1990	Kulynych et al, 1996	Roy et al, 1998 Jacobsen et al, 1996[mW]	Range Total:-15 to 6% Ant: -33 to 6% Post:-14 to 7%
Anterior (ant) STG	Yes	Marsh et al, 1997 Pearlson et al, 1997[L] McCarley et al, 1993[L] Shenton et al, 1992[L]	Pearlson et al, 1997[R] Shenton et al, 1992[R]	Jacobsen et al, 1996[m]	Sex × diagnosis[c] Total: 0% (2) Ant: N/A (0) Post: N/A (0)
	No	Pearlson et al, 1997[L]	Barta et al, 1997 Pearlson et al, 1997[R] DeLisi et al, 1994	Kulynych et al, 1996 Jacobsen et al, 1996[mW]	
Posterior (post) STG	Yes	Marsh et al, 1997 Pearlson et al, 1997[L] McCarley et al, 1993[L] Shenton et al, 1992[L] Hajek et al, 1997	Menon et al, 1995 Shenton et al, 1992[R]	Pearlson et al, 1997[R] Jacobsen et al, 1996[mW]	Side × diagnosis[d] Total: 10% (10) Ant: 40% (5), L > R Post: 50% (5), L > R

Table 1.5 continued

| Structure | Decreased in schizophrenia | | Increased in schizophrenia | Summary of findings |
	Adjusted[a] Significant ($p \leq 0.05$)	Trend ($p > 0.05$)		
No	Pearlson et al, 1997[L]	Kulynych et al, 1996; Menon et al, 1995	Pearlson et al, 1997[R]; Jacobsen et al, 1996[mW]	All trend ($p > 0.05$) except [w]($p \leq 0.05$)

*Many of the studies include some subjects with schizophreniform or schizoaffective disorder.

[L]Left; [R]right; [M]male; [F]female; N/A, result not available.

[a]Adjusted, i.e. whether controlled for height, head size, intracranial volume, or other relevant structure, by ratio, regression, or covariation; [b] % volume difference in schizophrenia; [c]% of studies finding a significant interaction (total number of studies); [d]% of studies finding a significant interaction (total number of studies); [e] Prefrontal; [f]premotor; [g]dorsolateral prefrontal; [h]ventrolateral prefrontal; [i]dorsomedial prefrontal; [j]orbitofrontal; [k]deficit syndrome cases; [l]non-deficit syndrome cases; [m]child-onset cases; [n]first-episode cases; [o]chronic patients; [p]anterior; [q]posterior; [v]amygdala–anterior hippocampus; [w]hallucinated schizophrenics; [x]non-hallucinated schizophrenics.

gender with diagnosis, with greater reduction of temporal lobe volume in the male cases in both studies, but only significantly so on the right side in one (Bogerts *et al.*, 1990*a*) and the left side in the other (Bryant *et al.*, 1999). The issue of asymmetry in schizophrenia is particularly relevant for the temporal lobe, and is discussed in Chapter 6.

Within the temporal lobe, the medial and lateral (neocortical) regions are functionally distinct, and each has been the subject of many structural investigations in schizophrenia. They are now considered in turn.

Medial temporal lobe

The medial temporal lobe comprises hippocampus, parahippocampal gyrus, and amygdala (Chapter 2). In agreement with several postmortem studies (Table 1.1), MRI findings taken overall indicate a reduction in the volumes of the amygdala–hippocampal complex in schizophrenia. This reduction has not been universally reported, although there are methodological problems in measuring volumes of these structures which may contribute to this. For example, it has been difficult to separate the amygdala from the anterior hippocampus, necessitating a combined volume to be measured; this is unsatisfactory especially since the two structures may be differentially affected (Altshuler *et al.*, 1998). It is also difficult to distinguish the most posterior portion of the hippocampus leading to truncated volumes being taken as representative. This assumption may be incorrect given evidence of shortening of the hippocampi in schizophrenia, even when smaller brain size has been controlled for (Bogerts *et al.*, 1991; Fukuzako *et al.*, 1996). Once hippocampal length was controlled for in the study of Fukuzako *et al.* (1996), there was no significant difference in hippocampal volume in the subjects with schizophrenia. Whether or not it is due to a linear reduction in size or a reduction in all dimensions, smaller hippocampi in schizophrenia seem to be a substantial finding, with most studies reporting absolute size as being less than controls.

A recent meta-analysis by Nelson *et al.* (1998) confirmed the presence of bilateral reduction in hippocampal volume in schizophrenia (by 4 per cent) which was increased when the amygdala was included within the structure measured (8 per cent reduction). In accord with Table 1.5, Nelson *et al.* (1998) found no consistent effect of laterality. The median reduction in the hippocampus, amygdala, and both taken together is of the order of 8 per cent in Table 1.5. Despite the findings of Nelson *et al.* (1998) that the measured reduction was not apparently in excess of any overall reduction in global grey matter volumes, controlling for total brain size slightly improves the distribution of significant findings (Table 1.5) and since the reduction in hippocampal volume is about twice that of overall brain volume, it cannot be ruled out that the hippocampi/medial temporal lobes are preferentially affected in schizophrenia.

Advances in the resolution achieved with MRI and the computer modelling of complex shapes show promise for the examination of hippocampal structure. Csernansky *et al.* (1998) used a template transformation procedure to illustrate shape differences in the hippocampi in schizophrenia. Their technique was able to discriminate between the patient and control groups, and successfully classified 80 per cent of subjects. The shape deformities in schizophrenia were localised, being limited to the lateral aspect of the head and the medial aspect of the hippocampal body bilaterally, regions of the hippocampus which send projections to the prefrontal cortex.

Medial temporal lobe cortical areas have also been studied with MRI. Significant volume reductions have been observed in the parahippocampal gyrus by Shenton *et al.* (1992) and McCarley *et al.* (1993). Pearlson *et al.* (1997) found this only to be the case for female subjects whilst others (DeLisi *et al.*, 1988; Woodruff *et al.*, 1997*b*; Hirayasu *et al.*, 1998; Havermans *et al.*, 1999) have found no decreases in this area. Where observed, reductions have been bilateral and of a median size of 7 per cent. Pearlson *et al.* (1997) also reported an 11 per cent reduction in the volume of the entorhinal cortex (anterior parahippocampal gyrus) bilaterally which was significant although it only remained so on the left side after controlling for total brain volume. Nasrallah *et al.* (1997) failed to demonstrate any volume reductions in the entorhinal cortex. Postmortem studies of parahippocampal and entorhinal size are also equivocal (Table 1.1 and Chapter 2).

Lateral temporal lobe

Interest in the lateral temporal lobes in schizophrenia centres upon the superior temporal gyrus (STG). This structure is adjacent to the Sylvian fissure, which was reported as enlarged in size in CT studies. The posterior left STG forms part of Wernicke's area and thus is involved in language processing; it also contains the auditory association cortex within the planum temporale.

Shenton *et al.* (1991) first reported a reduced STG volume in schizophrenia. The decrease was on the left, although where hemisphere effects have been examined subsequently, only one of 10 studies has reported an asymmetrical reduction from the left STG. The issue of asymmetrical alterations of STG structures in schizophrenia is discussed further in Chapter 6. The reductions in STG volume in schizophrenia appear to be greater in the posterior portion (median 8 per cent) compared with a 5 per cent reduction overall. However, as for the temporal lobe volume reductions generally, it is not yet clear if the STG is preferentially affected. There is, however, a suggestion in Table 1.5 that more significant results are reported in those studies which have controlled for intracranial or cerebral volume.

Several correlations between STG volume and the clinical features of schizophrenia have been identified. STG volume has been correlated inversely with severity of thought disorder in the posterior (Shenton *et al.*, 1992) and medial (Menon *et al.*, 1995) portions of this gyrus, inversely with hallucinations in the left anterior STG (Barta *et al.*, 1990, but not Havermans *et al.*, 1999), inversely with positive psychotic symptoms (Marsh *et al.*, 1997), but positively with delusions in the left posterior STG (Menon *et al.*, 1995). These various correlations suggest a relationship between symptom profile and the STG in schizophrenia, though clearly its nature and specificity needs further investigation.

Subcortical structures

MRI has for the first time allowed the *in vivo* study of subcortical structures. There continue to be problems in identifying the boundaries of these regions, but acceptable inter-rater reliabilities have been achieved in some studies.

Caudate nucleus

Stratta *et al.* (1997), Keshavan *et al.* (1998), and Shihabuddin *et al.* (1998) all found signif-icant reductions in caudate volumes, the latter study controlling for brain size. Conversely, increases were reported by Breier *et al.* (1992), Buchanan *et al.* (1993), and Bryant *et al.* (1999) in the left caudate, and by Frazier *et al.* (1996) bilaterally (the latter two studies controlling for brain size). Several other studies found no significant differences either in absolute caudate volumes (Chakos *et al.*, 1994; Rossi *et al.*, 1994; Corey-Bloom *et al.*, 1995; Stratta *et al.*, 1997) or when controlling for overall brain or intracranial size (Jernigan *et al.*, 1991; Chakos *et al.*, 1994; Corey-Bloom *et al.*, 1995; Flaum *et al.*, 1995; Lawrie *et al.*, 1999). The median volume difference between schizophrenic subjects and normal controls is therefore ~0 per cent (range –13 to +14 per cent).

A somewhat clearer picture emerges when neuroleptic medication is taken into account (Chapter 15). MRI studies of neuroleptic-naive subjects find caudate volumes to be unal-tered or decreased compared to controls (Keshavan *et al.*, 1998; Shihabuddin *et al.*, 1998), and follow-up of neuroleptic-treated patients has shown increases in caudate size over time which are reversible to some degree upon withdrawal. Chakos *et al.* (1994) followed up 29 first-episode patients and 10 controls over 18 months and found a significant 5.7 per cent increase in total caudate volumes in the patient group, compared with a non-signifi-cant 1.6 per cent reduction in the controls. Keshavan *et al.* (1994), in a 1-year follow-up of 11 first-episode psychotic patients, reported a significant 12 per cent increase in left and 18 per cent increase in right caudate volumes. Gur *et al.* (1998b), although somewhat at odds with these findings in reporting that previously treated patients tended to have smaller caudate volumes than neuroleptic-naive patients, who in turn had non-significantly smaller volumes than the normal controls, reported significant positive correlations between caudate volumes and neuroleptic dose. They also found that caudate volume correlated with severity of negative symptoms in previously treated, and severity of hallucinations in neuroleptic-naive, schizophrenic subjects. Corson *et al.* (1999) followed up a group of patients with schizophrenia spectrum disorders treated with typical or atypical neuroleptics over 2 years. Typical neuroleptics were associated with increased caudate volumes, whilst atypical drugs tended to have the opposite effect.

Other basal ganglia nuclei

No clear picture has emerged regarding the size of other basal ganglia structures in schiz-ophrenia from the MRI studies (nor postmortem; Table 1.1), and again the possibility of neuroleptic effects on the findings must be borne in mind (Corson *et al.*, 1999). Lenticular volumes were found to be increased in schizophrenia in one study (Jernigan *et al.*, 1991) but not in others (Rossi *et al.*, 1994; Corey-Bloom *et al.*, 1995; Lawrie *et al.*, 1999). Putamen volumes in schizophrenia have been reported as increased bilaterally (Frazier *et al.*, 1996; Shihabuddin *et al.*, 1998), on the right only (Elkashef *et al.*, 1994), and as unchanged (Rossi *et al.*, 1994; Stratta *et al.*, 1997; Keshavan *et al.*, 1998). The globus pallidus has shown increased volumes in two studies (Elkashef *et al.*, 1994; Frazier *et al.*, 1996) but not in two others (Kelsoe *et al.*, 1988; Woods *et al.*, 1996). Nucleus accumbens volumes are reportedly unaltered in schizophrenia (Rossi *et al.*, 1994; Stratta *et al.*, 1997).

Thalamus

The thalamus has long been proposed as a site of pathology in schizophrenia (see Chapter 13), though as with the postmortem studies (Table 1.1), the MRI evidence remains inconclusive, partly because for a number of reasons the thalamus is a difficult structure to image (Chapter 7).

Several of the MRI studies suggest decreased thalamic size in schizophrenia. Using a novel technique, Andreasen et al. (1994a) reported the thalamus and surrounding white matter to be the sites of specific regional abnormalities in schizophrenia. This group had also found a reduction of thalamic area (Andreasen et al., 1990), and Flaum et al. (1995), Frazier et al. (1996), Goldstein et al. (1996), and Staal et al. (1998) all reported thalamic volume reductions in schizophrenia. However, there have been several failures to replicate this finding (Jernigan et al., 1991; Buchsbaum et al., 1996; Portas et al., 1998; Arciniegas et al., 1999; Hazlett et al., 1999; Lawrie et al., 1999). Staal et al. (1998) examined the patients' unaffected siblings and found their thalamic volumes to be intermediate between the patient and control groups, and statistically different from both. In late-onset schizophrenia, Corey-Bloom et al. (1995) found a trend reduction in thalamic size. Gur et al. (1998b) compared neuroleptic-naive and previously treated schizophrenic patients, and found a trend ($p = 0.08$) reduction in the thalamic volumes of the former group compared with their normal controls. They also reported that thalamic volume correlated positively with neuroleptic dose.

The median reduction of thalamic volume in schizophrenia is ~5 per cent but was 17 per cent in a study of childhood-onset cases (Frazier et al., 1996). A possible relation with age of onset is supported by Jeste et al. (1998), who found that thalamic volume remained a significant predictor of age of onset of schizophrenia in combination with a neuropsychological test of abstraction and caudate volume, in a multiple regression analysis which controlled for age, duration of illness, and neuroleptic dose. No gender-specific effect on thalamic volume was found in three studies (Flaum et al., 1995; Buchsbaum et al., 1996; Arciniegas et al., 1999) and no hemisphere effect found in five (Flaum et al., 1995; Buchsbaum et al., 1996; Frazier et al., 1996; Arciniegas et al., 1999; Hazlett et al., 1999).

Posterior fossa structures

Cerebellum

CT was unable to image posterior fossa structures adequately and therefore the cerebellum was neglected in schizophrenia research until the advent of MRI. Subsequently whilst both functional (see Chapter 7) and structural (Katsetos et al., 1997) research has been carried out, it remains limited. Aylward et al. (1994) found a non-significant 3 per cent reduction in total cerebellar area in schizophrenia, and similar non-significant reductions in anterior and lobar areas on midline sagittal slices. Jacobsen et al. (1997a) examined children with schizophrenia and reported a significant reduction in the mid-sagittal area. Nasrallah et al. (1991) identified significantly larger cerebellar vermis areas, particularly in schizophrenic subjects with no history of perinatal insult.

Volumetric measures, though generally more accurate, have also been conflicting. Andreasen et al. (1994b) reported a trend ($p = 0.09$) of 1 per cent reduction in cerebellar

volume. Jacobsen *et al.* (1997*c*) found decreased volumes of the vermis and inferior posterior lobe in childhood-onset schizophrenia, but no total cerebellar volume reductions when
brain volume was controlled for. Nopoulos *et al.* (1997*a*) controlling for height, and Sharma
et al. (1998) controlling for height and brain volume, also found no significant differences
in cerebellar volumes in schizophrenia. Levitt *et al.* (1999), controlling for intracranial
volume, reported a significantly enlarged vermis as a result of increased vermal white
matter. Rossi *et al.* (1993) found an unchanged vermis : cerebrum ratio in schizophrenia,
but a reduced ratio in male compared with female patients. However, other studies show
no consistent gender effects on cerebellar volume in schizophrenia (Andreasen *et al.*, 1994*b*;
Flaum *et al.*, 1995; Nopoulos *et al.*, 1997*a*).

Brainstem

Imaging the brainstem was problematic with CT due to bone artefacts. Although this is
not a concern for MRI, only one such study has examined this area in schizophrenia.
Aylward *et al.* (1994) used sagittal slices and found no significant differences in medulla,
pons, or midbrain area in schizophrenia. There was a 13 per cent increase in area of the
fourth ventricle which remained significant after controlling for intracranial area.

Midline abnormalities

Corpus callosum

Relatively early formulations hypothesised that schizophrenia may be due to abnormalities
of interhemispheric communication. Initial postmortem studies provided some support for
corpus callosum (CC) alterations in schizophrenia (Table 1.1). Rosenthal and Bigelow
(1972) reported an increased thickness (width) of the CC, and subsequently that this occurred
only in a subgroup of cases with an early age of onset (Bigelow *et al.*, 1983). However,
Brown *et al.* (1986) found no difference in CC thickness in schizophrenia. Results from
comparable MRI studies have also been conflicting (see Woodruff *et al.*, 1993). Nasrallah
et al. (1986) reported a significant increase in thickness in the anterior and middle parts
of the CC in females with schizophrenia. In their own study, Woodruff *et al.* (1993) found
a reduction in anterior CC width in schizophrenia which was accounted for by comparisons between males only. Raine *et al.* (1990), in their study of right-handed subjects, found
that the normal gender difference in CC thickness was reversed, the CC being thicker in
female schizophrenics and thinner in male schizophrenics. Similar results were seen in a
psychiatric control group indicating that these abnormalities may not be specific to schizophrenia. Decreased CC length in schizophrenia has been reported (Woodruff *et al.*, 1993),
a variable which Colombo *et al.* (1994) found correlated with DSM IIIR axis V scores (a
general assessment of functioning) and age of onset. In contrast, Uematsu and Kaiya (1988)
reported positive correlations between elongation of the anterior CC and a number of poor
prognostic indicators.

Measurements of CC area have also led to conflicting results. Larger anterior and middle
CC areas (Nasrallah *et al.* 1986), larger anterior CC areas in male patients only (Colombo
et al., 1994), smaller CC areas (Kelsoe *et al.*, 1988; Rossi *et al.*, 1989, 1990; Stratta *et al.*,
1989; Woodruff *et al.* 1993), smaller CC areas in female patients only (Hoff *et al.*, 1994),

and no differences in CC area in schizophrenia (Mathew *et al.*, 1985; Machiyama *et al.*, 1987; Smith *et al.*, 1987; Kelsoe *et al.*, 1988; Uematsu and Kaiya, 1988; Hauser *et al.*, 1989; Casanova *et al.*, 1990; Raine *et al.*, 1990; Woodruff *et al.*, 1997*a*) have all been reported. Günther *et al.* (1991) reported a significantly increased CC : brain area ratio in type I but not type II schizophrenia. Despite the apparent inconsistencies, a meta-analysis of MRI studies showed that CC size is reduced in schizophrenia (Woodruff *et al.*, 1995), with a small mean effect size from the 11 studies included of –0.185 (p = 0.019). Few positive studies have controlled for brain size, although Woodruff *et al.* (1993) did so and their finding of reduced CC area in schizophrenia remained significant (see also Highley *et al.*, 1999*a*). In contrast Jacobsen *et al.* (1997*b*), in a study of childhood-onset schizophrenia, reported enlarged CC areas after controlling for total brain volume, primarily due to increased areas in the isthmus and rostral portion of the CC. In the largest study to date (Tibbo *et al.*, 1998), 79 schizophrenic subjects were compared with 65 controls. All were male and most were right handed. Controlling for height, a significant 5 per cent reduction in CC area in schizophrenia was observed. The reduction correlated inversely with negative symptoms. In their meta-analysis, Woodruff *et al.* (1995) also calculated effect sizes for the CC : brain area ratio and CC length. Neither differed significantly between patients and controls.

More sophisticated shape analysis techniques are now being used which may help clarify the status of the CC in schizophrenia. No overall differences in the shape or orientation of the CC in schizophrenia was found in a recent study (Tibbo *et al.*, 1998).

Total or partial agenesis of the CC in schizophrenia has been described in case reports and case series (Lewis *et al.*, 1988; Swayze *et al.*, 1990*b*; Degreef *et al.*, 1992*b*; David *et al.*, 1994). The CC develops embryologically in intimate relationship to the hippocampal formation, fornix, septum pellucidum, and cingulate gyrus. In individuals with callosal agenesis, abnormalities have also been found to occur in the development of these limbic structures (Swayze *et al.*, 1990*b*).

Septum pellucidum

The septum pellucidum is a midline membrane inferior to the CC, comprising two leaflets next to each other. Sometimes the leaflets are separated by a midline fluid space, called cavum septum pellucidum (CSP). Rarely, this is large and, if it extends posteriorly, is known as a cavum vergae. The occurrence of CSP in schizophrenia was first reported by Lewis and Mezey (1985) in six male patients whose illness followed early developmental impairments. The observation has been replicated a number of times (Degreef *et al.*, 1992*b*; DeLisi *et al.*, 1993; Jurjus *et al.*, 1993*b*; Scott *et al.*, 1993; Daviss *et al.*, 1994; Shioiri *et al.*, 1996; Nopoulos *et al.*, 1997*b*).

The reported incidence of CSP in normal populations varies greatly, from 0.15 to 85 per cent, and in schizophrenic patients from 15 to 58 per cent (Nopoulos *et al.*, 1997*b*). The disparity relates both to the difficulty defining clinically significant CSP, and the resolution of the technique used. Minor CSP have long been considered a normal variant. Degreef *et al.* (1992*b*) reported an MRI study (using 3.1 mm contiguous slices) in which 21 per cent of schizophrenic patients but only 2 per cent of controls had CSP, and in a concomitant postmortem study the figures were 61 and 31 per cent, respectively.

Small or equivocal lesions were excluded, and the same criteria used for both studies. Other researchers using MRI have included all sizes of CSP (often using the scale of Jurjus *et al.* (1993*b*); 0 = absent, 1 = equivocal or questionable, 2 = small, 3 and above = moderate to large) but have used variable slice thicknesses or gaps in their scans. Using 5 mm slices/5 mm gaps, Scott *et al.* (1993) and Jurjus *et al.* (1993*b*) reported CSP in 15 and 25 per cent of schizophrenic subjects, and in 5 and 19 per cent of controls, respectively. DeLisi *et al.* (1993), using 5 mm slices/2 mm gaps, found a prevalence of CSP in schizophrenia of 45 per cent and in controls of 30 per cent. Nopoulos *et al.* (1997*b*), using 1.5 mm contiguous slices, found a higher overall incidence amongst males (67 per cent) than females (46 per cent), but an equal incidence in controls (59 per cent) and subjects with schizophrenia (58 per cent). However, the latter had a significantly higher incidence of large (> 6 mm) CSP (21 per cent) than controls (3 per cent). The patients with large CSPs were all male. Finally, in treatment-resistant childhood-onset schizophrenia, Nopoulos *et al.* (1998*a*) reported a significant increase in the frequency of CSP > 6 mm (12 per cent) compared with the controls (1 per cent).

Shioiri *et al.* (1996) examined the specificity of CSP to schizophrenia by comparison with bipolar disorder and major depression. For grade 3 to 4 CSP, only the schizophrenic subjects had an increased incidence (12 per cent compared with 1 per cent). When all sizes of CSP were included, the prevalence in bipolar disorder (7 per cent) was higher than in the controls (1 per cent; $p < 0.05$) and non-significantly lower than that in schizophrenia (17 per cent; $p < 0.10$). CSP was not observed in any patient with major depression. Kwon *et al.* (1998) defined CSP by its appearance on four or more 1.5 mm contiguous coronal MRI slices and reported a higher frequency in schizophrenia (30 per cent) than normal controls (10 per cent; $p = 0.05$). Psychotic affective disorder and schizotypal personality disorder groups were intermediate between these values, and did not differ significantly from normal controls.

It is not clear what the functional consequences of large CSP are, although adjacent limbic system structures may be affected (Lewis and Mezey, 1985). Kwon *et al.* (1998) demonstrated an inverse correlation between degree of CSP and hippocampal volume. Jurjus *et al.* (1993*b*) found no relationship between CSP and clinical severity of schizophrenia, whereas Fukuzako and Kodama (1998) reported a significant relationship with poor outcome, and Kirkpatrick *et al.* (1997) related the degree of CSP with both ethnicity and severity of thought disorder.

Pineal gland abnormalities

Nieto and Nieto (1987) described sclerosis and gliosis in the pineal gland of 27 schizophrenic patients at postmortem. Using CT, Sandyk and Kay (1990) and Sandyk (1993) reported an association of pineal calcification with earlier onset of illness and the subsequent development of tardive dyskinesia; Sandyk (1993) also related degree of pineal calcification with severity of thought disorder. In an MRI study, Rajarethinam *et al.* (1995) found no difference in pineal gland volume in schizophrenia or schizophreniform disorder compared with control subjects.

Other neurodevelopmental and acquired lesions

Lewis (1989), Gerwitz *et al.* (1994), and Lawrie *et al.* (1997) have reviewed the wide range of neurodevelopmental or acquired brain abnormalities observed in some patients with psychosis. They include infarctions, post-traumatic changes, tumours, basal ganglia calcification, arachnoid cysts, venous angiomas, colloid and pineal cysts, cavum vergae, enlargement of the superior cerebellar cistern, enlarged cisterna magnae, and coarctation of the frontal horns. Inspection of large series of CT and MRI scans suggest that the frequency of unequivocal focal abnormalities in schizophrenia is ~4 to 12 per cent, whilst the rate in normal subjects is ~2 to 4 per cent, though there are negative studies (Jurjus *et al.*, 1993*a*; Symonds *et al.*, 1997). It is unclear how these specific lesions, present in a minority of individuals, relate to the quantitative alterations in cerebral and ventricular size demonstrable in groups of subjects with schizophrenia. Honer *et al.* (1995*b*) found no relationship between observed neurodevelopmental abnormalities and cortical sulcal enlargement in CT scans from 80 schizophrenics, although when other psychotic subjects were included (total n = 164) there was a trend inverse relationship between these two factors (p = 0.06).

Subcortical signal hyperintensities

Subcortical signal hyperintensities have been detected using MRI in a number of groups, including healthy young subjects, and have been associated with ageing, cerebrovascular disease, degenerative disorders, and late-life depression. They are not increased in frequency in schizophrenia (Johnstone *et al.*, 1986; Bartzokis *et al.*, 1991; Harvey *et al.*, 1993; Lawrie *et al.*, 1997), including in elderly subjects with early- or late-onset illness (Krull *et al.*, 1991; Corey-Bloom *et al.*, 1995). However, larger foci (Bartzokis *et al.*, 1991) and a greater brain area occupied by foci (Persaud *et al.*, 1997) have been reported in schizophrenia compared to controls. Swayze *et al.* (1990*a*) suggested that one result of birth anomalies might be periventricular haemorrhage or infarction resulting in the presence of small focal regions of signal hyperintensity. This was in accord with the finding of Persaud *et al.* (1997) that the greater area occupied by focal hyperintensities was seen in the schizophrenic subjects with a history of definite obstetric complications compared to those without.

Grey matter heterotopias

Grey matter heterotopias (GMHs) are collections of normal neurons abnormally located within the white matter secondary to an arrest of radial migration. They are clearly neurodevelopmental in origin (Chapter 11). Nopoulos *et al.* (1995*a*) described two patients who presented with symptoms of schizophrenia, but had no neurological abnormalities and otherwise normal scans, who demonstrated evidence of GMH. They suggested that such patients may be displaying gross manifestations of neuronal migration arrest as reported microscopically in schizophrenia (Akbarian *et al.*, 1993; see Chapters 3 and 8). In a larger series, however, Nopoulos *et al.* (1998*b*) found only one further case of GMH in 55 patients and none amongst controls.

Abnormalities of cortical gyrification

Southard (1915) described abnormalities in the gyrification of the temporal lobes in schizophrenia and similar observations have been made in some but not all recent postmortem studies (Table 1.1). Three-dimensional surface rendering with MRI has allowed this question to be addressed *in vivo,* but findings have been mixed. Kikinis *et al.* (1994) using both qualitative and quantitative analysis of temporal lobe sulcogyral patterns in schizophrenia reported a more vertical sulcal orientation in the left, and to a lesser extent the right, temporal lobe compared with controls. They also demonstrated sulci which were interrupted due to gyri coursing across them, again more marked on the left side. Part of the difficulty in taking these findings further has been the need for a reliable method of quantifying sulcal abnormalities. This is particularly important as the inter-rater reliabilities for the ratings in Kikinis *et al.* (1994) ranged from 0.39 to 0.78. Other researchers have also attempted a qualitative approach with negative findings and poor levels of inter-rater agreement (Noga *et al.*, 1996). Highley *et al.* (1998) examined photographs of lateral views of postmortem brains and using a quantitative technique failed to demonstrate any abnormal orientation of temporal lobe sulci in schizophrenia. However, they did report a bilateral increase in sulcal density compared to the controls.

The disadvantage of surface rendering in attempting to analyse gyral abnormalities is that over 70 per cent of the cortical surface area is hidden. Other methods have therefore been developed to attempt to assess the shape of the cortical surface. The gyrification index (GI) was originally a postmortem technique which has proven a useful measure in the field of epilepsy. The GI is the ratio of the total to the superficially exposed cortical surface as determined from linear measurements in coronal sections. Kulynych *et al.* (1997) found a significantly lower GI in schizophrenia (mean GI = 2.64, SD 0.11) than in controls (mean 2.80, SD 0.17, $p < 0.03$). The implied reduction in cortical folding was seen in both frontal and posterior cortex, suggesting a generalised effect. Other researchers have concentrated on the grey/white matter boundary, which is easier to discern with MRI, using fractal techniques to examine the complexity of cortical folding. Bullmore *et al.* (1994) found that, compared to controls, schizophrenic subjects had a non-significantly reduced grey/white matter boundary complexity, whereas bipolar disorder subjects had a significantly more complex grey/white matter boundary.

Structural abnormalities as part of a neural network

Most studies examine brain structures in isolation whilst looking at group effects and clinical correlates. The brain however is a highly interconnected neural network and abnormalities in one region may reflect abnormalites in a connected region. There have been a few tentative attempts to examine the inter-relatedness of various regional brain volumes. Breier *et al.* (1992) reported increased right frontal/hippocampal volume correlations in schizophrenia. Wible *et al.* (1995) also found that volumes of frontal and temporal lobe structures were more intercorrelated in schizophrenia. In particular, in their patient group, the anterior amygdala–hippocampal complex accounted for most of the variance in prefrontal lobe volumes. Woodruff *et al.* (1997*b*) examined the correlation coefficients between volumes of selected brain regions in 42 male schizophrenics and 43 male controls. The patients had a bilateral reduction of frontotemporal correlations and a left-sided reduction in frontohippocampal and temporoparahippocampal correlations, but an increased correlation between the volumes of the ventrolateral and dorsolateral prefrontal cortices.

Colombo *et al.* (1993) combined their schizophrenia and control groups (total $n = 36$) in a factor analysis of MRI-derived brain area measurements and extracted six factors accounting for 79 per cent of the variance. Factor 1 represented temporal lobe and total cerebral areas; factor 2, anterior and total right temporal horn areas; factor 3, total ventricular and left temporal horn areas; factors 4 and 5, hippocampal areas; and factor 6, posterior temporal horn areas. The two groups did not differ on any of these factor scores. Tien *et al.* (1996) studied MRI images from 44 schizophrenics and 60 controls and factor analysed 24 regional brain volumes, producing five factors in each group. Only the first two factors were similar in both groups, representing caudate/striatum and hippocampus/parahippocampal gyrus. The third normal factor, which represented amygdala/superior temporal gyrus, was not evident in the schizophrenics. The remaining factors in both groups were difficult to interpret but were labelled as entorhinal cortex and heteromodal association cortex. In controls, some of the factors intercorrelated ($r < 0.34$): basal ganglia with hippocampal, temporal, and heteromodal association cortex, and temporal with hippocampal and entorhinal cortex. There were lesser correlations in schizophrenia, the highest being between basal ganglia and hippocampus ($r = -0.26$) and heteromodal association cortex ($r = -0.21$). Kawasaki *et al.* (1997) factor analysed volumes derived from MRI scans of temporal lobe structures in schizophrenia and identified four uncorrelated factors (left and right STG and anterior and posterior medial temporal lobe) which together accounted for 87 per cent of the variance. This study lacked a control group for comparison.

The results and validity of such analyses should be treated with caution because of the problem of low subject to variable ratios, and the lack of an underlying hypothesis. However, they do illustrate the use of multivariate techniques to try to understand better the nature of brain abnormalities in schizophrenia.

Timing and progression of structural abnormalities

MRI studies of first-episode patients have shown ventricular enlargement (Degreef *et al.*, 1991, 1992*a*; DeLisi *et al.*, 1991*a,b*; Nopolous *et al.*, 1995*b*; Lim *et al.*, 1996*c*) and decreased cortical volume (Lim *et al.*, 1996*c*; Gur *et al.*, 1998*a*; Zipursky *et al.*, 1998*a*) of the same order as seen in chronic schizophrenia. Other data suggest that these abnormalities are seen in unaffected relatives at high risk of, and hence perhaps prior to, schizophrenia (Lawrie *et al.*, 1999). The findings support the notion, developed primarily on the basis of earlier CT findings, that the structural brain changes of schizophrenia are static, non-progressive abnormalities present at the onset of, and by implication before, the illness (Lewis, 1989; Vita *et al.*, 1997; see Chapter 8). However, longitudinal studies are required to address this question properly. This was problematic with CT and early MRI studies because they were prone to substantial measurement artefact. Whilst more recent volumetric studies are more reliable, the technical difficulties of re-registering within-subject scans to detect minor changes over time are still considerable.

Degreef *et al.* (1991) and DeLisi *et al.* (1991*b*, 1992) found no overall change in ventricular size at 2-year follow-up, but DeLisi *et al.* (1991*b*, 1992) did report that some patients had ventricular enlargement in excess of 20 per cent and that the degree of enlargement correlated inversely with the duration of hospital admission over the follow-up period. DeLisi *et al.* (1995, 1997) subsequently reported a significant increase in the left lateral ventricle : brain ratio in their 4-and 5-year follow-ups of the same cohort, though there was no absolute change in ventricular size and therefore the finding may simply reflect a concurrent change in brain volume. DeLisi *et al.* (1991*a,b*) also found a reduction from baseline in temporal lobe volume, particularly on the left, in their chronic schizophrenic sample, and a decreased right temporal lobe volume after 2 years in the first-episode sample. Further analysis of this cohort showed no significant differences from controls in the rate of change in caudate, temporal lobe, or hippocampal volumes, but reductions from baseline in right and left hemisphere volumes, right cerebellar volume, and area of the isthmus of the CC, and a significant increase in left lateral ventricle volume (DeLisi *et al.*, 1997). Gur *et al.* (1998*a*) followed up a cohort of patients (half of whom were in their first episode of psychosis at baseline) over 30 months with repeat MRI scans. Compared with controls, the schizophrenic subjects had greater reductions with time in left frontal lobe volume, less temporal lobe volume reduction, and no difference in brain volume.

A somewhat contrasting pattern of changes with time has been reported in the cohort of childhood-onset schizophrenia studied by Rapoport and colleagues. At 2-year follow-up, Jacobsen *et al.* (1998) found a reduced volume of right temporal lobe, superior temporal gyrus bilaterally, right anterior superior temporal gyrus, and left hippocampus, compared to age-matched controls. The findings persisted when controlling for cerebral volume at baseline and follow-up. At an average 4.3-year follow-up, brain volume was reduced significantly by 5.5 per cent, compared with 1.2 per cent in the controls, accounted for by an 8 per cent reduction in grey matter volume with no change in white matter (Rapaport *et al.*, 1999). The grey matter loss affected frontal, parietal, and temporal, but not occipital, lobes. This cohort also provide the strongest challenge to the view of static morphological change in the ventricular system in schizophrenia, since at 2-year follow-up there was a significant enlargement in ventricular volume in the children with schizophrenia (+19 per cent; $p < 0.001$) compared to controls, and also a greater reduction in thalamic area (Rapoport *et al.*, 1997).

The acknowledged heterogeneity of schizophrenia, for example in age of onset, may, together with the methodological problems, be responsible for these divergent findings. Indeed, although group means may show no change, there are frequently individuals who show considerable progressive ventricular enlargement which cannot be accounted for purely by measurement error and normal physiological fluctuation in ventricular size. Nair *et al.* (1997) followed up a small number of patients over 2 to 3 years with serial MRI scans and found that the overall rate of ventricular enlargement was three times that in normal controls. The distribution of results was non-normal, with a subgroup of patients having a rate of expansion over five times higher than the controls. Attempts have been made to distinguish these subgroups on clinical and other grounds (Nair *et al.*, 1997). In a CT study with an average 5-year follow-up, Davis *et al.* (1998) also reported heterogeneity, with a poorer outcome 'Kraepelinian' subgroup showing greater ventricular enlargement than the 'non-Kraepelinian' subjects, who did not differ from the controls.

Despite the complexities of the data, progressive brain changes do appear to be a real feature of schizophrenia, at least in some patients, and must be taken into account in neurodevelopmental hypotheses of the disorder (Chapter 8).

Diagnostic specificity of the findings

A number of volumetric imaging studies have compared schizophrenia with other psychotic and affective disorders.

Jones et al. (1994) in a large series of consecutively admitted patients found that those diagnosed with schizophrenia or schizoaffective disorder were more likely to have both increased lateral and third ventricles, whilst those cases diagnosed with affective psychoses were more likely to have increased third ventricle volumes only. Elkis et al. (1995) performed meta-analyses of the CT and MRI literature concerning ventricular and sulcal CSF spaces in affective disorder and schizophrenia. They concluded that patients with affective disorder also have significant if moderate enlargement of both these CSF spaces, but that studies which have directly compared the disorders show significantly more ventriculomegaly in schizophrenia, albeit with a small composite effect size ($d = -0.20$). They were unable to perform a meta-analysis of sulcal prominence in affective disorder versus schizophrenia as only three CT studies had examined this question and their results were inconclusive. However, Harvey et al. (1994) demonstrated significant increases in both cortical CSF and Sylvian fissure volumes bilaterally in schizophrenia compared with bipolar disorder.

A meta-analysis of brain size in bipolar disorder by Hoge et al. (1999) did not demonstrate any reduction from controls, in contrast to the similar meta-analysis of schizophrenia by Ward et al. (1996) discussed above. Nevertheless, alterations in regional brain volumes have been reported in bipolar disorder compared both to schizophrenia and healthy controls. Rossi et al. (1991) found significant bilateral reductions in whole and medial temporal lobe areas on coronal MRI scans in schizophrenia but not bipolar disorder. Altshuler et al. (1998) and Roy et al. (1998) reported no differences between these disorders on overall temporal lobe volume, whilst Harvey et al. (1994) reported increased left temporal lobe grey matter volumes in their bipolar disorder group. The study of Altshuler et al. (1998) did find that, compared to healthy controls, the schizophrenic subjects had reduced hippocampal volumes whereas the bipolar disorder subjects had enlarged amygdala volumes. Hirayasu et al. (1998) measured temporal lobe structures in first-episode schizophrenia, affective psychosis, and controls, and found smaller left superior temporal gyrus and left posterior amygdala–hippocampal volumes in the schizophrenics compared to both comparison groups. However, Velakoulis et al. (1999) reported significant reductions in left hippocampal volumes in both first-episode schizophrenia and first-episode affective disorder. Schlaepfer et al. (1994) demonstrated that bipolar disorder was not associated with any loss of heteromodal association cortex grey matter volume, in contrast to their schizophrenic subjects. Finally, Sullivan et al. (1998) compared schizophrenics with alcoholics and normal controls, and found that both patient groups had significant grey matter volume deficits but only the alcoholics had white matter volume deficits. In addition, whilst the schizophrenics had preferential frontal and anterior temporal grey matter deficits, the alcoholic subjects showed more homogeneous cortical grey matter loss.

These findings together suggest that the magnitude and/or localization of cerebral and ventricular pathology may be different in schizophrenia compared with affective disorders and alcoholism.

Conclusions and future directions

Methodological issues for future studies

MRI has opened up new opportunities for the understanding of schizophrenia from a structural perspective. However, the study of brain abnormalities in the disorder is still hindered by insufficient knowledge of the normal determinants of brain structure (e.g. its heritability; Bartley *et al.*, 1997). In the absence of a full understanding of these issues, the selection of patients and controls for future research needs to be very closely examined. Sound epidemiological principles are required for both groups for results to be properly generalisable. In terms of patient selection this would ideally involve the follow-up of a birth cohort to avoid selection bias, although in practice first-episode patients are more feasible. Recruitment should involve consecutively ascertained incident cases from a geographically designated catchment area. Control subjects should be drawn in an unbiased fashion from the same population. Exclusion criteria need to be vigorously argued for, and equivalent in both groups. Cases and controls need to be adequately matched at least on age, sex, ethnicity, and parental socioeconomic status, and scanned prospectively and concurrently. The functioning of control subjects should be established using the same measures applied to assess the patients. Both super-normal populations and undeclared pathology in control subjects is to be avoided (Olson *et al.*, 1993). Concerning experimental and statistical design, *a priori* hypotheses should be well defined, multivariate analyses are preferable to multiple testing, covariates are preferable to ratio measures, and multiple linear regression is desirable to clarify which brain areas, if any, are particularly affected in schizophrenia.

Clearly such stringent research methodology is not possible with postmortem brain samples and high quality MRI is the only currently available tool which can in any way replace direct observation of the brain. Image analysis has now reached a stage where consensus must be reached on the delineation of cortical structures from consistently located surface rendered sulci rather than midline structures. If midline structures are to be used to delineate cortical regions, reliable re-registration of images is essential in order to reduce the effects of parallax. Unbiased stereological image analysis techniques are advisable (Barta *et al.*, 1997; Chapter 14). Shape analysis packages which allow for the examination of multiple modes of structural variation are also likely to reduce spurious results from multiple testing. Recent applications such as statistical parametric maps are a welcome step in this direction (Friston *et al.*, 1996; Wright *et al.*, 1999), although still open to artefact. Brain averaging through other morphometric approaches are a recent innovation which shows considerable promise (Arndt *et al.*, 1996; DeQuardo *et al.*, 1996; Haller *et al.*, 1997; Tibbo *et al.*, 1998; Buckley *et al.*, 1999)

Perhaps most importantly, the effect sizes of most of the variables studied, ventricular volume excepted, have been very small. Most published studies, with numbers in each group of on average 32 subjects, are insufficiently powered to discriminate between patient and control groups, a fact well established by the meta-analysis of Ward *et al.* (1996) for overall brain size. This is also a significant problem with postmortem research (Chapter 14). Recruitment of sufficient subjects to avoid type II errors is likely to require multicentre collaborative research, which in itself introduces new problems particularly with MRI scanner standardisation between centres.

Conclusions

Despite these problems and their implications (discussed in Chapter 13), there is an emerging consensus, helped in part by a number of careful systematic reviews of the neuroimaging literature. People with schizophrenia have relatively smaller brains than normal age- and sex-matched subjects. The finding of ventricular enlargement is well replicated. Although ventricular size varies considerably in the normal population, affected individuals have consistently larger ventricles than their unaffected siblings, suggesting that when a proportion of the normal genetic variance in the population is controlled for, the findings are robust (Suddath *et al.*, 1990; Noga *et al.*, 1996). The unaltered white matter volumes suggest that ventriculomegaly may reflect reduced volumes of certain adjacent subcortical nuclei. For instance, reduction in thalamic volumes have been reported in a number of studies and may be the cause of third ventricle enlargement.

A widespread reduction in cortical (including hippocampal) volume in schizophrenia has also been extensively replicated. The loss of volume is present at illness onset, is of the order of 4 per cent, affects grey rather than white matter, and appears, unlike ventriculomegaly, to be specific to schizophrenia rather than to major mental disorder generally. The grey matter reduction seems most evident in heteromodal association cortex although it may affect the entire cortex to a lesser extent The STG is a particular area of interest and future attempts to examine structural correlates of positive psychotic symptoms should clarify its importance in the genesis of these. Ventricular enlargement does not correlate with cortical grey matter reduction or sulcal enlargement, providing indirect evidence suggestive of different aetiological mechanisms. There is a loss of the normal cerebral asymmetry, with temporal lobe structures being most affected (Chapter 6).

High-risk and family studies show that some of the structural abnormalities observed in schizophrenia are also present in non-psychotic relatives with or without other schizophrenia spectrum disorders (Harrison, 1999). Ventricles are larger in schizophrenic probands than in their unaffected siblings (Weinberger *et al.*, 1981; Delisi *et al.*, 1986; Sharma *et al.*, 1998) although the latter (Weinberger *et al.*, 1981; but not DeLisi *et al.*, 1986) and the schizotypal offspring of schizophrenic patients (Schulsinger *et al.*, 1984; but not Cannon *et al.*, 1994) in turn have larger ventricles than healthy subjects from unaffected families. Both schizophrenics and their schizotypal relatives show comparable degrees of cortical sulcal volume increase compared with healthy relatives and normal control subjects (Cannon *et al.*, 1994; Honer *et al.*, 1995*a*). It is unclear whether cortical grey matter volume is reduced in unaffected or schizotypal relatives of people with schizophrenia.

In total, the current structural imaging evidence supports the hypothesis that schizophrenia is a largely genetic, neurodevelopmental disorder of the cerebral cortex (Chapter 8). Ventricular enlargement may represent the aftermath of early neuroenvironmental risk factors, perhaps with a progressive element in the most severely affected patients, which acts in conjunction with a genetic diathesis represented by cortical changes, to produce the full schizophrenia phenotype. The findings of the MRI and CT studies provide a context in which the current attempts to reveal the microscopic pathology of schizophrenia, described in subsequent chapters, can and should be interpreted.

References

Akbarian S, Bunney WE, Potkin SG *et al.* (1993) Altered distribution of nicotinamide-adenine dinucleotide phosphate-diaphorase cells in frontal lobe of schizophrenics implies disturbance of cortical development. *Archives of General Psychiatry* **50**, 169–177.

Altshuler LL, Casanova MF, Goldberg TE and Kleinman JE (1990) The hippocampus and parahippocampus in schizophrenic, suicide, and control brains. *Archives of General Psychiatry* **47**, 1029–1034.

Altshuler LL, Bartzokis G, Grieder T, Curran J and Mintz J (1998) Amygdala enlargement in bipolar disorder and hippocampal reduction in schizophrenia: An MRI study demonstrating neuroanatomic specificity. *Archives of General Psychiatry* **55**, 663–664.

Alzheimer A (1897) Beitrage zur pathologischen Anatomie der Hirnrinde und zur anatomischen Grundlage einer Psychosen *Monatsschrift Psychiatrie und Neurologie* **2**, 82–120.

Andreasen NC, Ehrhardt JC, Swayze VW *et al.* (1990) Magnetic resonance imaging of the brain in schizophrenia. The pathophysiologic significance of structural abnormalities. *Archives of General Psychiatry* **47**, 35–44.

Andreasen NC, Flaum MA, Swayze VW *et al.* (1993) Intelligence and brain structure in normal individuals. *American Journal of Psychiatry* **150**, 130–134.

Andreasen NC, Arndt S, Swayze V *et al.* (1994*a*) Thalamic abnormalities in schizophrenia visualized through magnetic resonance image averaging. *Science* **266**, 294–298.

Andreasen NC, Flashman L, Flaum M *et al.* (1994*b*) Regional brain abnormalities in schizophrenia measured with magnetic resonance imaging. *Journal of the American Medical Association* **272**, 1763–1769.

Arciniegas D, Rojas DC, Teale P, Sheeder J, Sandberg E and Reite M (1999) The thalamus and the schizophrenia phenotype: failure to replicate reduced volume. *Biological Psychiatry* **45**, 1329–1335.

Arndt S, Cohen G, Alliger RJ, Swayze VW and Andreasen NC (1991) Problems with ratio and proportion measures of imaged cerebral structures. *Psychiatry Research* **40**, 79–89.

Arndt S, Rajarethinam R, Cizadlo T, O'Leary D, Downhill J and Andreasen NC (1996) Landmark based registration and measurement of magnetic resonance images: a reliability study. *Psychiatry Research* **67**, 145–154.

Arnold SE, Gur RE, Shapiro RM *et al.* (1995) Prospective clinicopathologic studies of schizophrenia: accrual and assessment of patients. *American Journal of Psychiatry* **152**, 731–737.

Aylward EH, Reiss A, Barta PE *et al.* (1994) Magnetic resonance imaging measurement of posterior fossa structures in schizophrenia. *American Journal of Psychiatry* **151**, 1448–1452.

Baaré WFC, Hulshoff Pol HE, Hijman R, Mali WPT, Viergever MA and Kahn RS (1999) Volumetric analysis of frontal lobe regions in schizophrenia: Relation to cognitive function and symptomatology. *Biological Psychiatry* **45**, 1597–1605.

Barr WB, Ashtari M, Bilder RM, Degreef G and Lieberman JA (1997) Brain morphometric comparison of first-episode schizophrenia and temporal lobe epilepsy. *British Journal of Psychiatry* **170**, 515–519.

Barta PE, Pearlson GD, Powers RE, Richards SS and Tune LE (1990) Auditory hallucinations and smaller superior temporal gyral volume in schizophrenia. *American Journal of Psychiatry* **147**, 1457–1462.

Barta PE, Pearlson GD, Brill LB *et al.* (1997) Planum temporale asymmetry reversal in schizophrenia: replication and relationship to gray matter abnormalities. *American Journal of Psychiatry* **154**, 661–667.

Bartley AJ, Jones DW and Weinberger DR (1997) Genetic variability of human brain size and cortical gyral patterns. *Brain* **120**, 257–269.

Bartzokis G, Garber HJ, Griswold VJ, Oldendorf WH, Mintz J and Marder SR (1991) T2 hyperintense foci on magnetic resonance images of schizophrenic patients and controls. *Psychiatry Research* **40**, 239–245.

Bilder RM, Wu H, Bogerts B *et al.* (1994) Absence of regional hemispheric volume asymmetries in first-episode schizophrenia. *American Journal of Psychiatry* **151**, 1437 1447.

Bigelow LB, Nasrallah HA and Rauscher FP (1983) Corpus callosum thickness in chronic schizophrenia. *British Journal of Psychiatry* **142**, 284–287.

Bogerts B, Hantsch J and Herzer M (1983) A morphometric study of the dopamine-containing cell groups in the mesencephalon of normals, Parkinsonian patients, and schizophrenics. *Biological Psychiatry* **18**, 951–969.

Bogerts B, Meertz E and Schonfeldt-Bausch R (1985) Basal ganglia and limbic system pathology in schizophrenia: a morphometric study of brain volume and shrinkage. *Archives of General Psychiatry* **42**, 784–791.

Bogerts B, Ashtari M, Degreef G, Alvir JM, Bilder RM and Lieberman JA (1990*a*) Reduced temporal limbic structure volumes on magnetic resonance images in first episode schizophrenia. *Psychiatry Research* **35**, 1–13.

Bogerts B, Falkai P, Haupts M *et al.* (1990*b*) Post-mortem volume measurements of limbic system and basal ganglia structures in chronic schizophrenics: initial results from a new brain collection. *Schizophrenia Research* **3**, 295–301.

Bogerts B, Falkai P and Greve B (1991) Evidence of reduced temporolimbic structure volumes in schizophrenia. *Archives of General Psychiatry* **48**, 956–957.

Bogerts B, Lieberman JA, Ashtari M *et al.* (1993) Hippocampus–amygdala volumes and psychopathology in chronic schizophrenia. *Biolological Psychiatry* **33**, 236–246.

Breier A, Buchanan RW, Elkashef A, Munson RC, Kirkpatrick B and Gellad F (1992) Brain morphology and schizophrenia. A magnetic resonance imaging study of limbic, prefrontal cortex, and caudate structures. *Archives of General Psychiatry* **49**, 921–926.

Brown R, Colter N, Corsellis N *et al.* (1986) Postmortem evidence of structural brain changes in schizophrenia: differences in brain weight, temporal horn area and parahippocampal gyrus compared with affective disorder. *Archives of General Psychiatry* **43**, 36–42.

Bruton CJ, Crow J, Frith CD, Johnstone EC, Owens DGC and Roberts GW (1990) Schizophrenia and the brain: a prospective clinico-neuropathological study. *Psychological Medicine* **20**, 285–304.

Bryant NL, Buchanan RW, Vladar K, Breier A and Rothman M (1999) Gender differences in temporal lobe structures of patients with schizophrenia: a volumetric MRI study. *American Journal of Psychiatry* **156**, 603–609.

Buchanan RW, Breier A, Kirkpatrick B *et al.* (1993) Structural abnormalities in deficit and nondeficit schizophrenia. *American Journal of Psychiatry* **150**, 59–65.

Buchanan RW, Vladar K, Barta PE and Pearlson GD (1998) Structural evaluation of the prefrontal cortex in schzophrenia. *American Journal of Pyschiatry* **155**, 1049–1055.

Buchsbaum MS, Someya T, Teng CY *et al.* (1996) PET and MRI of the thalamus in never-medicated patients with schizophrenia. *American Journal of Psychiatry* **153**, 191–199.

Buckley PF, Dean D, Bookstein FL *et al.* (1999) Three-dimensional magnetic resonance-based morphometrics and ventricular dysmorphology in schizophrenia. *Biological Psychiatry* **45**, 62–67.

Bullmore E, Brammer M, Harvey I, Persaud R, Murray R and Ron M (1994) Fractal analysis of the boundary between white matter and cerebral cortex in magnetic resonance images: a controlled study of schizophrenic and manic-depressive patients. *Psychological Medicine* **24**, 771–781.

Cannon TD, Mednick SA, Parnas J, Schulsinger F, Praestholm J and Vestergaard A (1994) Developmental brain abnormalities in the offspring of schizophrenic mothers. II: Structural brain characteristics of schizophrenia and schizotypal personality disorder. *Archives of General Psychiatry* **51**, 955–962.

Cannon TD, van Erp TGM, Huttunen M *et al.* (1998) Regional gray matter, white matter, and cerebrospinal fluid distributions in schizophrenic patients, their siblings and controls. *Archives of General Psychiatry* **55**, 1084–1091.

Casanova MF, Sanders RD, Goldberg TE *et al.* (1990) Morphometry of the corpus callosum in monozygotic twins discordant for schizophrenia: a magnetic resonance imaging study. *Journal of Neurology, Neurosurgery and Psychiatry* **53**, 416–421.

Chakos MH, Lieberman JA, Bilder RM *et al.* (1994) Increase in caudate nuclei volumes of first-episode schizophrenic patients taking antipsychotic drugs. *American Journal of Psychiatry* **151**, 1430–1436.

Colombo C, Abbruzzese M, Livian S *et al.* (1993) Memory functions and temporal-limbic morphology in schizophrenia. *Psychiatry Research* **50**, 45–56.

Colombo C, Bonfanti A and Scarone S (1994) Anatomical characteristics of the corpus callosum and clinical correlates in schizophrenia. *European Archives of Psychiatry and Clinical Neuroscience* **243**, 244–248.

Corey-Bloom J, Jernigan T, Archibald S, Harris MJ and Jeste DV (1995) Quantitative magnetic resonance imaging of the brain in late-life schizophrenia. *American Journal of Psychiatry* **152**, 447–449.

Corsellis JAN (1976) Psychoses of obscure pathology. In: Blackwood H and Corsellis JAN eds, *Greenfield's neuropathology* 3rd edn. London: Edward Arnold, pp. 903–915.

Corson PW, Nopoulos P, Miller DD, Arndt S and Andreasen NC (1999) Change in basal ganglia volume over 2 years in patients with schizophrenia: typical versus atypical neuroleptics. *American Journal of Psychiatry* **156**, 1200–1204.

Cowell PE, Kostianovsky DJ, Gur RC, Turetsky BI and Gur RE (1996) Sex differences in neuroanatomical and clinical correlations in schizophrenia. *American Journal of Psychiatry* **153**, 799–805.

Crow TJ (1980) Molecular pathology of schizophrenia. More than one disease process? *British Medical Journal* **280**, 66–68.

Crow TJ, Ball J, Bloom SR *et al.* (1989) Schizophrenia as an anomaly of development of cerebral asymmetry. *Archives of General Psychiatry* **46**, 1145–1150.

Csernansky JG, Joshi S, Wang L *et al.* (1998) Hippocampal morphometry in schizophrenia by high dimensional brain mapping. *Proceedings of the National Academy of Sciences* **95**, 11406–11411.

Daniel D, Goldberg T, Gibbons R and Weinberger D (1991) Lack of bimodal distribution of ventricular size in schizophrenia: a Gaussian mixture analysis of 1056 cases and controls. *Biological Psychiatry* **30**, 887–903.

Dauphinais ID, DeLisi LE, Crow TJ *et al.* (1990) Reduction in temporal lobe size in siblings with schizophrenia: a magnetic resonance imaging study. *Psychiatry Research* **35**, 137–147.

David AS, Wacharasindhu A and Lishman WA (1994) Severe psychiatric disturbance and abnormalities of the corpus callosum: review and case series. *Journal of Neurology Neurosurgery and Psychiatry* **56**, 85–93.

Davis KL, Buchsbaum MS, Shihabuddin L *et al.* (1998) Ventricular enlargement in poor-outcome schizophrenia. *Biological Psychiatry* **43**, 783–93.

Daviss SR, Bolden R and Conley RC (1994) Cavum septum pellucidum in MR images of treatment-resistant and treatment-responsive schizophrenic subjects. *Schizophrenia Research* **11**, 138.

Degreef G, Ashtari M, Wu HW, Borenstein M, Geisler S and Lieberman J (1991) Follow up MRI study in first episode schizophrenia. *Schizophrenia Research* **5**, 204–206.

Degreef G, Ashtari M, Bogerts B *et al.* (1992a) Volumes of ventricular system subdivisions measured from magnetic resonance images in first-episode schizophrenic patients. *Archives of General Psychiatry* **49**, 531–537.

Degreef G, Bogerts B, Falkai P *et al.* (1992b) Increased prevalence of the cavum septum pellucidum in magnetic resonance scans and post-mortem brains of schizophrenic patients. *Psychiatry Research: Neuroimaging* **45**, 1–13.

DeLisi LE, Goldin LR, Hamovit JR, Maxwell ME, Kurtz D and Gershon ES (1986) A family study of the association of increased ventricular size with schizophrenia. *Archives of General Psychiatry* **43**, 148–153.

DeLisi LE, Dauphinais ID and Gershon ES (1988) Perinatal complications and reduced size of brain limbic structures in familial schizophrenia. *Schizophrenia Bulletin* **14**, 185–191.

DeLisi LE, Hoff AL, Schwartz JE *et al.* (1991a) Brain morphology in first-episode schizophrenic-like psychotic patients: a quantitative magnetic resonance imaging study. *Biological Psychiatry* **29**, 159–175.

DeLisi LE, Stritzke PH, Holan V *et al.* (1991*b*) Brain morphological changes in 1st episode cases of schizophrenia: are they progressive? *Schizophrenia Research* **5**, 206–208.

DeLisi LE, Stritzke P, Riordan H *et al.* (1992) The timing of brain morphological changes in schizophrenia and their relationship to clinical outcome. *Biological Psychiatry* **31**, 241–254.

DeLisi LE, Hoff AL, Kushner M and Degreef G (1993) Increased prevalence of cavum septum pellucidum in schizophrenia. *Psychiatry Research: Neuroimaging* **50**, 193–199.

DeLisi LE, Hoff AL, Neale C and Kushner M (1994) Asymmetries in the superior temporal lobe in male and female first-episode schizophrenic patients: measures of the planum temporale and superior temporal gyrus by MRI. *Schizophrenia Research* **12**, 19–28.

DeLisi LE, Tew W, Xie S *et al.* (1995) A prospective follow-up study of brain morphology and cognition in first-episode schizophrenic patients: preliminary findings. *Biological Psychiatry* **38**, 349–360.

DeLisi LE, Sakuma M, Tew W, Kushner M, Hoff AL and Grimson R (1997) Schizophrenia as a chronic active brain process: a study of progressive brain structural change subsequent to the onset of schizophrenia. *Psychiatry Research* **74**, 129–140.

DeQuardo JR, Bookstein FL, Green WDK, Brunberg JA and Tandon R (1996) Spatial relationships of neuroanatomic landmarks in schizophrenia. *Psychiatry Research* **67**, 81–91.

Elkashef AM, Buchanan RW, Gellad F, Munson RC and Breier A (1994) Basal ganglia pathology in schizophrenia and tardive dyskinesia: an MRI quantitative study. *American Journal of Psychiatry* **151**, 752–755.

Elkis H, Friedman L, Wise A and Meltzer HY (1995) Meta-analyses of studies of ventricular enlargement and cortical sulcal prominence in mood disorders. Comparisons with controls or patients with schizophrenia. *Archives of General Psychiatry* **52**, 735–746.

Falkai P and Bogerts B (1986) Cell loss in the hippocampus of schizophrenics. *European Archives of Psychiatry and Neurological Science* **236**, 154–161.

Falkai P, Bogerts B and Rozumek M (1988) Limbic pathology in schizophrenia: the entorhinal region—a morphometric study. *Biological Psychiatry* **24**, 515–521.

Flaum M, Andreasen NC, Swayze VW, O'Leary DS and Alliger RJ (1994) IQ and brain size in schizophrenia. *Psychiatry Research* **53**, 243–257.

Flaum M, Swayze VW, O'Leary DS *et al.* (1995) Effects of diagnosis, laterality, and gender on brain morphology in schizophrenia. *American Journal of Psychiatry* **152**, 704–714.

Flor-Henry P (1969) Psychosis and temporal lobe epilepsy. *Epilepsia* **10**, 363–395.

Frazier JA, Giedd JN, Hamburger SD *et al.* (1996) Brain anatomic magnetic resonance imaging in childhood-onset schizophrenia. *Archives of General Psychiatry* **53**, 617–624.

Friston KJ, Frith CD, Fletcher P, Liddle PF and Frackowiak RS (1996) Functional topography: multidimensional scaling and functional connectivity in the brain. *Cerebral Cortex* **6**, 156–164.

Fukuzako H and Kodama S (1998) Cavum septum pellucidum in schizophrenia. *Biological Psychiatry* **43**, 467.

Fukuzako H, Fukazako T, Hashiguchi T *et al.* (1996) Reduction in hippocampal formation volume is caused mainly by its shortening in chronic schizophrenia: assessment by MRI. *Biological Psychiatry* **39**, 938–945.

Gewirtz G, Squires-Wheeler E, Sharif Z and Honer WG (1994) Results of computerised tomography during first admission for psychosis. *British Journal of Psychiatry* **164**, 789–795.

Goldstein JM, Seidman LJ, Goodman JM *et al.* (1996) The impact of sex on cognition and structural brain abnormalities in schizophrenia. *Biological Psychiatry* **39**, 575.

Günther W, Petsch R, Steinberg R *et al.* (1991) Brain dysfunction during motor activation and corpus callosum alterations in schizophrenia measured by cerebral blood flow and magnetic resonance imaging. *Biological Psychiatry* **29**, 535–555.

Gur RE, Mozley PD, Resnick SM *et al.* (1991) Magnetic resonance imaging in schizophrenia. I. Volumetric analysis of brain and cerebrospinal fluid. *Archives of General Psychiatry* **48**, 407–412.

Gur RE, Mozley PD, Shtasel DL *et al.* (1994) Clinical subtypes of schizophrenia: differences in brain and CSF volume. *American Journal of Psychiatry* **151**, 343–350.

Gur RE, Cowell P, Turetsky BI *et al.* (1998a) A follow-up magnetic resonance imaging study of schizophrenia: relationship of neuroanatomical changes to clinical and neurobehavioural measures. *Archives of General Psychiatry* **55**, 145–152.

Gur RE, Maany V, Mozley PD, Swanson C, Bilker W and Gur RC (1998b) Subcortical MRI volumes in neuroleptic-naive and treated patients with schizophrenia. *American Journal of Psychiatry* **155**, 1711–1717.

Haller JW, Banerjee A, Christensen GE *et al.*(1997) Three-dimensional hippocampal MR morphometry with high dimensional transformation of a neuroanatomic atlas. *Radiology* **202**, 504–510.

Harrison PJ (1999) Brains at risk of schizophrenia. *Lancet* **353**, 3–4.

Harvey I, McGuffin P, Williams M and Toone BK (1990) The ventricle–brain ratio (VBR) in functional psychoses: an admixture analysis. *Psychiatry Research* **35**, 61–69.

Harvey I, Ron MA, Du Boulay G, Wicks D, Lewis SW and Murray RM (1993) Reduction of cortical volume in schizophrenia on magnetic resonance imaging. *Psychological Medicine* **23**, 591–604.

Harvey I, Persaud R, Ron MA, Baker G and Murray RM (1994) Volumetric MRI measurements in bipolars compared with schizophrenics and healthy controls. *Psychological Medicine* **24**, 689–699.

Hauser P, Dauphinais ID, Berrettini W, DeLisi LE, Gelernter J and Post RM (1989) Corpus callosum dimensions measured by magnetic resonance imaging in bipolar affective disorder and schizophrenia. *Biological Psychiatry* **26**, 659–668.

Havermans R, Honig A, Vuurman EFPM *et al.* (1999) A controlled study of temporal lobe structure volumes and P300 responses in schizophrenic patients with persistent auditory hallucinations. *Schizophrenia Research* **38**, 151–158.

Hazlett EA, Buchsbaum MS, Byne W *et al.* (1999) Three-dimensional analysis with MRI and PET of the size, shape, and function of the thalamus in the schizophrenia spectrum. *American Journal of Psychiatry* **156**, 1190–1199.

Heckers S, Heinsen H, Heinsen YC and Beckmann H (1990) Limbic structures and lateral ventricle in schizophrenia: a quantitative post mortem study. *Archives of General Psychiatry* **47**, 1016–1022.

Heckers S, Heinsen H, Heinsen YC and Beckmann H (1991) Cortex, white matter and basal ganglia in schizophrenia: a volumetric postmortem study. *Biological Psychiatry* **29**, 556–566.

Highley JR, Esiri MM, McDonald B, Cooper SJ and Crow TJ (1998) Temporal-lobe length is reduced, and gyral folding is increased in schizophrenia: a post-mortem study. *Schizophrenia Research* **34**, 1–12.

Highley JR, Esiri MM, McDonald B, Cortina-Borja M, Herron BM and Crow TJ (1999*a*) The size and fibre composition of the corpus callosum with respect to gender and schizophrenia: a post-mortem study. *Brain* **122**, 99–110.

Highley JR , Esiri MM, McDonald B, Roberts HC, Walker MA and Crow TJ (1999*b*) The size and fiber composition of the anterior commissure with respect to gender and schizophrenia. *Biological Psychiatry* **45**, 1120–1127.

Highley JR, McDonald B, Walker MA, Esiri MM and Crow TJ (1999*c*) Schizophrenia and temporal lobe asymmetry. A post-mortem stereological study of tissue volume. *British Journal of Psychiatry* **175**, 127–134.

Hirayasu Y, Shenton ME, Salisbury DF *et al.* (1998) Lower left temporal lobe MRI volumes in patients with first-episode schizophrenia compared with psychotic patients with first-episode affective disorder and normal subjects. *American Journal of Psychiatry* **155**, 1384–1391.

Hoff AL, Riordan H, O'Donnell D *et al.* (1992) Anomalous lateral sulcus asymmetry and cognitive function in first-episode schizophrenia. *Schizophrenia Bulletin* **18**, 257–272.

Hoff AL, Neal C, Kushner M and DeLisi LE (1994) Gender differences in corpus callosum size in first-episode schizophrenics. *Biological Psychiatry* **35**, 913–919.

Hoge EA, Friedman L and Schulz SC (1999) Meta-analysis of brain size in bipolar disorder. *Schizophrenia Research* **37**, 177–181.

Honer WG, Bassett AS, Squires-Wheeler E *et al.* (1995*a*) The temporal lobes, reversed asymmetry and the genetics of schizophrenia. *Neuroreport* **7**, 221–224.

Honer WG, Squires-Wheeler E, Smith GN, Sharif Z, Chan S and Gewirtz G (1995*b*) Developmental abnormalities and cortical sulcal enlargement in psychosis. *Schizophrenia Research* **16**, 121–125.

Jacobsen LK, Giedd JN, Vaituzis AC *et al.* (1996) Temporal lobe morphology in childhood-onset schizophrenia. *American Journal of Psychiatry* **153**, 355–361.

Jacobsen LK, Giedd JN, Berquin PC *et al.* (1997*a*) Quantitative morphology of the cerebellum and fourth ventricle in childhood-onset schizophrenia. *American Journal of Psychiatry* **154**, 1663–1669.

Jacobsen LK, Giedd JN, Rajapakse JC *et al.* (1997*b*) Quantitative magnetic resonance imaging of the corpus callosum in childhood onset schizophrenia. *Psychiatry Research: Neuroimaging* **68**, 77–86.

Jacobsen LK, Giedd JN, Tanrikut C *et al.* (1997*c*) Three dimensional cortical morphometry of the planum temporale in childhood onset schizophrenia. *American Journal of Psychiatry* **154**, 685–687.

Jacobsen KJ, Giedd JN, Castellanos FX *et al.* (1998) Progressive reduction of temporal lobe structures in childhood-onset schizophrenia. *American Journal of Psychiatry* **155**, 678–685.

Jakob H and Beckmann H (1986) Prenatal development disturbances in the limbic allocortex in schizophrenics. *Journal of Neural Transmission* **65**, 303–326.

Jernigan TL, Zisook S, Heaton RK, Moranville JT, Hesselink JR and Braff DL (1991) Magnetic resonance imaging abnormalities in lenticular nuclei and cerebral cortex in schizophrenia. *Archives of General Psychiatry* **48**, 881–890.

Jeste DV and Lohr JB (1989) Hippocampal pathologic findings in schizophrenia. A morphometric study. *Archives of General Psychiatry* **46**, 1019–1024.

Jeste DV, McAdams LA, Palmer BW *et al.* (1998) Relationship of neuropsychological and MRI measures to age of onset of schizophrenia. *Acta Psychiatrica Scandinavia* **98**, 156–164.

Johnstone EC, Crow TJ, Frith CD, Husband J and Kreel L (1976) Cerebral ventricular size and cognitive impairment in chronic schizophrenia. *Lancet* **ii**, 924–926.

Johnstone EC, Crow TJ, Macmillan JF, Owens DG, Bydder GM and Steiner RE (1986) A magnetic resonance study of early schizophrenia. *Journal of Neurology, Neurosurgery and Psychiatry* **49**, 136–139.

Jones PB, Harvey I, Lewis SW *et al.* (1994) Cerebral ventricle dimensions as risk factors for schizophrenia and affective psychosis: an epidemiological approach to analysis. *Psychological Medicine* **24**, 995–1011.

Jurjus GJ, Nasrallah HA, Brogan M and Olson SC (1993*a*) Developmental brain anomalies in schizophrenia and bipolar disorder: a controlled MRI study. *Journal of Neuropsychiatry and Clinical Neuroscience* **5**, 375–378.

Jurjus GJ, Nasrallah HA, Olson SC and Schwarzkopf SB (1993*b*) Cavum septum pellucidum in schizophrenia, affective disorder and healthy controls: a magnetic resonance imaging study. *Psychological Medicine* **23**, 319–322.

Katsetos CD, Hyde TM and Herman MM (1997) Neuropathology and the cerebellum in schizophrenia—an update: 1996 and future directions. *Biological Psychiatry* **42**, 213–224.

Kawasaki Y, Maeda Y, Urata K *et al.* (1993) A quantitative magnetic resonance imaging study of patients with schizophrenia. *European Archives of Psychiatry and Clinical Neurosciences* **242**, 268–272.

Kawasaki Y, Maeda Y, Higashima M *et al.* (1997) Reduced auditory P300 amplitude, medial temporal lobe reduction and psychopathology in schizophrenia. *Schizophrenia Research* **26**, 107–115.

Kelsoe JR, Cadet JL, Pickar D and Weinberger DR (1988) Quantitative neuroanatomy in schizophrenia. A controlled magnetic resonance imaging study. *Archives of General Psychiatry* **45**, 533–541.

Keshavan MS, Bagwell WW, Haas GL, Sweeney JA, Schooler NR and Pettegrew JW (1994) Changes in caudate volume with neuroleptic treatment. *Lancet* **344**, 1434.

Keshavan MS, Rosenberg D, Sweeney JA and Pettegrew JW (1998) Decreased caudate volume in neuroleptic-naive psychotic patients. *American Journal of Psychiatry* **155**, 774–778.

Kikinis R, Shenton ME, Gerig G *et al.* (1994) Temporal lobe sulco-gyral pattern anomalies in schizophrenia: an *in vivo* MR three-dimensional surface rendering study. *Neuroscience Letters* **182**, 7–12.

Kirkpatrick B, Litman D, Kim JW, Vladar K, Breier A and Buchanan RW (1997) Failure of fusion of the septum pellucidum and the heterogeneity of schizophrenia. *Journal of Nervous and Mental Diasease* **185**, 639–641.

Kraepelin E (1896) *Psychiatrie, ein lehrbuch für studierende und ärzte*, 5th edn. Leipzig: Barth.

Kraepelin E (1919) *Dementia praecox and paraphrenia*. In: Robertson GM ed., translated by Barclay RM and Krieger RE (1971). New York: Huntington.

Krull AJ, Press G, Dupont R, Harris MJ and Jeste DV (1991) Brain imaging in late-onset schizophrenia and related psychoses. *International Journal of Geriatric Psychiatry* **6**, 651–658.

Kulynych JJ, Vladar K, Jones DW and Weinberger DR (1996) Superior temporal gyrus volume in schizophrenia: a study using MRI morphometry assisted by surface rendering. *American Journal of Psychiatry* **153**, 50–56.

Kulynych JJ, Luevani LF, Jones DW and Weinberger DR (1997) Cortical abnormality in schizophrenia: an *in vivo* application of the gyrification index. *Biological Psychiatry* **41**, 995–999.

Kwon JS, Shenton ME, Hirayasu Y *et al.* (1998) MRI study of cavum septi pellucidi in schizophrenia, affective disorder, and schizotypal personality disorder. *American Journal of Psychiatry* **155**, 509–515.

Lauriello J, Hoff A, Wieneke MH *et al.* (1997) Similar extent of brain dysmorphology in severely ill women and men with schizophrenia. *American Journal of Psychiatry* **154**, 819–825.

Lawrie SM and Abukmeil SS (1998) Brain abnormality in schizophrenia. A systematic and quantitative review of volumetric magnetic resonance imaging studies. *British Journal of Psychiatry* **172**, 110–120.

Lawrie SM, Abukmeil SS, Chiswick A, Egan V, Santosh CG and Best JJK (1997) Qualitative cerebral morphology in schizophrenia: a magnetic resonance imaging study and systematic literature review. *Schizophrenia Research* **25**, 155–166.

Lawrie SM, Whalley H, Kestelman JN *et al.* (1999) Magnetic resonance imaging of brain in people at high risk of developing schizophrenia. *Lancet* **353**, 30–33.

Lesch A and Bogerts B (1984) The diencephalon in schizophrenia: Evidence for reduced thickness of the periventricular grey matter. *European Archives of Psychiatry and Neurological Sciences* **234**, 212–219.

Levitt JJ, McCarley RW, Nestor PG *et al.* (1999) Quantitative volumetric MRI study of the cerebellum and vermis in schizophrenia: clinical and cognitive correlates. *American Journal of Psychiatry* **156**, 1105–1107.

Lewis SW (1989) Congenital risk factors for schizophrenia. *Psychological Medicine* **19**, 5–13.

Lewis SW (1990) Computerised tomography in schizophrenia 15 years on. *British Journal of Psychiatry* (Suppl. 9), 16–24.

Lewis SW and Mezey GC (1985) Clinical correlates of septum pellucidum cavities: An unusual association with psychosis. *Psychological Medicine* **15**, 43–54.

Lewis SW, Reveley MA, David AS and Ron MA (1988) Agenesis of the corpus callosum and schizophrenia: a case report. *Psychological Medicine* **18**, 341–347.

Liddle PF and Morris DL (1991) Schizophrenic syndromes and frontal lobe performance. *British Journal of Psychiatry* **158**, 340–345.

Lim KO, Harris D, Beal M *et al.* (1996*a*) Gray matter deficits in young onset schizophrenia are independent of age of onset. *Biological Psychiatry* **40**, 4–13.

Lim KO, Sullivan EV, Zipursky RB and Pfefferbaum A (1996*b*) Cortical gray matter volume deficits in schizophrenia: a replication. *Schizophrenia Research* **20**, 157–164.

Lim KO, Tew W, Kushner M, Chow K, Matsumoto B and DeLisi LE (1996*c*) Cortical gray matter volume deficit in patients with first-episode schizophrenia. *American Journal of Psychiatry* **153**, 1548–1553.

Lim KO, Hedehus M, Mosely M, de Crespigny A, Sullivan EV and Pfefferbaum A (1999) Compromised white matter tract integrity in schizophrenia inferred from diffusion tensor imaging. *Archives of General Psychiatry* **56**, 367–374.

Lohr J and Jeste DV (1988) Locus ceruleus morphometry in aging and schizophrenia. *Acta Psychiatrica Scandinavica* **77**, 689–697.

McCarley RW, Shenton ME, O'Donnell BF *et al.* (1993) Auditory P300 abnormalities and left posterior superior temporal gyrus volume reduction in schizophrenia. *Archives of General Psychiatry* **50**, 190–197.

Machiyama Y, Wanatabe Y and Machiyama R (1987) Cerebral dynamics, laterality and psychopathology. In: Takahashi R, Flor-Henry P, Gruzelier J and Niwa S, eds. *Cerebral dynamics, laterality and psychopathology.* Hakone, Japan: Elsevier Science Publishers, pp. 411–412.

Marsh L, Suddath RL, Higgins N and Weinberger DR (1994) Medial temporal lobe structures in schizophrenia: relationship of size to duration of illness. *Schizophrenia Research* **11**, 225–238.

Marsh L, Harris D, Lim KO *et al.*(1997) Structural magnetic resonance imaging abnormalities in men with severe chronic schizophrenia and an early age at clinical onset. *Archives of General Psychiatry* **54**, 1104–1112.

Marsh L, Lim KO, Hoff AL *et al.* (1999) Severity of schizophrenia and magnetic resonance imaging abnormalities: a comparison of state and veterans hospital patients. *Biological Psychiatry* **45**, 49–61.

Mathalon DH, Sullivan EV, Rawles JM and Pfefferbaum A (1993) Correction for head size in brain-imaging measurements. *Psychiatry Research* **50**, 121–139.

Mathew RJ, Partain CL, Prakash R, Kulkarni MV, Logan TP and Wilson WH (1985) A study of the septum pellucidum and corpus callosum in schizophrenia with MR imaging. *Acta Psychiatrica Scandinavia* **72**, 414–421.

Menon RR, Barta PE, Aylward EH *et al.* (1995) Posterior superior temporal gyrus in schizophrenia: grey matter changes and clinical correlates. *Schizophrenia Research* **16**, 127–135.

Morice R and Delahunty A (1996) Frontal/executive impairments in schizophrenia. *Schizophrenia Bulletin* **22**, 125–137.

Morrison-Stewart SL, Williamson PC, Corning WC, Kutcher SP, Snow WG and Merskey H (1992) Frontal and non-frontal lobe neuropsychological test performance and clinical symptomatology in schizophrenia. *Psychological Medicine* **22**, 353–359.

Nair TR, Christensen JD, Kingsbury SJ, Kumar NG, Terry WM and Garver DL (1997) Progression of cerebroventricular enlargement and the subtyping of schizophrenia. *Psychiatry Research* **74**, 141–150.

Nasrallah HA, Andreasen NC, Coffman JA *et al.* (1986) A controlled magnetic resonance imaging study of corpus callosum thickness in schizophrenia. *Biological Psychiatry* **21**, 274–82 .

Nasrallah HA, Schwarzkopf SB, Olson SC and Coffman JA (1991) Perinatal brain injury and cerebellar vermal lobules I–X in schizophrenia. *Biological Psychiatry* **29**, 567–574.

Nasrallah HA, Sharma S and Olson SC (1997) The volume of the entorhinal cortex in schizophrenia: a controlled MRI study. *Progress in Neuropsychopharmacology and Biological Psychiatry* **21**, 1317–1322.

Nelson MD, Saykin AJ, Flashman LA and Riordan HJ (1998) Hippocampal volume reduction in schizophrenia as assessed by magnetic resonance imaging: A meta-analytic study. *Archives of General Psychiatry* **55**, 433–440.

Nieto A and Nieto D (1987) The red nucleus, the substantia nigra and the pineal gland responsible for mental illness. *International Journal of Neuroscience* **32**, 277–278.

Noga JT, Bartley AJ, Jones DW, Torrey EF and Weinberger DR (1996) Cortical gyral anatomy and gross brain dimensions in monozygotic twins discordant for schizophrenia. *Schizophrenia Research* **22**, 27–40.

Nopoulos PC, Flaum M, Andreasen NC and Swayze VW (1995*a*) Gray matter heterotopias in schizophrenia. *Psychiatry Research* **61**, 11–14.

Nopoulos P, Torres I, Flaum M, Andreasen NC, Ehrhardt JC and Yuh WT (1995*b*) Brain morphology in first-episode schizophrenia. *American Journal of Psychiatry* **152**, 1721–1723.

Nopoulos P, Flaum M and Andreasen NC (1997*a*) Sex differences in brain morphology in schizophrenia. *American Journal of Psychiatry* **154**, 1648–1654.

Nopoulos P, Swayze V, Flaum M, Ehrhardt JC, Yuh WT and Andreasen NC (1997*b*) Cavum septi pellucidi in normals and patients with schizophrenia as detected by magnetic resonance imaging. *Biological Psychiatry* **41**, 1102–1108.

Nopoulos PC, Giedd JN, Andreasen NC and Rapoport JL (1998*a*) Frequency and severity of enlarged cavum septum pellucidi in childhood-onset schizophrenia. *American Journal of Psychiatry* **155**, 1074–1079.

Nopoulos P, Swayze V, Flaum M and Andreasen NC (1998*b*) Incidence of ectopic gray matter in patients with schizophrenia and healthy control subjects studied with MRI. *Journal of Neuropsychiatry and Clinical Neuroscience* **10**, 351–353.

O'Callaghan E, Buckley P, Redmond O *et al.* (1992) Abnormalities of cerebral structure in schizophrenia on magnetic resonance imaging: interpretation in relation to the neurodevelopmental hypothesis. *Journal of the Royal Society of Medicine* **85**, 227–231.

Olson SC, Bornstein RA, Schwarzkopf SB and Nasrallah HA (1993) Are controls in schizophrenia research 'normal'? *Annals of Clinical Psychiatry* **5**, 1–5.

Pakkenberg B (1987) Post-mortem study of chronic schizophrenic brains. *British Journal of Psychiatry* **151**, 744–752.

Pakkenberg B (1990) Pronounced reduction of total neuron number in mediodorsal thalamic nucleus and nucleus accumbens in schizophrenics. *Archives of General Psychiatry* **47**, 1023–1028.

Pearlson GD, Tune LE, Wong DF *et al.* (1993) Quantitative D2 dopamine receptor PET and structural MRI changes in late-onset schizophrenia. *Schizophrenia Bulletin* **19**, 783–795.

Pearlson GD, Petty RG, Ross CA and Tien AY (1996) Schizophrenia: A disease of heteromodal association cortex? *Neuropsychopharmacology* **14**, 1–17.

Pearlson GD, Barta PE, Powers RE *et al.* (1997) Medial and superior temporal gyrus volumes and cerebral asymmetry in schizophrenia versus bipolar disorder. *Biological Psychiatry* **41**, 1–14.

Persaud R, Russow H, Harvey I *et al.* (1997) Focal signal hyperintensities in schizophrenia. *Schizophrenia Research* **27**, 55–64.

Plum F (1972) Prospects for research on schizophrenia. 3. Neurophysiology, neuropathological findings. *Neuroscience Research Program Bulletin* **10**, 384–388.

Portas CM, Goldstein JM, Shenton ME *et al.* (1998) Volumetric evaluation of the thalamus in schizophrenic male patients using magnetic resonance imaging. *Biological Psychiatry* **43**, 649–659.

Raine A, Harrison GN, Reynolds GP, Sheard C, Cooper JE and Medley I (1990) Structural and functional characteristics of the corpus callosum in schizophrenics, psychiatric controls, and normal controls. A magnetic resonance imaging and neuropsychological evaluation. *Archives of General Psychiatry* **47**, 1060–1064.

Raine A, Lencz T, Reynolds GP *et al.* (1992) An evaluation of structural and functional prefrontal deficits in schizophrenia: MRI and neuropsychological measures. *Psychiatry Research* **45**, 123–137.

Rajarethinam R, Gupta S and Andreasen NC (1995) Volume of the pineal gland in schizophrenia, an MRI study. *Schizophrenia Research* **14**, 253–255.

Rapoport JL, Giedd J, Kumra S *et al.* (1997) Childhood-onset schizophrenia: progressive ventricular change during adolescence. *Archives of General Psychiatry* **54**, 897–903.

Rapoport JL, Giedd JN, Blumenthal J *et al.* (1999) Progressive cortical change during adolescence in childhood-onset schizophrenia. *Archives of General Psychiatry* **56**, 649–654.

Raz S and Raz N (1990) Structural brain abnormalities in the major psychoses: a quantitative review of the evidence from computerized imaging. *Psychological Bulletin* **108**, 93–108.

Rosenthal R and Bigelow LB (1972) Quantitative brain measurements in chronic schizophrenia. *British Journal of Psychiatry* **121**, 259–264.

Rossi A, Stratta P, Gallucci M, Passariello R and Casacchia M (1989) Quantification of corpus callosum and ventricles in schizophrenia with nuclear magnetic resonance imaging: a pilot study. *American Journal of Psychiatry* **146**, 99–101.

Rossi A, Stratta P, D'Albenzio L *et al.* (1990) Reduced temporal lobe as in schizophrenia: preliminary evidence from a controlled multiplanar magnetic resonance imaging study. *Biological Psychiatry* **27**, 61–68.

Rossi A, Stratta P, Di Michele V *et al.* (1991) Temporal lobe structure by magnetic resonance in bipolar affective disorders and schizophrenia. *Journal of Affective Disorders* **21**, 19–22.

Rossi A, Stratta P, Mancini F, de Cataldo S and Casacchia M (1993) Cerebellar vermal size in schizophrenia: a male effect. *Biological Psychiatry* **33**, 354–357.

Rossi A, Stratta P, Mancini F *et al.* (1994) Magnetic resonance imaging findings of amygdala–anterior hippocampus shrinkage in male patients with schizophrenia. *Psychiatry Research* **52**, 43–53.

Roy PD, Zipursky RB, Saint-Cyr JA, Bury A, Langevin R and Seeman MV (1998) Temporal horn enlargement is present in schizophrenia and bipolar disorder. *Biological Psychiatry* **44**, 418–422.

Sandyk R and Kay SR (1990) Pineal calcification in schizophrenia. Relationship to age of onset and tardive dyskinesia. *Schizophrenia Research* **5**, 85–86.

Sandyk R (1993) The relationship of thought disorder to third ventricle width and calcification of the pineal gland in chronic schizophrenia. *International Journal of Neuroscience* **68**, 53–59.

Schlaepfer TE, Harris GJ, Tien AY *et al.* (1994) Decreased regional cortical gray matter volume in schizophrenia. *American Journal of Psychiatry* **151**, 842–848.

Schulsinger F, Parnas J, Petersen ET *et al.* (1984) Cerebral ventricular size in the offspring of schizophrenic mothers. A preliminary study. *Archives of General Psychiatry* **41**, 602–606.

Schwarzkopf SB, Nasrallah HA, Olson SC, Bogerts B, McLaughlin JA and Mitra T (1991) Family history and brain morphology in schizophrenia: an MRI study. *Psychiatry Research* **40**, 49–60.

Scott TF, Price TR, George MS, Brillman J and Rothfus W (1993) Midline cerebral malformations and schizophrenia. *Journal of Neuropsychiatry and Clinincal Neuroscience* **5**, 287–293.

Selemon LD, Rajkowska G and Goldman-Rakic PS (1995) Elevated neuronal density in prefrontal area 46 in brains from schizophrenic patients: application of a three-dimensional stereological counting method. *Journal of Comparative Neurology* **392**, 402–412.

Shan-Ming Y, Flor-Henry P, Dayi C, Tiangi L, Shuguang Q and Zenxiang M (1985) Imbalance of hemisphere functions in the major psychoses: a study of handedness in the peoples republic of China. *Biological Psychiatry* **20**, 906–917.

Sharma T, Lancaster E, Lee D *et al.* (1998) Brain changes in schizophrenia: Volumetric MRI study of families multiply affected with schizophrenia—the Maudsley Family Study 5. *British Journal of Psychiatry* **173**, 132–138.

Shenton ME, Kikinis R, McCarley RW, Metcalf D, Tieman J and Jolesz FA (1991) Application of automated MRI volumetric measurement techniques to the ventricular system in schizophrenics and normal controls. *Schizophrenia Research* **5**, 103–113.

Shenton ME, Kikinis R, Jolesz FA *et al.* (1992) Abnormalities of the left temporal lobe and thought disorder in schizophrenia. A quantitative magnetic resonance imaging study. *New England Journal of Medicine* **327**, 604–612.

Shihabuddin L, Buschbaum MS, Hazlett EA *et al.* (1998) Dorsal striatal size, shape, and metabolic rate in never-medicated and previously medicated schizophrenics performing a verbal learning task. *Archives of General Psychiatry* **55**, 235–243.

Shioiri T, Oshitani Y, Kato T *et al.* (1996) Prevalence of cavum septum pellucidum detected by MRI in patients with bipolar disorder, major depression and schizophrenia. *Psychological Medicine* **26**, 431–434.

Smith RC, Baumgartner R and Calderon M (1987) Magnetic resonance imaging studies of the brains of schizophrenic patients. *Psychiatry Research* **20**, 33–46.

Southard EE (1915) On the topographical distribution of cortex lesions and anomalies in dementia praecox with some account of their functional significance: IV. Clinical and anatomical analysis of twenty-five cases of dementia praecox, being a random selection. *American Journal of Insanity* **71**, 603–671.

Staal WG, Hulshoff Pol HE, Schnack H, van der Schot AC and Kahn RS (1998) Partial volume decrease of the thalamus in relatives of patients with schizophrenia. *American Journal of Psychiatry* **155**, 1784–1786.

Stratta P, Rossi A, Gallucci M, Amicarelli I, Passariello R and Casacchia M (1989) Hemispheric asymmetries and schizophrenia: a preliminary magnetic resonance imaging study. *Biological Psychiatry* **25**, 275–284.

Stratta P, Mancini F, Mattei P, Daneluzzo E, Casacchia M and Rossi A (1997) Association between striatal reduction and poor Wisconsin card sorting test performance in patients with schizophrenia. *Biological Psychiatry* **42**, 816–820.

Suddath RL, Casanova MF, Goldberg TE, Daniel DG, Kelsoe JR and Weinberger DR (1989) Temporal lobe pathology in schizophrenia: a quantitative magnetic resonance imaging study. *American Journal of Psychiatry* **146**, 464–472.

Suddath RL, Christison GW, Torrey EF, Casanova MF and Weinberger DR (1990) Anatomical abnormalities in the brains of twins discordant for schizophrenia. *New England Journal of Medicine* **322**, 842–845.

Sullivan EV, Mathalon DH, Lim KO, Marsh L and Pfefferbaum A (1998) Patterns of regional cortical dysmorphology distinguishing schizophrenia and chronic alcoholism. *Biological Psychiatry* **43**, 118–131.

Swayze VW, Andreasen NC, Alliger RJ, Ehrhardt JC and Yuh WT (1990*a*) Structural brain abnormalities in bipolar affective disorder. Ventricular enlargement and focal signal hyper-intensities. *Archives of General Psychiatry* **47**, 1054–1059.

Swayze VW, Andreasen NC, Ehrhardt JC, Yuh WTC, Alliger RJ and Cohen GA (1990*b*) Developmental abnormalities of the corpus callosum in schizophrenia. *Archives of Neurology* **47**, 805–808.

Swayze VW, Andreasen NC, Alliger RJ, Yuh WT and Ehrhardt JC (1992) Subcortical and temporal structures in affective disorder and schizophrenia: a magnetic resonance imaging study. *Biological Psychiatry* **31**, 221–240.

Symonds LL, Olichney JM, Jernigan TL, Corey-Bloom J, Healy JF and Jeste DV (1997) Lack of clinically significant gross structural abnormalities in MRIs of older patients with schizophrenia and related psychoses. *Journal of Neuropsychiatry and Clinical Neuroscience* **9**, 251–258.

Tibbo P, Nopoulos P, Arndt S and Andreasen NC (1998) Corpus callosum shape and size in male patients with schizophrenia. *Biological Psychiatry* **44**, 405–412.

Tien AY, Eaton WW, Schlaepfer TE *et al.* (1996) Exploratory factor analysis of MRI brain structure measures in schizophrenia. *Schizophrenia Research* **19**, 93–101.

Turetsky B, Cowell PE, Gur RC, Grossman RI, Shtasel DL and Gur RE (1995) Frontal and temporal lobe brain volumes in schizophrenia. Relationship to symptoms and clinical subtype. *Archives of General Psychiatry* **52**, 1061–1070.

Uematsu M and Kaiya H (1988) The morphology of the corpus callosum in schizophrenia. An MRI study. *Schizophrenia Research* **1**, 391–398.

van Horn JD and McManus IC (1992) Ventricular enlargement in schizophrenia. A meta-analysis of studies of the ventricle : brain ratio (VBR). *British Journal of Psychiatry* **160**, 687–697.

Velakoulis D, Pantelis C, McGorry PD *et al.* (1999) Hippocampal volume in first-episode psychoses and chronic schizophrenia. *Archives of General Psychiatry* **56**, 133–140.

Vita A, Dieci M, Giobbio GM, Tenconi F and Invernizzi G (1997) Time course of cerebral ventricular enlargement in schizophrenia supports the hypothesis of its neurodevelopmental nature. *Schizophrenia Research* **23**, 25–30.

Vogeley K, Hobson T, Scheider-Axmann T, Honer WG, Bogerts B and Falkai P (1998) Compartmental volumetry of the superior temporal gyrus reveals sex differences in schizophrenia—a post-mortem study. *Schizophrenia Research* **31**, 83–87.

Ward KE, Friedman L, Wise A and Schulz SC (1996) Meta-analysis of brain and cranial size in schizophrenia. *Schizophrenia Research* **22**, 197–213.

Weinberger DR, Torrey EF, Neophytides AN and Wyatt RJ (1979) Structural abnormalities in the cerebral cortex of chronic schizophrenic patients. *Archives of General Psychiatry* **36**, 935–939.

Weinberger DR, DeLisi LE, Neophytides AN and Wyatt RJ (1981) Familial aspects of CT scan abnormalities in chronic schizophrenic patients. *Psychiatry Research* **4**, 65–71.

Weinberger DR, Wagner RL and Wyatt RJ (1983) Neuropathological studies of schizophrenia: A selective review. *Schizophrenia Bulletin* **9**, 193–212.

Whitworth AB, Honeder M, Kremser C *et al.* (1998) Hippocampal volume reduction in male schizophrenic patients. *Schizophrenia Research* **31**, 73–81.

Wible CG, Shenton ME, Hokama H *et al.* (1995) Prefrontal cortex and schizophrenia. A quantitative magnetic resonance imaging study. *Archives of General Psychiatry* **52**, 279–288.

Woodruff PW, Pearlson GD, Geer MJ, Barta PE and Chilcoat HD (1993) A computerized magnetic resonance imaging study of corpus callosum morphology in schizophrenia. *Psychological Medicine* **23**, 45–56.

Woodruff PW, McManus IC and David AS (1995) Meta-analysis of corpus callosum size in schizophrenia. *Journal of Neurology, Neurosurgery and Psychiatry* **58**, 457–461.

Woodruff PW, Phillips ML, Rushe T, Wright IC, Murray RM and David AS (1997*a*) Corpus callosum size and inter-hemispheric function in schizophrenia. *Schizophrenia Research* **23**, 189–196.

Woodruff PWR, Wright IC, Shuriquie N *et al.* (1997*b*) Structural brain abnormalities in male schizophrenics reflect fronto-temporal dissociation. *Psychological Medicine* **27**, 1257–1266.

Woods BT and Yurgelun-Todd D (1991) Brain volume loss in schizophrenia: when does it occur and is it progressive? *Schizophrenia Research* **5**, 202–204.

Woods BT, Yurgelun-Todd D, Goldstein JM, Seidman LJ and Tsuang MT (1996) MRI brain abnormalities in chronic schizophrenia: one process or more? *Biological Psychiatry* **40**, 585–596.

Wright IC, Ellison ZR, Sharma T, Friston KJ, Murray RM and McGuire PK (1999) Mapping of grey matter changes in schizophrenia. *Schizophrenia Research* **35**, 1–14.

Zaidel DW, Esiri MM and Harrison PJ (1997) The hippocampus in schizophrenia: lateralized increase in neuronal density and altered cytoarchitectural asymmetry. *Psychological Medicine* **27**, 703–713.

Zipursky RB, Lim KO, Sullivan EV, Brown BW and Pfefferbaum A (1992) Widespread cerebral gray matter volume deficits in schizophrenia. *Archives of General Psychiatry* **49**, 195–205.

Zipursky RB, Marsh L, Lim KO *et al.* (1994) Volumetric MRI assessment of temporal lobe structures in schizophrenia. *Biological Psychiatry* **35**, 501–516.

Zipursky RB, Seeman MV, Bury A, Langevin R, Wortzman G and Katz R (1997) Deficits in gray matter volume are present in schizophrenia but not bipolar disorder. *Schizophrenia Research* **26**, 85–92.

Zipursky RB, Lambe EK, Kapur S and Mikulis DJ (1998*a*) Cerebral gray matter volume deficits in first episode psychosis. *Archives of General Psychiatry* **55**, 540–546.

Zipursky RB, Zhang-Wong J, Lambe EK, Bean G and Beiser M (1998*b*) MRI correlates of treatment response in first episode psychosis. *Schizophrenia Research* **30**, 81–90.

2 Hippocampal Pathology

Steven E. Arnold

The hippocampal formation has been a region of extensive clinical investigation in schizophrenia and also the most commonly studied region in postmortem research (Shapiro, 1993; Arnold and Trojanowski, 1996). There are a number of reasons to justify this. Clinicians have long noted similarities between the symptoms of schizophrenia and those of the schizophrenia-like organic psychoses associated with temporal lobe epilepsy, temporal lobe tumors, and cerebrovascular lesions, herpes encephalitis, and neurodegenerative diseases such as Alzheimer's disease and frontotemporal degenerative dementias which have particular predilections for the hippocampal region (Davison, 1983). In addition, early clinical neurobiological investigators described enlarged temporal horns in schizophrenia using pneumoencepholgraphy (Jacobi and Winkler, 1929) while electroencephalographers frequently reported abnormal recordings from temporal electrodes (Ellingson, 1954).

In the modern era, neuropsychological studies have found that within the context of widespread or even global cognitive impairments, there are differential deficits in verbal and visual declarative memory which have been attributed to hippocampal dysfunction (Gruzelier *et al.*, 1988; Saykin *et al.*, 1991). Follow-up cognitive studies find that these deficits persist even after the more florid psychotic symptoms attenuate with treatment (Gur *et al.*, 1998). This stability suggests a static, perhaps neuroanatomical, abnormality in the hippocampal formation. Indeed, structural neuroimaging studies have identified selective volume deficits in the amygdalohippocampal region and parahippocampal gyrus in schizophrenia (Nelson *et al.*, 1998), though findings are controversial and some investigators report that the smaller volumes are not regionally selective (Chapters 1 and 13). Some neuroimaging researchers have tried to elucidate more specifically the role of neuroanatomical abnormalities of the hippocampal formation in schizophrenia by corre-lating volumetric measures with various symptoms and signs. For instance, poor performance on tests of verbal memory, abstraction, and categorization as well as positive symptoms have been reported to correlate with reduced size of ventromedial temporal lobe structures (Shenton *et al.*, 1992; Bogerts *et al.*, 1993; Nestor *et al.*, 1993). Similarly, studies employing PET and functional MRI (Chapter 7) have reported abnormal blood flow or metabolic activity in the hippocampal region and these also have been found to correlate with psychi-atric measures (Friston *et al.*, 1992; Saykin *et al.*, 1995; Schroder *et al.*, 1995; Silbersweig *et al.*, 1995).

Despite remaining controversies, the clinical research findings together provide ample justification for the attention that has been paid to the hippocampal formation in postmortem studies. Another reason that the hippocampal formation is an attractive region to examine is that its normal neuroanatomy and connectivity are well delineated. Thus, it is a good model system in which to identify subtle, disease-related morphological, cellular, and mole-cular differences. This chapter reviews the histopathological findings in the hippocampal formation in schizophrenia described over the last quarter century. While 'lesions' pathog-nomonic for schizophrenia still await identification, the progressive characterization of the numerous abnormalities that have been reported holds great promise.

Neuroanatomy of the normal hippocampal formation

The hippocampal formation is found in the ventromedial portion of the temporal lobe. As shown in Fig. 2.1, it is composed of the dentate gyrus, the hippocampus proper (i.e. ammonic subfields CA1 to CA4), subiculum, and entorhinal cortex (Rosene and Van Hoesen, 1987; Amaral and Insausti, 1990). The dentate gyrus is easily identified as a thin, wavy layer of highly compacted granule cells that stain intensely for Nissl substance. Within the hilus formed by the limbs of the dentate gyrus lies CA4. This is a cluster of polymorphic neurons that can be distinguished from the next subfield, CA3, by its looser organization and its 'doubling back' from the projected trajectory of CA3 into the hilus. Given its intrin-sically less organized appearance, the boundaries between CA4 and the polymorphic layer of the dentate gyrus can be difficult to determine. The cellular layers of both CA3 and CA2 are characterized as a continuous thin, condensed band of large, more intensely staining pyramidal cells of relatively uniform alignment. As it extends into the hilus of the dentate gyrus, the neuron layer of CA3 fans out but remains distinct until its border with CA4. The border of CA2 with CA1 is easily demarcated by an abrupt change in appearance. CA1 is a relatively broad layer of perpendicularly oriented pyramidal cells that are less densely packed than in CA2 and with slightly greater variability of orientation. In general, the neurons of CA1 are smaller in size than corresponding neurons in subiculum or in CA2 and CA3.

The subiculum rests in the superior aspect of the parahippocampal gyrus along the hippocampal fissure. It is composed of large and medium sized pyramidal cells intermixed with some stellate cells throughout, and horizontally oriented fusiform neurons in the deepest aspects adjacent to the angular bundle (white matter of the parahippocampal gyrus). The

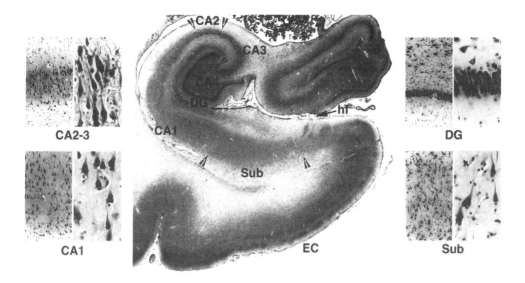

Fig. 2.1 Nissl-stained coronal section through the hippocampal formation and caudal portion of the entorhinal cortex (part of the parahippocampal gyrus). Insets at higher magnifications show the cytoarchitecture of the cellular layers of the subiculum (Sub), dentate gyrus (DG), CA1, and the border zone of CA2 and CA3. Left inset, x100; right, x400; hf, hippocampal fissure.

cells in the transition zone between CA1 and subiculum have been highlighted by some anatomists as comprising a distinct entity, the prosubiculum, with its own distinguishing cytoarchitectural, neurochemical, and connectional features. Others consider it part of the subiculum. The subiculum is distinguished from the presubiculum by contrasting its cells to the small pyramidal cells characteristic of the presubiculum's pyramidal cell layer, as well as the presence of the 'clouds' of small cells overlying the pyramidal cell layer of the presubiculum. Because of its various putative subdivisions, the subiculum is sometimes known as the subicular complex.

The entorhinal cortex is a periallocortex lying on the inferior and medial aspects of the anterior portion of the parahippocampal gyrus. It is easily distinguished cytoarchitecturally by its hallmark clusters of stellate neurons in layer II (pre-α cells) and the relatively acellular lamina dissecans constituting layer IV (see Fig. 2.3). Despite its unique appearance the entorhinal cortex is cytoarchitecturally and hodologically complex and has been named and subdivided according to several different schemes (Van Hoesen and Pandya, 1975; Braak, 1980; Amaral *et al.*, 1987; Insausti *et al.*, 1995).

The components of the hippocampal formation are integrated in an orderly connectional system that serves as a turnaround point for hierarchical streams of cortical processing and as a node for cortical–limbic–subcortical interactions. Afferent projections from association cortices in all four lobes converge on neurons in layer II and the superficial portion of layer III of the entorhinal cortex (Van Hoesen, 1982; Fig. 2.2). Axons from these neurons form the perforant pathway which projects to the outer molecular layer of the dentate gyrus and synapse on dendrites of granule cells. This pathway is the main, though not sole, conduit for information regarding sensory experience to enter the hippocampus. The granule cells' axons are known as mossy fibers (not to be confused with mossy cells, which are a separate hilar cell population) and project to neurons in CA4 and CA3. CA3 neurons then originate the Schaffer collateral projections to CA2 and especially CA1, and thence to the subiculum. Neurons within CA1 and subiculum send efferent projections back to the entorhinal cortex (layer V), and also directly to diverse cortical association areas in frontal, temporal, and parietal lobes, and to subcortical targets such as the amygdala, ventral striatum, and hypothalamus (Rosene and Van Hoesen, 1977; Amaral and Insausti, 1990). The circuit described here is excitatory, and is complemented by various inhibitory interneuron populations.

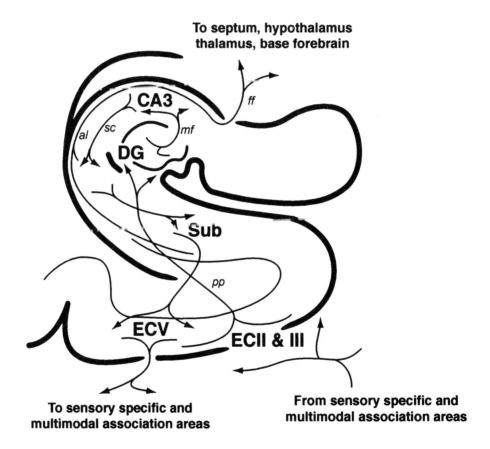

Fig. 2.2 Circuitry of the hippocampal formation. *al*, alveus; DG, dentate gyrus; ECII & III, layers II and III of the entorhinal cortex; ECV, layer V of entorhinal cortex; *ff*, fimbria-fornix; *mf*, mossy fibres; *pp*, perforant pathway; *sc*, Schaffer collaterals; Sub, subiculum.

Particularly important in linking the hippocampus with the rest of the brain are layers II and III of the entorhinal cortex which contain the principal afferent recipient neurons, and CA1, subiculum, and layer V of the entorhinal cortex which contain the principal efferent projection neurons that provide feedback connections to diverse cortical and subcortical brain regions. This extensive feedforward and feedback connectivity with much of the cerebrum puts the hippocampal formation in a nodal position to control or influence a wide variety of higher cognitive and emotional processes (Damasio, 1989). It is easy to see how abnormalities in the hippocampal formation could have far-reaching consequences in various neuropsychological processes that are awry in schizophrenia.

Gross morphometry of the hippocampal formation in schizophrenia

Quantitative gross anatomical studies of the postmortem brain have used similar planimetric and volumetric methods to those used in *in vivo* neuroimaging studies to measure the size of ventromedial temporal lobe structures. The principal studies are listed in Table 2.1. It is interesting that while MRI studies generally report smaller hippocampal and parahippocampal volumes, the postmortem findings are less consistent. There are a number of methodological variables that might explain these inconsistencies, such as the limited sample sizes of most postmortem studies, the methods of sampling cross-sectional profiles for area determination, or varying methods for determining boundaries of and within the hippocampus. In light of these constraints and the excellent and still improving resolution of structural MRI, it even may not be necessary to examine postmortem specimens for gross morphology at all.

Table 2.1 Gross postmortem measurements of the hippocampal formation in schizophrenia

Region/parameter	Finding	Positive reports of the finding	Negative reports of the finding
Hippocampal area or volume	Decreased	Bogerts *et al*, 1985 Jeste and Lohr 1989 Bogerts *et al*, 1990	Heckers *et al*, 1990, 1991 Altshuler *et al*,1990 Bruton *et al*, 1990 Benes *et al*, 1991
Parahippocampal area or volume	Decreased	Bogerts *et al*, 1985 Falkai *et al*, 1988	Colter *et al*, 1987
Parahippocampal cortical thickness	Decreased	Brown *et al*, 1986 Colter *et al*, 1987 Altshuler *et al*, 1990	

Hippocampal cytoarchitecture and neuronal morphometry in schizophrenia

Cytoarchitectural studies

Cytoarchitecture refers to the cellular composition and spatial arrangement of cells in a given brain region. Because cytoarchitecture is largely determined during fetal brain development, descriptions of cytoarchitectural abnormalities of the entorhinal cortex and hippocampus (Table 2.2) have played prominent roles in discussions of schizophrenia as a neurodevelopmental disorder (Chapter 8).

The entorhinal cortex has been a particularly interesting and controversial area of cytoarchitectural investigation in schizophrenia. Jakob and Beckmann (1986) first reported 'definite' qualitative cytoarchitectural abnormalities in superficial layers of the rostral entorhinal cortex in 20 of 64 patients with schizophrenia, and equivocal changes in another 22. These abnormalities consisted of poor development of layers II and III—also known as layers pre-α, pre-β, and pre-γ in the nomenclature of Braak (1980)—with atypically ordered neurons of differing size in layer II (pre-α) instead of the characteristic clustering of neurons into islands, a reduced number of neurons in the superficial portion of layer III (pre-β), and heterotopic groups of neurons belonging to layer II that instead were found in layer III. In addition, many of the neurons appeared smaller and there was poor development and a reduction in neuron numbers in layer IV (pre-α). Glial number and distribution appeared normal. The authors suggested that the findings were most consistent with an abnormality of neuronal migration occurring in the second trimester of gestation when the laminar pattern of the entorhinal cortex is set (Jakob and Beckmann, 1986, 1994).

Another study also qualitatively described the entorhinal cortex, in a sample of six patients (all postleucotomy) and 16 controls (including three postleucotomy and two post-thalamotomy for non-schizophrenic conditions) from the archival Yakovlev collection (Arnold *et al.*, 1991*b*). Case selection was determined by rigorous application of diagnostic criteria to chart review. Blind to diagnosis, raters reported various abnormalities in the rostral and intermediate portions of the entorhinal cortex in each of the schizophrenia individuals. These included bizarre invaginations of the normally smooth entorhinal surface with disruption of superficial cortical layers, poorly formed layer II neuron clusters with heterotopic displacement of neurons typical of layer II deep into layer III, paucity of neurons in superficial layers, and attenuation of deeper layers (Fig. 2.3). They suggested that such abnormalities were most consistent with disturbed cortical development and, because of the pivotal role that the entorhinal cortex plays in cortical–hippocampal connectivity, that disturbance of these connections could have far-reaching neuropsychological consequences.

These findings and conclusions have been influential for neurodevelopmental theorists of schizophrenia (Chapter 8) and have even helped spawn animal models which explore the effects of neonatal lesions of the entorhinal and hippocampal regions (Chapter 12). However, some other groups have not been able to confirm the initial findings. One of the chief criticisms is that the described abnormalities in schizophrenia just reflect the normal variability of cytoarchitectural appearance of the entorhinal cortex (Heinsen *et al.*, 1996). Certainly the cytoarchitecture of the entorhinal cortex is quite heterogeneous along its rostral–caudal axis and individual variability may be most prominent in the rostral subfields

Table 2.2 Cytoarchitectural and neuronal morphometric findings in the hippocampal formation in schizophrenia

Region/parameter	Finding	Positive reports of the finding	Negative reports of the finding
Cytoarchitecture			
Entorhinal cortex	Abnormal lamination and cellular disarray	Jakob and Beckmann, 1986, 1994; Falkai et al, 1988; Casanova et al, 1990; Arnold et al, 1991b; Arnold et al, 1997	Krimer et al, 1997; Akil and Lewis, 1997; Bernstein et al, 1998
Neuron Density and Number			
Hippocampal neuron density	Decreased	Falkai and Bogerts, 1986; Jeste and Lohr, 1989	Kovelman and Scheibel, 1984; Benes et al, 1991; Heckers et al, 1991; Arnold et al, 1995a; Zaidel et al, 1997a
Hippocampal neuron density	Decreased	Falkai and Bogerts, 1986	Heckers et al, 1991
Entorhinal cortex neuron density	Decreased	Falkai et al, 1988; Krimer et al, 1997	Heckers et al, 1991; Arnold et al, 1995a
Entorhinal cortex neuron number	Decreased	Falkai et al, 1988	Heckers et al, 1991
Neuron size			
Hippocampal neuron size	Decreased	Benes et al, 1991; Arnold et al, 1995a; Zaidel et al, 1997b	Christison et al, 1989 (CA 1 only); Benes et al, 1998
Entorhinal cortex neuron size	Decreased	Arnold et al, 1995a	
Neuron alignment			
Variability of alignment	Increased	Kovelman and Scheibel, 1984; Conrad et al, 1991; Jonsson et al, 1997	Altshuler et al, 1987; Benes et al, 1991; Arnold et al, 1995a; Zaidel et al, 1997b

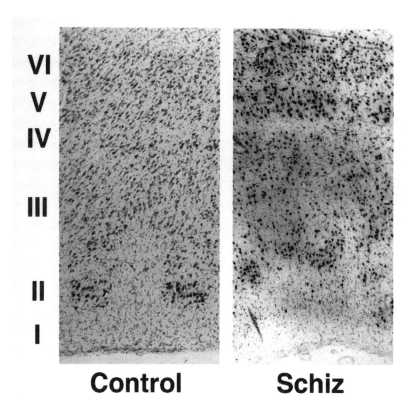

Fig. 2.3 Control and schizophrenic entorhinal cortex. Compared to the control, the entorhinal cortex in this 37-year-old male schizophrenic shows disorganization of superficial lamina with poorly formed and disorganized neuron clusters in layer II, a patchy appearance in layer III, and smaller neurons in layers II and III (x100).

where the purported abnormalities in schizophrenia were described. With an eye to such considerations, Akil and Lewis (1997) found no qualitative differences between 10 schizophrenic and 10 control subjects in entorhinal cytoarchitecture; neither did Krimer *et al.* (1997).

Another criticism of all these studies is that they are qualitative descriptions and thus vulnerable to substantial subjectivity on the part of the investigators. There have been three studies attempting to quantify spatial arrangement of neurons in the entorhinal cortex. In the same study mentioned above, Krimer *et al.* (1997) measured the volumes and positioning of individual layers of the entorhinal cortex and found no differences for these variables between schizophrenics and controls. Arnold *et al.* (1997) mapped the co-ordinates of neurons in layers II, III, and V of the rostral entorhinal cortex and used spatial point pattern analyses to compare their distributions in eight schizophrenics and eight matched controls. They reported subtle but statistically significant differences, with schizophrenics having an abnormally clustered dispersion of neurons and a reduced mean effective radius ('dead space') around neurons in layer III, increased mean effective radius in layer II, and no changes in layer V. Although they were not as obvious or dramatic, the findings were interpreted as roughly concordant with their previous qualitative findings mentioned above (Arnold *et al.*, 1991*b*). Finally, Bernstein *et al.* (1998) found layer II heterotopias at the same frequency in controls as in schizophrenics.

If cytoarchitectural abnormalities of the entorhinal cortex do occur in schizophrenia, the neurobiological basis is still unclear. Aberrant migration of nascent neurons from the ventricular zone to the cortex during fetal development has been the mechanism most heralded as the basis for the disturbed cytoarchitectural appearance. However, cytoarchitecture is determined by a complex orchestration of a host of developmental and degenerative processes (see Chapters 8 and 11) and a defect in any of these could affect the final neuronal arrangement. Migration, neuron enlargement and differentiation under the influence of intrinsic and extrinsic growth factors, programmed cell death during brain maturation, cell death with normal aging and intercurrent diseases, and the amounts and arrangements of innervating nerve fibres, as well as other components of the neuropil space separating neurons all contribute to the ultimate cytoarchitectural appearance of the entorhinal cortex postmortem. Which of these determinants might be responsible for the abnormalities that have been observed in at least some patients with schizophrenia is not yet known.

Neuronal density and number

Quantifying the number of neurons within the hippocampal region also has been of great interest. Here too, results are controversial. Given the nature of schizophrenia as a disease with remote or very protracted pathoetiologies and no obvious histopathological abnormalities to the naked eye in most cases, the methodology used to discern subtle differences in cell density or number is especially critical. Most studies of schizophrenia have assessed neuron *density* rather than the total number of neurons. This is problematic in that neuron loss may or may not be reflected in decreased neuron density. Commensurate shrinkage of the neuropil space as a component of the reference volume for the density measurement would tend to hide any true reduction in overall neuron number. Another methodological limitation is that most studies have used cell counting methods that do not account for under- or over-counting due to size, orientation, shape, or splitting of cells. Failure to account for these variables allows for substantial bias that may introduce variances of as much as 40 per cent from true counts (West, 1993). More modern methods such as the recently popularized stereological quantitation tools help to address these limitations and are beginning to be used by schizophrenia researchers (see Chapters 13 and 14).

Most studies have found no abnormalities in neuron density in the subfields of the hippocampus (Table 2.2), although one reported decreased density in CA3 and CA4 (Jeste and Lohr, 1989) and one found a lateralized *increase* in neuron density in right CA3 and CA1 (Zaidel *et al.*, 1997*a*). Two studies have estimated total neuron numbers in the hippocampus. While Falkai and Bogerts (1986) found no differences between schizophrenics and controls for neuron densities, total neuron numbers were decreased in all subfields because of the decreased volumes of the hippocampus found. In contrast, using stereological methods, Heckers *et al.* (1991) found no differences between schizophrenics and controls for either neuron density or total neuron estimates. More recently, Benes *et al.* (1998) used a spatial counting approach to measure the densities and total numbers of pyramidal and non-pyramidal neurons in the ammonic subfields in a schizophrenia sample and a small sample of manic-depressives. Compared to controls they found a selective reduction in density and total number of non-pyramidal neurons in CA2 in the schizophrenia group, but also the manic-depressive group.

Findings in the entorhinal cortex have been controversial as well. Several qualitative reports described decreased neuron densities therein (Jakob and Beckmann, 1986; Casanova *et al.*, 1990; Arnold *et al.*, 1991*b*). Of the quantitative studies (Table 2.2), three out of four reported no differences. A further study estimated total neuron number and reported a decrease which was primarily due to a smaller estimated volume of the entorhinal cortex (Falkai *et al.*, 1988).

Overall, the weight of the evidence indicates no substantial abnormality in overall neuron density in the hippocampal formation in schizophrenia, although the possibility of selective decreases in neuronal subpopulations is intriguing and potentially meaningful. Whether or not individuals with schizophrenia have abnormally few neurons overall in the hippocampal formation thus hinges on the reference volume for the region. As mentioned, MRI studies suggest strongly that the volumes are decreased in schizophrenia whereas the postmortem studies are less clear, albeit fewer in number, and smaller in scale. The issue remains unsettled.

Neuronal size and shape

Several studies have measured neuron size in the hippocampal region and findings have been relatively consistent. Benes *et al.* (1991) measured pyramidal neurons in the posterior hippocampus and found 13 to 18 per cent reductions in neuron size in CA1 to CA4 in schizophrenia compared to controls. Arnold *et al.* (1995*a*) similarly reported smaller neurons in the ammonic subfields, and in the subiculum (21 per cent) and layer II of the entorhinal cortex (14 per cent). They further measured neurons in primary motor and primary visual cortices to examine the regional specificity of findings for the hippocampal formation and noted no size differences between control and schizophrenia groups for these non-limbic regions. Zaidel *et al.* (1997*b*) also examined size and shape of neurons in the ammonic subfields with an additional eye to possible asymmetries (Chapter 6). They found significantly smaller neurons in left CA1 and CA2 and in right CA3, but without a significant reduction in subicular neuron size on either side. Shape was also measured and they found a significant elongation of neurons in the left subiculum and CA1, and right CA3. In contrast to these studies, Christison *et al.* (1989) reported no alterations in neuron size and shape, although this study measured only 12 neurons in CA1 in each of 17 schizophrenia cases. Benes *et al.* (1998) also found no differences in neuron size.

Overall, the above findings from several independent groups indicate cellular dystrophy in schizophrenia. The basis for this is not yet clear. The size of a neuron soma generally corresponds to the extent of neuronal processes (axons and dendritic arbors) that need to be metabolically supported by it (Chapter 11). Whether neuronal processes are attenuated in the hippocampal formation in schizophrenia is not known. Some recent preliminary Golgi studies (in neocortex) report decreased dendritic spine density (Aganova and Uranova, 1992; Lewis and Glantz, 1997; Garey *et al.*, 1998; Glantz and Lewis, 2000; see also Chapter 4).

At the molecular level, neuron size and shape are determined by several families of cytoskeletal proteins including neurofilament proteins, actins, tubulins, and microtubule associated proteins (MAP) (Burgoyne, 1991), which interact to construct the scaffolding of the cell body, dendritic and axonal diameters, and dendritic spine morphology. The neuronal cytoskeleton has been probed in schizophrenia. In a small qualitative immuno-histochemical study, Arnold *et al.* (1991*c*) used a panel of well-characterized antibodies to assess the expression of phosphorylated neurofilament triplet proteins, α- and β-tubulins, and MAP2, MAP5 (also known as MAP1B), and tau. They reported relatively specific deficits in the expression of MAP2 and MAP5 in the subiculum in five of six individuals with schizophrenia compared to controls, and a deficit in MAP2 in the entorhinal cortex in four of six. It is noteworthy that these are the same regions where neurons were particularly small (Arnold *et al.*, 1995*a*). Rosklija *et al.* (1995) independently examined subicular MAP2 in a much larger series of patients and confirmed the deficit in a third of their cases and in no normal controls. However, they questioned the disease specificity in that some patients with other neuropsychiatric conditions also showed decreased subicular MAP2. Their recent Golgi report of subicular dendritic abnormalities in both schizophrenia and mood disorder extends this evidence (Rosoklija *et al.*, 2000). Finally, Cotter *et al.* (1997) examined MAP2 in schizophrenia and found an increase in left-sided, non-phosphorylated MAP2 immunodensity in subiculum and CA1 while MAP2 immunoreactive neuron counts were similar to that of controls and there were no associated alterations in interneuronal distance or neuron orientation.

The point at which MAP2 or other cytoskeletal abnormalities fit in the neurobiological pathways that lead to schizophrenia is unclear. A direct relationship between MAP2 expression and neuronal morphology has not been reported. Furthermore, MAP2 expression is regulated by a number of factors such as *N*-methyl-D-aspartate (NMDA)-receptor agonists, serotonin, nerve growth factor, gangliosides, and both cyclic adenosine monophosphate (cAMP) and phosphoinositol second messenger systems (Sano *et al.*, 1990; Perez *et al.*, 1995; Halpain, 1996), and abnormalities in these or other mechanisms might be the primary culprits. Nonetheless, these preliminary cytoskeletal studies represent an important effort towards elucidating the molecular pathways that might culminate in neuronal morphological abnormalities in schizophrenia.

Neuron orientation

Orientation of neuronal processes is another aspect of neuronal morphology that has been investigated in schizophrenia, again with controversial findings. Investigators have examined how uniform the axis of orientation is for pyramidal neurons and their apical dendrites in the ammonic subfields of the hippocampus. Kovelman and Scheibel (1984) originally reported significantly greater variability (disarray) in pyramidal cell orientation in schizophrenics compared to controls. This finding was partially replicated by the same group (Conrad *et al.*, 1991). More recently a very small study reported a correlation between disarray and reduced neuronal density (Jonsson *et al.*, 1997). However, the attempts of other groups using both similar and different methods have all been negative (Altshuler *et al.*, 1987; Christison *et al.*, 1989; Benes *et al.*, 1991; Arnold *et al.*, 1995*a*; Zaidel *et al.*, 1997*b*).

If disorganization of pyramidal neurons is a feature of schizophrenia, it too could be due to a number of possibilities. One is a developmentally based neuronal migration disturbance, as originally proposed (Kovelman and Scheibel, 1984). Alternatively, the disarray could be a normal neuronal response to spatially or temporally abnormal afferent innervation (with neuron process growth responding to the trophic influences of abnormal afferent fibres). Another possibility is that there could be a defect in the expression or targeting of the cytoskeletal proteins necessary to establish neuronal processes and thus normal polarity.

Intrinsic and extrinsic hippocampal axonal innervation in schizophrenia

'Miswiring' of the brain is an important hypothetical construct for schizophrenia that holds that the unusual sensory and thought processes and cognitive deficits arise from aberrant patterns or fidelity of neuroanatomical connections (Frith and Done, 1988; Gray *et al.*, 1991; Stevens *et al.*, 1992; Benes, 1993). Studies of dendrites and synapses (Chapter 4) represent two avenues to investigate this hypothesis. Axonal innervation is another, though there have only been a few investigations concerning the hippocampal formation. In a preliminary study of the entorhinal cortex in four individuals with schizophrenia, Longson *et al.* (1996) reported that the density of small calibre glutamatergic vertical axons was increased compared to controls. Based on analogy to the known neuroanatomical circuits in other species, the authors proposed that this was due to increased extrinsic innervation from the amygdala (see Chapter 3). Akil *et al.*, (2000) recently reported a decrease in tyrosine-hydroxylase containing axons in the entorhinal cortex, suggestive of altered dopamine innervation in schizophrenia.

Two studies have examined the zinc-rich mossy fiber pathway in the hippocampus in schizophrenia, with conflicting findings. These investigations were prompted by the relationship between hippocampal zinc and learning and memory (Frederickson *et al.*, 1990; Guidolin *et al.*, 1992) and the possibility that the purported abnormalities in the entorhinal cortex in schizophrenia alter the innervation of the dentate gyrus granule cells, which in turn would lead to alterations of the mossy fiber pathway connecting them with CA3 and CA4 (Fig. 2.2). Such phenomena have been described in animals after experimental lesions (Steward, 1992). Goldsmith and Joyce (1995) reported that the optical density of Timm's stained mossy fibers was significantly decreased in the hilus of the dentate gyrus, CA4 and CA3 in their elderly schizophrenia sample compared to both normal elderly and Alzheimer's disease control cases. In contrast, Adams *et al.* (1995) found no differences between schizophrenia, normal control and psychiatric control groups. The basis for the discrepancy is unclear: cases in the latter study were somewhat younger, but otherwise the sample sizes, staining methods, and optical densitometric methods were almost identical.

Cognitive impairment, dementia, and investigations of neurodegeneration in schizophrenia

As described above, generalized cognitive impairment with preferential impairments in learning and memory is a prominent feature of schizophrenia, a pattern indicative of temporo-hippocampal dysfunction. The persistence of these deficits suggests a static encephalopathy compatible with either abnormal neurodevelopment (which might be consistent with the type of cytoarchitectural and neuronal morphometric findings described above) or a post-maturational neural injury. If either of these were indeed the case, the course of psychiatric and neuropsychological functioning should remain fairly stable throughout life. However, long-term longitudinal follow-up studies indicate substantial heterogeneity of outcome (Bleuler, 1968; Ciompi, 1980; Winokur *et al.* 1987; Carpenter and Kirkpatrick, 1988; Lindstrom, 1996). Some patients stabilize or even improve after their initial presentation, but others exhibit a slow but progressive deterioration.

The possibility of premature and/or progressive dementia and neurodegeneration in at least some patients with schizophrenia is an historically important hypothesis, first described by Morel (1860) and later Kraepelin (1919) who marked dementia praecox as a brain disorder and emphasized a chronic, deteriorating course over time with only a minority of patients showing recovery or remission. A neurodegenerative hypothesis has been supported by several recent longitudinal volumetric MRI studies which have found progressive brain atrophy in some patients (De Lisi *et al.*, 1995; Gur *et al.*, 1998; see Chapter 1). In addition, recent studies focusing on schizophrenia in late life have revealed a high frequency and sever-ity of cognitive and functional impairments. Davidson *et al.* (1995) examined a large, severely ill, institutionalized population of individuals with schizophrenia across the lifespan. They found a slow but steady decline in cognitive function with each decade, culminating in a severe dementia in the majority of elderly patients. Likewise, Arnold *et al.* (1995*b*) found that at least two-thirds of elderly, chronically institutionalized patients with schizophrenia met criteria for an additional diagnosis of dementia. Psychometric testing revealed a neuropsychological profile similar to that of Alzheimer's disease (Moberg *et al.*, 1995).

Diagnostic neuropathological examinations have failed to find any consistent explana-tions for the dementia in these deteriorated, elderly patients. The frequency of various neuropathological findings (e.g. lacunar infarcts, Alzheimer's disease, Parkinsons's disease, meningiomas, etc.) is perhaps slightly greater than that seen among a general, community-based elderly population (Bruton *et al.*, 1990; Arnold *et al.*, 1995*b*; Golier *et al.*, 1995), though even this may be an artefact of case collection (Chapter 14). Certainly, the partic-ular lesions are highly miscellaneous and most patients, even with severe dementia, are without abnormalities. This is remarkable, given that in community samples of individuals with dementia in late life, 50 to 60 per cent have Alzheimer's disease, 20 to 30 per cent have vascular dementia or a mixed Alzheimer's/vascular dementia, and 10 to 20 per cent have dementia due to a wide variety of other neurodegenerative, structural, or metabolic etiologies (Larson *et al.*, 1984).

To assess the possibility of a more subtle neurodegeneration or neural injury in schizo-phrenia, there have been a number of investigations quantifying various histopathological and immunocytochemical markers in schizophrenia. These include specific disease-related lesions such as neurofibrillary tangles, amyloid plaques, and Lewy bodies, as well as more general responses to any number of degenerative, infectious, traumatic, or other causes, including astrocytosis, microglial proliferation, and excessive ubiquitin expression. Beyond its purported role in schizophrenia, the hippocampal formation has been of special interest in these studies because of its selective vulnerability for these lesions (Chapter 11) For instance, the entorhinal cortex is the first and most severely affected region of the brain in Alzheimer's disease (Arnold et al., 1991a; Braak and Braak, 1991). The hippocampus and entorhinal cortex are also heavily involved in other degenerative diseases such as frontotemporal degenerative dementias, Lewy body diseases, and amyotrophic lateral sclerosis–dementia (Arnold et al., 1998). These quantitative studies have found no evidence of ongoing neurodegeneration or neural injury in schizophrenia, even among the most severely ill, elderly, and deteriorated. As summarized in Table 2.3, no abnormalities have been reported in the quantity of neurofibrillary tangles or senile plaques, nor concerning other disease-specific neurodegenerative lesions such as Lewy bodies, Pick bodies, or protease-resistant prions. In addition, no decreases in cholinergic activity, a neurochemical correlate of a number of neurodegenerative conditions, have been observed (Haroutunian et al., 1994). A recent meta-analysis also concluded that Alzheimer's disease was, despite some earlier suggestions, no commoner in schizophrenia than expected (Baldessarini et al., 1997). Similarly, quantitative studies have not identified any excess astrocytosis using either traditional histological staining or modern immunohistochemical methods (see Chapter 5).

Arnold et al. (1998) recently approached the issue of neurodegeneration in schizophrenia in a fairly comprehensive manner by quantifying six relevant markers in the hippocampus and other cortical regions in a sample of 23 elderly individuals with schizophrenia. The patients had been prospectively accrued, diagnosed by consensus according to standard criteria, and clinically characterized with a battery of assessment scales. All had been chronically hospitalized and two thirds had sufficient cognitive impairment to warrant an additional diagnosis of dementia. While this sample is not representative of schizophrenia at large, it was particu-

Table 2.3 Investigations of neurodegeneration and neural injury in the hippocampal formation in schizophrenia

Parameter	Finding	Reports of the finding	Reports not confirming finding
Quantation of Alzheimer's disease markers with focus on elderly patients with schizophrenia and dementia	No change	Purohit et al, 1993 Powchik et al, 1993 Casanova et al, 1993 Arnold et al, 1994, 1995a, 1998 Nizato et al, 1998	None
Other neurodegenerative disease markers (Lewy bodies, Pick bodies, ubiquitin, apolipoprotein E genotype, abnormal prion protein)	No change	Purohit et al, 1993 Arnold et al, 1995a, 1998, 1999	None

larly well suited for studies of neurodegeneration because of the severity, chronicity, advanced age, and poor outcome of the cases. Thus, if accumulated degenerative pathology were an aspect of schizophrenia, it should be more evident in this sample than in any other group.

Immunohistochemistry was used to label sensitively and specifically neurofibrillary tangles, senile plaques, Lewy bodies, glial fibrillary acidic protein-positive astrocytes, as well as resting and reactive microglia (brain macrophages) and dystrophic neurites (identified by their immunoreactivity for ubiquitin). The densities of these markers were quantified using non-biased stereological counting methods in the entorhinal cortex, subiculum, and CA1, as well as in mid-frontal, orbitofrontal, and calcarine cortices. There were no statistically significant differences between the schizophrenics and matched non-neuropsychiatric controls for any of the neurodegenerative markers in any region, while both groups exhibited far fewer lesions than an Alzheimer's disease 'positive control' group. Furthermore, within the schizophrenia sample there were no significant correlations between cognitive and psychiatric ratings and densities of any of the neuropathological markers. The investigators concluded that there was no significant histological evidence of neurodegeneration or ongoing neural injury in the cerebral cortex in schizophrenia beyond that seen in a normal control group, and that common age-related degenerative lesions could not account for the dementia observed.

Without evidence of conventional neurodegenerative pathology in schizophrenia, other factors must be considered in order to explain the deterioration and dementia that occurs in some patients. It remains a possibility that the effects of other normal age-related changes are amplified in the setting of presumably abnormal neural circuitry in schizophrenia. Thus, neurodevelopmental abnormalities may represent a state of decreased cerebral reserve with commensurately increased vulnerability to the cognitive toxicity of even small amounts of neural injury or neurodegenerative lesions that accompany aging. Accordingly, patients may demonstrate neuropsychological deficits prior to their first psychotic episode and relatively static deficits in short-term follow-up studies, but undergo a very slow decline over decades, as described by Davidson *et al.* (1995).

When considering the 'decreased cerebral reserve' hypothesis, it is interesting to note the topographical similarities between the brain regions with reported cytoarchitectural and neuronal morphometric abnormalities in schizophrenia and those that are most vulnerable to aging and the common neurodegenerative diseases, such as the entorhinal cortex. Given that initial studies find no correlations between the quantity of neurodegenerative markers and cognitive impairment in schizophrenia (Arnold *et al.*, 1998), it is possible there is a correlation between the baseline severity of neurodevelopmental abnormalities and the clinical features, including dementia. The task remains to better delineate the nature of such abnormalities.

Regional specificity of hippocampal neuropathological findings

Leaving aside the ongoing controversies about the neuroanatomical findings in schizophrenia (Chapter 13), one can question to what extent the reported abnormalities described here are anatomically specific for the hippocampal formation.

There have been no comparable studies of cytoarchitectural disorganization or neuronal malorientation of the kind described in the entorhinal cortex and hippocampus in other areas. Such studies would be of considerable interest. However, the hypothesis of abnormal neuronal migration in schizophrenia that derived from the entorhinal and hippocampal findings has been explored in other regions. Although their specific findings differ, both Akbarian *et al.* (1996) and Anderson *et al.* (1996) have reported a maldistribution of interstitial neurons in white matter subjacent to frontal and temporal lobe neocortices. These neurons are remnants of the cortical subplate which helps guide the migration of neurons and directs cortical innervation during fetal development. Abnormalities in the distribution of these neurons in both temporal and frontal lobes suggest that mechanisms of neuronal migration or programmed cell death during brain development may be disturbed throughout the brain.

Neuron density and number have been examined in other brain regions, including frontal cortices, basal ganglia, thalamus, cerebellum, and brainstem, and have been found to be variably decreased, unchanged, or increased (reviewed in Bogerts, 1993; Shapiro, 1993; Arnold and Trojanowski, 1996; see Chapter 3). Numerous methodological considerations are present among the studies and so, as with the hippocampus, we await more definitive data on this issue.

As with hippocampal pyramidal neurons, decreases in neuron size have been reported in several other areas: anterior cingulate cortex (Benes *et al.*, 1986), dorsolateral prefrontal cortex (Rajkowska *et al.*, 1998), substantia nigra (Bogerts *et al.*, 1983), locus coeruleus (Lohr and Jeste, 1988), and cerebellar Purkinje cells (Lohr and Jeste, 1986; Tran *et al.*, 1998), but not primary motor or calcarine cortices (Arnold *et al.*, 1995*a*). Most of these studies require confirmation, but it is interesting that the size abnormalities are especially present in brain regions important for cognitive and/or emotional processing. Finally, studies of neurodegenerative disease lesions have been negative in multiple other regions in addition to hippocampus (Arnold and Trojanowski, 1996).

In summary, it is difficult to know the extent to which cytoarchitectural and neuronal morphometric abnormalities are selective for the hippocampal formation. Considerably more work needs to be done. The neuropsychological profile of schizophrenia indicates widespread impairment, but with some special involvement of limbic, temporal, and frontal neural systems. Much attention from neurobiological researchers has rightfully focused on the neuroanatomy, neurochemistry, and functioning of regions within these systems. However, there are also numerous data indicating neurobiological abnormalities elsewhere. Diverse examples include visual backward masking abnormalities (which indicate lateral geniculate and/or primary visual cortex dysfunction; Green and Walker, 1986); abnormal compound motor evoked potentials observed with transcranial magnetic stimulation of the motor cortex (suggesting impaired primary corticospinal inhibition of motor responses or even peripheral nerve dysfunction; Puri *et al.*, 1996), and deviant patterns of cerebral activity rather than any region-specific deficits observed in PET activation studies (Schroder *et al.*, 1996). Thus, it is possible that some as yet undefined neurobiological abnormalities associated with schizophrenia are present widely throughout the nervous system. Perhaps the predominant symptoms of schizophrenia preferentially involve higher cognitive, emotional, and social domains because the underlying cellular and molecular abnormalities of the disorder become most eloquent in brain regions of high complexity or plasticity, or prolonged maturation.

Concluding remarks

We are now at a stage of neuropathological research where the methodological limitations that plagued past investigations—such as diagnostic uncertainties, poor clinical characterization, non-uniform tissue processing, and the capriciousness, poor sensitivity, and non-specificity of classical histological stains—have given way to diagnostic rigor, standardized methods of tissue processing, molecularly-specific labeling procedures, and computer-assisted quantitative analysis (Chapter 14). This places us in a far better position to identify changes in any number of neuronal proteins or mRNAs that could give rise to subtle histological abnormalities such as smaller size or altered spatial arrangement of neurons in the hippocampal formation.

In terms of understanding the pathoetiology of schizophrenia, findings in the hippocampus suggest neurodevelopmental abnormalities far more than neurodegenerative ones. Identifying and characterizing aberrant developmental mechanisms decades after they may have taken place remains a challenging task. Finally, it is highly unlikely that such histopathological and molecular abnormalities are exclusive to the hippocampal formation. Nonetheless, because of the pivotal role that this region plays in the neural systems subserving cognition and emotion, any abnormality present there would likely have far-reaching effects.

References

Adams CE, DeMasters BK, Freedman R (1995) Regional zinc staining in postmortem hippocampus form schizophrenic patients. *Schizophrenia Research* **18**,71–77.

Aganova EA, Uranova NA (1992) Morphometric analysis of synaptic contacts in the anterior limbic cortex in the endogenous psychoses. *Neuroscience and Behavioral Physiology* **22**, 59–65.

Akbarian S, Kim JJ, Potkin SG, Hetrick WP, Bunney WE, Jones EG (1996) Maldistribution of interstitial neurons in prefrontal white matter of the the brains of schizophrenic patients. *Archives of General Psychiatry* **53**, 425–436.

Akil M, Lewis DA (1997) Cytoarchitecture of the entorhinal cortex in schizophrenia. *American Journal of Psychiatry* **154**, 1010–1012.

Akil M, Edgar CL, Pierri JN *et al.* (2000) Decreased density of tyrosine hydroxylase-immunoreactive axons in the entorhinal cortex of schizophrenic subjects. *Biological Psychiatry* **47**, 361–370.

Altshuler LL, Conrad A, Kovelman JA, Scheibel A (1987) Hippocampal pyramidal cell orientation in schizophrenia. *Archives of General Psychiatry* **44**, 1094–1098.

Altshuler LL, Casanova MF, Goldberg TE, Kleinman JE (1990) The hippocampus and parahippocampus in schizophrenic, suicide, and control brains. *Archives of General Psychiatry* **44**, 1094–1098.

Amaral DG, Insausti R (1990) Hippocampal formation. In: Paxinos G, ed. *The human nervous system*. San Diego: Academic Press, pp. 711–755.

Amaral DG, Insausti R, Cowan WM (1987) The entorhinal cortex of the monkey: I. Cytoarchitectonic organization. *Journal of Comparative Neurology* **264**, 326–355.

Anderson SA, Volk DW, Lewis DA (1996) Increased density of microtubule associated protein 2-immunoreactive neurons in the prefrontal white matter of schizophenic subjects. *Schizophrenia Research* **19**, 111–119.

Arnold SE, Trojanowski JQ (1996) Recent advances in defining the neuropathology of schizophrenia. *Acta Neuropathologica* **92**, 217–231.

Arnold SE, Hyman BT, Flory J, Damasio AR, Hoesen GWV (1991*a*) The topographical and neuroanatomical distribution of neurofibrillary tangles and neuritic plaques in the cerebral cortex of patients with Alzheimer's disease. *Cerebral Cortex* **1**, 103–116.

Arnold SE, Hyman BT, Hoesen GWV, Damasio AR (1991*b*) Some cytoarchitectural abnormalities of the entorhinal cortex in schizophrenia. *Archives of General Psychiatry* **48**, 625–632.

Arnold SE, Lee VMY, Gur RE, Trojanowski JQ (1991*c*) Abnormal expression of two microtubule-associated proteins (MAP2 and MAP5) in specific subfields of the hippocampal formation in schizophrenia. *Proceedings of the National Academy of Sciences USA* **88**, 10850–10854.

Arnold SE, Franz BR, Trojanowski JQ (1994) Elderly patients with schizophrenia exhibit infrequent neurodegenerative lesions. *Neurobiology of Aging* **15**, 299–303.

Arnold SE, Franz BR, Gur RC et al. (1995*a*) Smaller neuron size in schizophrenia in hippocampal subfields that mediate cortical–hippocampal interactions. *American Journal of Psychiatry* **152**, 738–748.

Arnold SE, Gur RE, Shapiro RM et al. (1995*b*) Prospective clinicopathological studies of schizophrenia: Accrual and assessment. *American Journal of Psychiatry* **152**, 731–737.

Arnold SE, Han L-Y, Ruscheinsky DD (1997) Further evidence of cytoarchitectural abnormalities of the entorhinal cortex in schizophrenia using spatial point pattern analyses. *Biological Psychiatry* **42**, 639–647.

Arnold SE, Trojanowski JQ, Gur RE, Han L Y, Choi C (1998) Absence of neurodegeneration and neural injury in the cerebral cortex in a sample of elderly patients with schizophrenia. *Archives of General Psychiatry* **55**, 225–232.

Arnold SE, Trojanowski JQ, Parchi P (1999) Protease resistant prion proteins are not present in sporadic 'poor outcome' schizophrenia. *Journal of Neurology, Neurosurgery, and Psychiatry* **66**, 90–92.

Baldessarini RJ, Hegarty JD, Bird ED, Benes FM (1997) Meta-analysis of postmortem studies of Alzheimer's disease-like neuropathology in schizophrenia. *American Journal of Psychiatry* **154**, 1180–1182.

Benes FM (1993) Neurobiological investigations in cingulate cortex of schizophrenic brain. *Schizophrenia Bulletin* **19**, 537–549.

Benes FM, Davidson J, Bird ED (1986) Quantitative cytoarchitectural studies of the cerebral cortex of schizophrenics. *Archives of General Psychiatry* **43**, 31–35.

Benes FM, Sorensen I, Bird ED (1991) Reduced neuronal size in posterior hippocampus of schizophrenic patients. *Schizophrenia Bulletin* **17**, 597–608.

Benes FM, Kwok EW, Vincent SL, Todtenkopf MS (1998) A reduction of nonpyramidal cells in sector CA2 of schizophrenics and manic depressives. *Biological Psychiatry* **44**, 88–97.

Bernstein H-G, Krell D, Baumann B *et al.* (1998) Morphometric studies of the entorhinal cortex in neuropsychiatric patients and controls: clusters of heterotopically displaced lamina II neurons are not indicative of schizophrenia. *Schizophrenia Research* **33**, 125–132.

Bleuler M (1968) A 23-year longitudinal study of 208 schizophrenics and impressions in regard to the nature of schizophrenia. In: Rosenthal D, Kety SS, eds. *The transmission of schizophrenia*. New York: Pergamon Press, pp. 3–12.

Bogerts B (1993) Recent advances in the neuropathology of schizophrenia. *Schizophrenia Bulletin* **19**, 431–445.

Bogerts B, Hantsch J, Herzer M (1983) A morphometric study of the dopamine-containing cell groups in the mesencephalon of normals, Parkinson patients, and schizophrenics. *Biological Psychiatry* **18**, 951–969.

Bogerts B, Meertz E, Schonfeldt-Bausch R (1985) Basal ganglia and limbic system pathology in schizophrenia. *Archives of General Psychiatry* **42**, 784–791.

Bogerts B, Falkai P, Haupts M *et al.* (1990) Post-mortem volume measurements of limbic system and basal ganglia structures in chronic schizophrenics. Initial results from a new brain collection. *Schizophrenia Research* **3**, 295–301.

Bogerts B, Lieberman JA, Ashtari M *et al.* (1993) Hippocampus–amygdala volumes and psychopathology in chronic schizophrenia. *Biological Psychiatry* **33**, 236–246.

Braak H (1980) *Architectonics of the human telencephalic cortex*. Berlin: Springer.

Braak H, Braak E (1991) Neuropathological staging of Alzheimer-related changes. *Acta Neuropathologica* **82**, 239–259.

Brown R, Colter N, Corsellis JAN *et al.* (1986) Postmortem evidence of structural brain changes in schizophrenia. *Archives of General Psychiatry* **43**, 36–42.

Bruton CJ, Crow TJ, Frith CD, Johnstone EC, Owens DGC, Roberts GW (1990) Schizophrenia and the brain: a prospective clinico-neuropathological study. *Psychological Medicine* **20**, 285–304.

Burgoyne RD (1991) *The neuronal cytoskeleton*. New York: Wiley-Liss.

Carpenter WT, Kirkpatrick B (1988) The heterogeneity of the long-term course of schizophrenia. *Schizophrenia Bulletin* **14**, 515–542.

Casanova MF, Carosella N, Kleinman JE (1990) Neuropathological findings in a suspected case of childhood schizophrenia. *Journal of Neuropsychiatry and Clinical Neuroscience* **2**, 313–319.

Casanova MF, Carosella NW, Gold JM, Kleinman JE, Weinberger DR, Powers RE (1993) A topographical study of senile plaques and neurofibrillary tangles in the hippocampi of patients with Alzheimer's disease and cognitively impaired patients with schizophrenia. *Psychiatry Research* **49**, 41–62.

Christison GW, Casanova MF, Weinberger DR, Rawlings R, Kleinman JE (1989) A quantitative investigation of hippocampal pyramidal cell size, shape, and variability of orientation in schizophrenia. *Archives of General Psychiatry* **46**, 1027–1032.

Ciompi L (1980) Catamnestic long-term study on the course of life and aging of schziophrenics. *Schizophrenia Bulletin* **6**, 606–618.

Colter N, Battal S, Crow TJ, Johnstone EC, Brown R, Bruton C (1987) White matter reduction in the parahippocampal gyrus of patients with schizophrenia. *Archives of General Psychiatry* **44**, 1023.

Conrad AJ, Abebe T, Austin R, Forsythe S, Scheibel AB (1991) Hippocampal pyramidal cell disarray in schizophrenia as a bilateral phenomenon. *Archives of General Psychiatry* **48**, 413–417.

Cotter D, Kerwin R, Doshi B, Martin CS, Everall IP (1997) Alterations in hippocampal non-phosphorylated MAP2 protein expression in schizophrenia. *Brain Research* **765**, 238–246.

Damasio AR (1989) Time-locked multiregional retroactivation: a systems-level proposal for the neural substances of recall and recognition. *Cognition* **33**, 25–62.

Davidson M, Harvey PD, Powchik P *et al.* (1995) Severity of symptoms in chronically insti-tutionalized geriatric schizophrenic patients. *American Journal of Psychiatry* **152**, 197–207.

Davison K (1983) Schizophrenia-like psychoses associated with organic cerebral disorders: a review. *Psychiatric Developments* **1**, 1–34.

DeLisi LE, Tew W, Xie SH *et al.* (1995) A prospective follow-up study of brain morphology and cognition in first-episode schizophrenic patients—preliminary findings. *Biological Psychiatry* **38**, 349–360.

Ellingson RJ (1954) The incidence of EEG abnormality among patients with mental disor-ders of apparently nonorganic origin, a critical review. *American Journal of Psychiatry* **111**, 263–285.

Falkai P, Bogerts B (1986) Cell loss in the hippocampus of schizophrenics. *European Archives of Psychiatry and Neurological Sciences* **236**, 154–161

Falkai P, Bogerts B, Rozumek M (1988) Limbic pathology in schizophrenia: the entorhinal region—a morphometric study. *Biological Psychiatry* **24**, 515–521.

Frederickson RE, Frederickson CJ, Danscher G (1990) *In situ* binding of bouton zinc reversibly disrupts performance on a spatial memeory task. *Behavioral Brain Research* **38**, 25–33.

Friston KJ, Liddle PF, Frith CD, Hirsch SR, Frackowiak RS (1992) The left medial temporal region and schizophrenia. A PET study. *Brain* **115**, 367–382.

Frith CD, Done DJ (1988) Towards a neuropsychology of schizophrenia. *British Journal of Psychiatry* **152**, 437–443.

Garey LJ, Ong WY, Patel TS *et al.* (1998) Reduced dendritic spine density on cerebral cortical pyramidal neurons in schizophrenia. *Journal of Neurology, Neurosurgery and Psychiatry* **65**, 446–453.

Glantz LA, Lewis DA (2000) Decreased dendritic spine density on prefrontal cortical pyra-midal neurons in schizophrenia. *Archives of General Psychiatry*, **57**, 65–73.

Goldsmith SK, Joyce JN (1995) Alterations in hippocampal mossy fiber pathway in schiz-ophrenia and Alzheimer's disease. *Biological Psychiatry* **37**, 122–126.

Golier JA, Davidson M, Haroutunian V *et al.* (1995) Neuropathological study of 101 elderly schizophrenics: Preliminary findings. *Schizophrenia Research* **15**, 120.

Gray JA, Feldon J, Rawlins JNP, Helmsley DR, Smith AD (1991) The neuropsychology of schizophrenia. *Behavioral Brain Sciences* **14**, 1–84.

Green M, Walker E (1986) Symptom correlates of vulnerability to backward masking in schizophrenia. *American Journal of Psychiatry* **143**, 181–186.

Gruzelier J, Seymour K, Wilson J (1988) Impairments on neuropsychological tests of temporohippocampal and frontohippocampal functions and word fluency in remitting schizophrenic and affective disorders. *Archives of General Psychiatry* **45**, 623–629.

Guidolin D, Polato P, Venturin G *et al.* (1992) Correlation between zinc level in mossy fibers and spatial memory in aged rats. *Annals of the New York Academy of Sciences* **673**, 187–193.

Gur RE, Cowell P, Turetsky BI *et al.* (1998) A follow-up MRI study of schizophrenia: Relationship of neuroanatomic changes with clinical and neurobehavioral measures. *Archives of General Psychiatry* **55**, 145–152.

Halpain S (1996) Dynamic regulation of MAP2 in living neurons. *Journal of Neurochemistry* **66**, S33.

Haroutunian V, Davidson M, Kanof PD *et al.* (1994) Cortical cholinergic markers in schizophrenia. *Schizophrenia Research* **12**, 137–144.

Heckers S, Heinsen H, Heinsen YC, Beckmann H (1990) Limbic structures and lateral ventricle in schizophrenia: a quantitative postmortem study. *Archives of General Psychiatry* **47**, 1016–1022.

Heckers S, Heinsen H, Geiger B, Beckmann H (1991) Hippocampal neuron number in schizophrenia. A stereological study. *Archives of General Psychiatry* **48**, 1002–1008.

Heinsen H, Grossman E, Rub U *et al.* (1996) Variability in the human entorhinal region may confound neuropsychiatric diagnoses. *Acta Anatomica* **157**, 226–237.

Insausti R, Tunon T, Sobreviela T, Insausti AM, Gonzalo LM (1995) The human entorhinal cortex: A cytoarchitectonic analysis. *Journal of Comparative Neurology* **355**, 171–198.

Jacobi W, Winkler H (1929) Untersuchungen des liquor cerebrospinalis mit dem zeisschen spektographan fur chemiker. *Deutche Zeitschrift fur Nervenh* **111**, 5–18.

Jakob H, Beckmann H (1986) Prenatal developmental disturbances in the limbic allocortex in schizophrenics. *Journal of Neural Transmission* **65**, 303–326.

Jakob H, Beckmann H (1994) Circumscribed malformation and nerve cell alterations in the entorhinal cortex of schizophrenics. Pathogenetic and clinical aspects. *Journal of Neural Transmission* **98**, 83–106.

Jeste DV, Lohr JB (1989) Hippocampal pathologic findings in schizophrenia: a morphometric study. *Archives of General Psychiatry* **46**, 1019–1024.

Jonsson SAT, Luts A, Guldberg-Kjaer N, Brun A (1997) Hippocampal pyramidal cell disarray correlates negatively to cell number: implications for the pathogenesis of schizophrenia. *European Archives of Psychiatry and Clinical Neurosciences* **247**, 120–127.

Kovelman JA, Scheibel AB (1984) A neurohistological correlate of schizophrenia. *Biological Psychiatry* **19**, 1601–1621.

Kraepelin E (1919) *Dementia praecox and paraphrenia*. Edinburgh: Livingstone.

Krimer LS, Herman MM, Saunders RC *et al.* (1997) A qualitative and quantitative analysis of the entorhinal cortex in schizophrenia. *Cerebral Cortex* **7**, 732–739.

Larson EB, Reifler BV, Featherstone HJ, English DR (1984) Dementia in elderly outpatients: A prospective study. *Annals of Internal Medicine* **100**, 417–423.

Lewis DA, Glantz LA (1997) Specificity of decreased spine density on layer III pyramidal cells in schizophrenia. *Schizophrenia Research* **24**, 39.

Lindstrom LH (1996) Clinical and biological markers for outcome in schizophrenia. *Neuropsychopharmacology* **14**, 23S–26S.

Lohr JB, Jeste DV (1986) Cerebellar pathology in schizophrenia? A neuronometric study. *Biological Psychiatry* **21**, 865–875.

Lohr JB, Jeste DV (1988) Locus ceruleus morphometry in aging and schizophrenia. *Acta Psychiatrica Scandinavica* **77**, 689–697.

Longson D, Deakin JFW, Benes FM (1996) Increased density of entorhinal glutamate-immunoreactive vertical fibers in schizophrenia. *Journal of Neural Transmission* **103**, 503–507.

Moberg PJ, Mahr R, Gibney M *et al.* (1995) Neuropsychological functioning in elderly patients with schizophrenia and Alzheimer's disease. *Journal of the International Neuropsychological Society* **1**, 132.

Morel BA (1860) *Maladies mentales.* Paris: Masson.

Nelson MD, Saykin AJ, Flashman LA, Riordan HJ (1998) Hippocampal volume reduction in schizophrenia as assessed by magnetic resonance imaging: a meta-analytic study. *Archives of General Psychiatry* **55**, 433–440.

Nestor PG, Shenton ME, McCarley RW *et al.* (1993) Neuropsychological correlates of MRI temporal lobe abnormalities in schizophrenia. *American Journal of Psychiatry* **150**, 1849–1855.

Niizato K, Arai T, Kuroki N, Kase KSI, Ikeda K (1998) Autopsy study of Alzheimer's disease brain pathology in schizophrenia. *Schizophrenia Research* **31**, 177–184.

Perez J, Mori S, Caivano M *et al.* (1995) Effects of fluvoxamine on the protein phosphorylation system associated with rat neuronal microtubules. *European Neuropsychopharmacology,* **5**, 65–69.

Powchik P, Davidson M, Nemeroff CB *et al.* (1993) Alzheimer's-disease-related protein in geriatric schizophrenic patients with cognitive impairment. *American Journal of Psychiatry* **150,** 1726–1727.

Puri BK, Davey NJ, Ellaway PH, Lewis SW (1996) An investigation of motor function in schizophrenia using transcranial magnetic stimulation of the motor cortex *British Journal of Psychiatry* **169**, 690–695.

Purohit DP, Davidson M, Perl DP *et al.* (1993) Severe cognitive impairment in elderly schizophrenic patients: A clinicopathological study. *Biological Psychiatry* **33**, 255–260.

Rajkowska G, Selemon LD, Goldman-Rakic PS (1998) Neuronal and glial somal size in the prefrontal cortex: a postmortem morphometric study of schizophrenia and Huntington disease. *Archives of General Psychiatry* **55**, 215–224.

Rosene DL, Van Hoesen GW (1977) Hippocampal efferents reach widespread areas of cerebral cortex and amygdala in the rhesus monkey. *Science* **198**, 315–317.

Rosene DL, Van Hoesen GW (1987) The hippocampal formation of the primate brain. In: Jones EG, Peters A, eds. *Cerebral cortex.* Volume 6, *Further aspects of cortical function, including hippocampus.* New York: Plenum, pp. 345–456.

Rosoklija G, Kaufman MA, Liu D *et al.* (1995) Subicular MAP-2 immunoreactivity in schizophrenia. *Society for Neuroscience Abstracts* **21**, 2126.

Rosoklija G, Toomayan G, Ellis SP *et al.* (2000) Structural abnormalities of subicular dendrites in subjects with schizophrenia and mood disorders. *Archives of General Psychiatry,* **57**, 349–356.

Sano M, Katoh-Semba R, Kitajima S, Sato C (1990) Changes in levels of microtubule-associated proteins in relation to the outgroth of neurites form PC12D celss, a forskolin- and nerve growth factor-responsive subline of PC12 pheochromocytoma cells. *Brain Research* **510**, 269–276.

Saykin AJ, Gur RC, Gur RE *et al.* (1991) Neuropsychological function in schizophrenia: selective impairment in memory and learning. *Archives of General Psychiatry* **48**, 618–624.

Saykin AJ, Riordan HJ, Weaver JB *et al.* (1995) Memory activation in schizophrenia— preliminary observations using functional magnetic resonance imaging (FMRI). *Schizophrenia Research* **15**, 97.

Schroder J, Buchsbaum MS, Siegel BV, Geider FJ, Niethammer R (1995) Structural and functional correlates of subsyndromes in chronic schizophrenia. *Psychopathology* **28**, 38–45.

Schroder J, Buchsbaum MS, Siegel BV *et al.* (1996) Cerebral metabolic activity correlates of subsyndromes in chronic schizophrenia. *Schizophrenia Research* **19**, 41– 53.

Shapiro RM (1993) Regional neuropathology in schizophrenia: Where are we? Where are we going? *Schizophrenia Research* **10**, 187–239.

Shenton ME, Kikinis R, Jolesz FA (1992) Abnormalities of the left temporal lobe and thought disorder in schizophrenia: A quantitative magnetic resonance imaging study. *New England Journal of Medicine* **327**, 604–612.

Silbersweig DA, Stern E, Frith C *et al.* (1995) A functional neuroanatomy of hallucina- tions in schizophrenia. *Nature* **378**, 176–179.

Stevens JR, Casanova M, Poltorak M, Germain L, Buchan GC (1992) Comparison of immunocytochemical and Holzer's methods for detection of acute chronic gliosis in human postmortem material. *Journal of Neuropsychiatry and Clinical Neurosciences* **4**, 168–173.

Steward O (1992) Lesion-induced synapse reorganization in the hippocampus of cats: Sprouting of entorhinal, commisural/associational, and mossy fiber projections after unilateral entorhinal cortex lesions, with comments on the normal organization of these pathways. *Hippocampus* **2**, 247–268.

Tran KD, Smutzer GS, Doty RL, Arnold SE (1998) Reduced Purkinje cell size in the cere- bellar vermis of elderly patients with schizophrenia. *American Journal of Psychiatry* **155**, 1288–1290.

Van Hoesen GW (1982) The parahippocampal gyrus. New observations regarding its cortical connections in the monkey. *Trends in Neurosciences* **5**, 345–350.

Van Hoesen GW, Pandya DN (1975) Some connection of the entorhinal (area 28) and perirhinal (area 35) cortices of the rhesus monkey. I. Temporal lobe afferents. *Brain Research* **95**, 1–24.

West MJ (1993) New stereological methods for counting neurons. *Neurobiology of Aging* **14**, 287–293.

Winokur G, Pfohl B, Tsuang M (1987) A 40-year follow-up of hebephrenic-catatonic schiz- ophrenia. In: Miller N, Cohen G, eds. *Schizophrenia and aging*. New York: Guilford Press, pp. 52–60.

Zaidel DW, Esiri MM, Harrison PJ (1997*a*) The hippocampus in schizophrenia: Lateralized increase in neuronal density and altered cytoarchitectural asymmetry. *Psychological Medicine* **27**, 703–713.

Zaidel DW, Esiri MM, Harrison PJ (1997*b*) Size, shape, and orientation of neurons in the left and right hippocampus: Investigations of normal asymmetries and alterations in schizophrenia. *American Journal of Psychiatry* **154**, 812–818.

3 Cortical Pathology: a New Generation of Quantitative Microscopic Studies

Francine M. Benes

> 'Where have all the graveyards gone?
> Gone to flowers everyone!'
> (Pete Seeger)

In the past 15 years, a wide variety of approaches have been adopted to the study of the neuropathology of schizophrenia. The quest has been given new hope as increasingly sensitive and quantifiable microscopic techniques, such as cell counting, immunocytochemistry, receptor binding autoradiography, and *in situ* hybridization have been applied. Exciting possibilities have begun to develop regarding the underlying histopathology of the cerebral cortex in schizophrenia; however, caution is needed because of the preliminary nature of all the results.

The first section deals with stereomorphometric studies which have the important strength of providing a broad vista as to how the corticolimbic system may be altered. Such studies have generally had the straightforward goal of determining if shrinkage and neuronal loss are features of schizophrenia; but, as the reader will see, the path created in pursuit of an answer to this question has not been a smooth and untroubled one, even though important clues have emerged. In the next three sections, cytochemical results from studies of the GABA, glutamate, and dopamine systems are used to address the fundamental question of whether there are changes in these neurotransmitter systems and, if so, whether the pattern suggests specific ways in which corticolimbic circuitry is affected in schizophrenia. An important corollary issue considered is whether there is evidence of excitotoxicity. The review concludes by discussing whether the neurodevelopmental hypothesis of schizophrenia (Chapter 8) is compatible with the observed cortical pathology. Hopefully, the reader will gain an appreciation of the complex nature of microscopic studies of schizophrenia and the fact that they are themselves in a developmental phase, one that offers great promise for eventually unravelling the riddle of the neuropathology of this disorder (Benes, 1995a).

Stereomorphometric studies

Contemporary microscopic approaches, in conjunction with structural imaging (Chapter 1) have assessed the size of various brain regions in schizophrenia. Amongst other alterations, several groups have provided evidence for a reduction in the volume of limbic structures (see Table 2.1 in Chapter 2). It is important to emphasize that volume changes may occur as a result of different histopathological processes, some irreversible but some reversible in nature (Benes, 1993a). The presence of volume loss does not necessarily indicate that neuronal cell death has occurred. To rule in, or rule out, the presence of neuronal degeneration, detailed cell counting is required. In keeping with the size reductions, several studies have detected a loss of neurons in prefrontal cortex, anterior cingulate cortex (Benes et al., 1986, 1991a), and primary motor cortex (Benes et al., 1986), as well as in hippocampal and parahippocampal regions (Chapter 2). The mediodorsal thalamus (Dom, 1976; Pakkenberg, 1990) and nucleus accumbens (Pakkenberg, 1990) in schizophrenia have also been found to have fewer neurons consonant with a decreased volume. Nevertheless, a reduction in either the density or total numbers of neurons is also not sufficient to prove that a degenerative process, such as that seen in Alzheimer's disease, has occurred. To confirm this, it is generally accepted that a gliotic reaction would be present, i.e. glial cell proliferation and hypertrophy (Chapter 11), so it is noteworthy that studies which have systematically evaluated glial cells in various regions have found no evidence for a gliotic reaction (Benes et al, 1986; see Chapter 5). One study has demonstrated a significant increase of astrocytes positive for glial fibrillary acidic protein in elderly schizophrenics who were demented (Arnold et al., 1996). This finding points to the importance of viewing histopathological changes in schizophrenia with respect to the entire lifecycle (Benes, 1988). While the absence of gliosis in schizophrenia as a whole provides a compelling argument that a 'typical' pattern of neuronal death does not ordinarily play a role in this disorder, there is still a possibility that an excitotoxic process may have occurred and account for the lower density of neurons (see below).

Our ability to understand the significance of neuronal loss without gliosis has been complicated by the fact that several recent cell counting studies have not demonstrated a reduction in the number of neurons, in both the prefrontal cortex (Akbarian et al., 1995b; Selemon et al., 1995) and the hippocampal formation (Chapter 2). One study surveyed the 'entire cortical mantle' and found no change in the total number of neurons (Pakkenberg, 1993). There are many different methodological factors that could potentially contribute to the differences in findings (Chapters 13 to 15). These include sample heterogeneity, the tissue preparation, the brain regions investigated, and the cell counting methodology employed. In this respect, the most commonly employed methodology uses a two-dimensional approach to assess the numbers of cells in a single x–y plane and expresses the data as a density, i.e. number of cells per unit area of tissue. A strength of two-dimensional cell counting is the fact that large microscopic fields are routinely analyzed using a 25x objective, and each and every neuron in a column of cerebral cortex that is approximately 0.3 mm wide is counted. However, such an approach can yield erroneous data when there are differences in the size of cells: smaller cells in one group will result in an underestimate of cell density, while cells that are larger will produce an overestimate (Weibel, 1979), unless a mathematical correction is applied (Abercrombie, 1946). Some investigators believe that such *post hoc* calculations are not accurate (Williams and Rakic, 1988; Coggeshall and Lekan, 1996) and that three-dimensional cell counting techniques are required to obtain unbiased density estimates (Gundersen *et al.*, 1988). The reader is referred to a recent review, which concluded that none of these factors can adequately explain the variety of positive and negative findings that have been reported in schizophrenia (Benes, 1997*a*; see also Chapter 14). For example, neuronal loss has been found with both two-dimensional (Colon, 1972; Benes *et al.*, 1986, 1991*a*) and three-dimensional (Pakkenberg, 1990) methods; negative results are also divided between two-dimensional (Benes *et al.*, 1991*b*; Akbarian *et al.*, 1995*b*; Arnold *et al.*, 1995) and three-dimensional (Heckers *et al.*, 1991; Pakkenberg, 1993) counting methods. Instead, anatomical heterogeneity may be of greater relevance. For example, neuronal loss has been reported in Brodmann areas 10 and 24 (Colon, 1972; Benes *et al.*, 1986, 1991*a*), with negative results for area 9 and 46 (Akbarian *et al.*, 1995*b*; Selemon *et al.*, 1995, 1998).

Cortical neuropil in schizophrenia

Complementing the neuronal counting studies, recent investigations have suggested that there may be significant changes in the neuropil of the dorsolateral prefrontal cortex (Brodmann areas 9 and 46) in schizophrenia, specifically a decrease in neuropil volume (Selemon *et al.*, 1995, 1998). Such an alteration, though subtle and non-specific, could nevertheless contribute to abnormal functioning of these areas (Chapter 11). If the volume of the cortical mantle is reduced, but the total number of neurons is unchanged, then it is reasonable to conclude that there is a reduction in the space surrounding the neuronal cell bodies (Selemon *et al.*, 1995, 1998). The neuropil contains a variety of cellular processes that include (a) dendrites and their spines; (b) synaptic terminals; (c) axons and their collateral branches that are both intrinsic (i.e. from within the same region) and extrinsic (i.e. from other cortical and subcortical regions); (d) glia and their processes; and (e) arteries, arterioles, capillaries, and venous sinuses. In the case of the vasculature, there have been no studies to date that have examined the distribution of this tissue compartment in the cortex of schizophrenic brain. Concerning glial elements, the density of these cells is either unchanged or decreased in schizophrenia (see above). As for axonal fibers in schizophrenia, these processes may also show no change in number, since two studies have failed to detect a difference in their density in the prefrontal cortex (Benes *et al.*, 1992*a*; Benes 1993). A reasonable hypothesis is that the decreased cortical volume in areas 9 and 46 could be related to a decrease of dendritic processes in these regions (Selemon and Goldman-Rakic, 1999; Fig. 3.1).

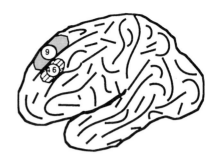

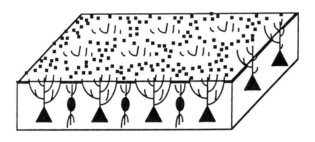

Normal

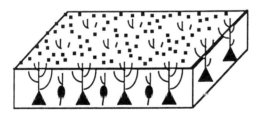

Schizophrenic

Fig. 3.1 A schematic diagram depicting the 'reduced neuropil' hypothesis of schizophrenia. The diagram shows a block of normal (upper) and schizophrenic (lower) dorsolateral prefrontal cortex. In schizophrenia, the total number of neurons is unchanged; however, there is a decrease in the volume of the tissue, that can be best explained by a contraction of the neuropil surrounding the neuronal cell bodies. (Reproduced with permission from Selemon and Goldman-Rakic, 1999.)

One final possibility must, however, be considered: a decrease of neuropil could be related to a loss of synapses (Chapter 4). Consistent with this idea is the report of decreased synaptophysin immunoreactivity in dorsolateral prefrontal cortex (Glantz and Lewis, 1997). However, in another study, synaptophysin and other presynaptic terminal proteins were found to be increased in the cingulate cortex, with no change in the frontal, temporal, or parietal cortices (Gabriel *et al.*, 1997). These latter data again suggest regional hetero-geneity, with an increase of synaptic complexes in the neuropil of some cortical areas, such as the cingulate, but decreases in others such as the prefrontal cortex and hippocampal formation (Chapter 4). Increased levels of growth associated protein 43 (GAP43), a protein implicated in synaptic development and plasticity, have been reported in associational cortices in schizophrenia (Perrone-Bizzozero *et al.*, 1996). This could potentially contribute to an abnormal sprouting of axon terminals in this region proposed to occur in the disorder (Stevens, 1992). It is important to point out, however, that altered levels of synaptic proteins can occur in the absence of changes in the number of synapses. Accordingly, the above findings might represent changes restricted to the functional regulation of these proteins in axon terminals.

Overall, there are probably alterations in the organization of cortical neuropil in schizophrenia. However, these changes, like those for neuronal number, may vary from one area to another and reflect alterations of neural circuitry that are dependent upon the specific patterns of connectivity and functional organization that are present in each region (Chapter 10).

Findings in layer II

In an attempt to gain insight into how a reduction in the number of neurons may have arisen in the anterior cingulate cortex in schizophrenia (Benes *et al.*, 1986), a stereomor-phometric analysis was developed to analyze the spatial arrangement of neurons (Benes and Bird, 1987). The data suggested that schizophrenics might have smaller and more widely separated neuronal clusters in layer II of anterior cingulate cortex than those in normal controls (Benes and Bird, 1987); no change was seen in the dorsolateral prefrontal cortex (area 10). This observation prompted the development of a model in which the expanded cell-free zones lying between the anterior cingulate layer II clusters in schizo-phrenia contain increased numbers of associative afferent fibers. Support for this model came from a blinded study using polyclonal antibodies against phosphorylated epitopes of the neurofilament protein NFP200K cytoskeletal subunit to visualize axons (Majocha *et al.*, 1985). An increased density of vertical, but not horizontal, axons was found in layer II and upper portions of IIIa in schizophrenia (Benes *et al.*, 1987). A subsequent study also found an increase of vertical axons in superficial laminae of the entorhinal region (Benes *et al.*, 1992*a*), but not in prefrontal cortex (Benes, 1993*a*). The entorhinal finding is noteworthy given that alterations of neuronal clusters in layer II (pre-α layer) of that region have also been reported (see Chapter 2).

Changes in schizophrenia compared with affective disorder

The first suggestion that a loss of interneurons might be present in schizophrenia came in a doctoral dissertation from the Karolinska Institute which reported a decrease in the number of small neurons in the dorsomedial and pulvinar nuclei of the thalamus (Dom, 1976; Dom *et al.*, 1981). Later, a similar change was noted in the anterior cingulate and prefrontal cortices (Benes *et al.*, 1991*a*), with subjects who had superimposed mood disturbances showing a more striking decrease than those without. This raised the possibility that GABAergic cell loss might show a stronger association with affective disorder than with schizophrenia. Interestingly, a replicative study in which subjects with bipolar disorder (manic depression) were included as a comparison group showed a similar pattern, with the bipolar cases having approximately a 30 per cent decrease compared to 16 per cent in the schizophrenics (Vincent *et al.*, 1997). It is noteworthy that another study in which tyrosine hydroxylase (TH)-immunoreactive fibers were analyzed (see below) was found in a *post hoc* analysis to also show an 18 per cent reduction in the density of interneurons in layer II of anterior cingulate cortex (Benes, 1998). A meta-analysis of the three studies (Todtenkopf and Benes, 1998) indicates that the reduction in the density of interneurons in layer II of anterior cingulate cortex was 16 per cent in schizophrenia ($n = 25$ cases), 25 per cent in schizoaffective disorder ($n = 18$), and 30 per cent in bipolar disorder ($n = 12$). Taken together, these data suggest that there is a loss of interneurons in affective disorder, perhaps greater than that which occurs in schizophrenia. In a recent study of the hippocampal formation, a decrease in the number of non-pyramidal neurons was observed in sector CA2; however, here the change was the same in schizophrenia and bipolar disorder (Benes *et al.*, 1998). Based on these results, it has been postulated that a loss of GABAergic neurons might be related to a factor, such as stress, that both disorders share to an equivalent degree. Why there should be a greater change in anterior cingulate cortex but not in hippocampus in bipolar disorder than in schizophrenia is difficult to explain; it is conceivable that each disorder involves region-specific alterations of neural circuitry that impact on GABAergic neurons to a differing extent.

The cortical GABA system

Roberts (1972) first proposed that schizophrenia might involve a defect in GABAergic neurotransmission, and it is reasonable to conceptualize that a loss of GABAergic inhibitory cells in association cortex in schizophrenia could result in profound disturbances in central information processing and provide a neurobiological basis for the defective central filtering observed in the disorder (Detre and Jarecki, 1971). The decreased density of interneurons described above is consistent with this possibility, and with other empirical data showing increased ^{3}H-muscimol binding (Hanada *et al.*, 1987), decreased glutamate decarboxylase (GAD) activity (Bird *et al.*, 1979), and decreased GABA uptake in the frontal cortex (Simpson *et al.*, 1989); a decrease of GABA uptake has also been observed in the amygdala (Reynolds *et al.*, 1990). More recently, a reduction of neurons immunoreactive for the calcium binding protein parvalbumin has been demonstrated in the cingulate cortex (Beasley and Reynolds, 1996). Since this peptide appears to be preferentially associated with interneurons believed to be inhibitory basket cells (Conde *et al.*, 1994), these latter results are in keeping with the idea that GABA cell loss could be a feature of schizophrenia (although it is possible that the amount of parvalbumin present within a normal number of cells had fallen below the level of detection). Another study reported an increase in the density of neurons immunoreactive for calbindin in the dorsolateral prefrontal cortex, but no change in those containing a third calcium binding protein, calretinin (Daviss and Lewis, 1995). It is becoming increasingly clear that our understanding of how the GABA system is disturbed in schizophrenia must take into account the fact that there are many different types of non-pyramidal neurons that use GABA as a neurotransmitter, and that each may show a unique pattern of change (Chapter 10).

Consistent with the cell counting study (Benes *et al.*, 1991*a*), a marked up-regulation of GABA$_A$ receptor binding activity has been observed in layer II and, to a lesser exent, layer III of both the anterior cingulate (Benes *et al.*, 1992*b*) and prefrontal (Benes *et al.*, 1996*b*) cortices in schizophrenia. The fact that the changes were most marked in layer II where the decreased density of non-pyramidal cells has also been most striking is in keeping with the idea that a decrease of GABAergic cells and/or activity has given rise to a compensatory up-regulation of the GABA$_A$ receptor. It is noteworthy that a similar pattern has been observed in the hippocampal formation, where the reduction of non-pyramidal cell density was seen in CA2 (Benes *et al.*, 1998) and where increased GABA$_A$ receptor binding was found in CA2 and CA3 (Benes *et al.*, 1996*a*, 1997*b*). The cellular distribution of the increased GABA$_A$ receptor binding is quite different, however, in the cortex compared with hippocampus (Fig. 3.2): in prefrontal cortex, the receptor was selectively up-regulated on pyramidal neurons, a pattern that is in line with a reduction of inhibitory GABAergic inputs to these cells; in the hippocampal formation, on the other hand, the up-regulation of the GABA$_A$ receptor in CA3 in schizophrenia was found on non-pyramidal neurons. This latter pattern suggests that there may be a reduction of disinhibitory GABAergic activity (i.e. GABA cells providing inhibitory input to other GABA cells), in this sector in schizophrenia. It is not clear why such a difference in cellular distribution would occur, but it may reflect the unique pattern of intrinsic connectivity in the cortex compared to the hippocampus.

The GABA$_A$ receptor complex also contains a high affinity site for binding benzodiazepine compounds. A recent study demonstrated that there was an up-regulation of the GABA$_A$ site, but not the benzodiazepine receptor in the hippocampus in schizophrenia (Benes *et al.*, 1997*b*); exposure to benzodiazepines was carefully evaluated and found not to account for the lack of difference with respect to this receptor. A study from another laboratory did detect a decrease of benzodiazepine receptor binding activity in the hippocampus of schizophrenics (Squires *et al.*, 1993); however, they did not consider exposure to benzodiazepines in the interpretation of the results. Increased GABA$_A$ receptor but not benzodiazepine receptor binding raises the possibility that regulation of these sites may be uncoupled in schizophrenia. It is noteworthy that a similar uncoupling phenomenon has recently been identified for Purkinje neurons in the cerebellum of the staggerer mouse mutant, with mRNA for both the β_2 and γ_2 subunits being markedly decreased in early postnatal life (Luntz-Leybman *et al.*, 1995). Certain heteromeric combinations of subunits are associated with the GABA receptor complex, but it is the γ_2 isoform that is necessary for benzodiazepine receptor binding activity (Wisden *et al.*, 1992; Rabow *et al.*, 1995). Accordingly, it will be essential to know whether expression of the γ_2 isoform is altered in schizophrenia or whether an anomalous isoform has been substituted. In the dorsolateral prefrontal cortex (area 9), the expression of mRNAs for the common α, β and γ subunit isoforms showed no differences between schizophrenics and controls (Akbarian *et al.*, 1995*a*). It is important to emphasize, however, that the mRNA content of a cell does

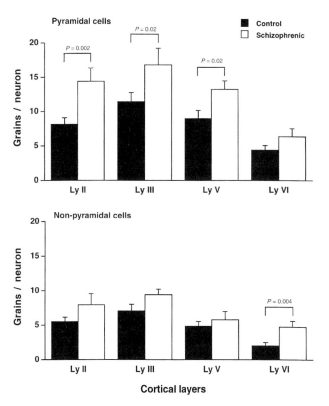

Fig. 3.2 High resolution studies of GABA$_A$ receptor binding in various layers of the prefrontal cortex from normal controls (solid bars) and schizophrenic subjects (open bars). There is a marked increase of GABA$_A$ receptor binding in layers II, III and V of the schizophrenics, but no change in layer VI. These changes are thought to represent a compensatory up-regulation of this receptor in response to a loss of GABAergic cells and/or activity in this and other regions of the corticolimbic system. The data do not exclude the possibility, however, that the GABA receptor complex may be genetically abnormal in schizophrenia and that the increase of binding to the GABA$_A$ site might represent a primary defect. (Adapted from Benes *et al.*, 1996*b*.)

not necessarily reflect the synthesis, post-translational modification, and degradation of biologically active protein. Moreover, since there are different isoforms of each subunit (Rabow *et al.*, 1995), it is possible that a unique permutation of isoforms is present in schizophrenia which was not detected using the cDNAs employed by Akbarian *et al.* (1995*a*).

The cortical glutamate system

Evidence for a disturbance of glutamatergic function in schizophrenia has come from both microscopic and biochemical studies (Benes, 1996; Tamminga, 1998). The emphasis here is on the former; however, some neurochemical findings will be mentioned in the context of how they may relate to the histological findings of volume shrinkage and neuronal cell loss via an excitotoxic injury.

An increased number of vertical fibers in the upper layers of anterior cingulate cortex in schizophrenia is mentioned above. Since the NFP200K antibody non-specifically visualizes different types of axons, regardless of their site of origin or their neurotransmitter phenotype, an alternative strategy was used which could help identify the fibers that were increased. Since the fibers might be incoming associative axons, a monoclonal antibody against a glutamate–glutaraldehyde conjugate was employed, because these inputs are believed to use glutamate as their transmitter (Conti *et al.*, 1988). Using this antibody in a blinded study, the density of vertical fibers with a small calibre (1–2 μm) in layers II and upper portions of IIIa was found to be much higher (80 per cent) in anterior cingulate gyrus, but no different in prefrontal cortex, in schizophrenia (Benes *et al.*, 1992*a*). Thus, these data not only provided a replication of the earlier findings using the immunolocalization of NFP200K, but also suggested that the increased vertical fibers were glutamatergic.

Layer II of the anterior cingulate gyrus receives glutamatergic afferents from several sources. Some of the vertical fibers could be intrinsic in nature and arise from pyramidal neurons in layer V (Martin, 1984) and Martinotti cells found in layers V and VI (Fairen *et al.*, 1982) that project axon collaterals vertically towards layer I. While the neurotransmitter employed by Martinotti cells is not as yet known, that for pyramidal cells is thought to be glutamate (Monaghan and Cotman, 1985; Conti *et al.*, 1988) and most associative fibers originate from pyramidal neurons in superficial layers of the cortex (Jones, 1984). It is also possible that the increased vertical fibers could be subcortical in origin. For example, the anterior, dorsomedial, and interstitial thalamic nuclei all project to anterior cingulate cortex (Bentoviglio *et al.*, 1993), with the anterior nucleus being the primary source of thalamocortical afferents to layer I. Another potential source of the increased vertical axons detected in schizophrenia may be the amygdala, which sends a massive projection from the basolateral nucleus to layer II (Van Hoesen *et al.*, 1993). It is noteworthy that prefrontal cortex does not receive an appreciable projection from the amygdala (Van Hoesen *et al.*, 1993), and if the amygdala were the source of the vertical fibers in anterior cingulate cortex, this differential distribution could help to explain why increases were detected in anterior cingulate but not prefrontal cortex (Benes *et al.*, 1992*a*). Consistent with this possibility is the preliminary evidence that glutamate-immunoreactive fibers may also be increased in schizophrenia in superficial layers of the entorhinal cortex (Longson *et al.*, 1996) to which the accessory basal nucleus of the amygdala sends a substantial projection (Amaral *et al.*, 1992). Interestingly, the antibody used to visualize these fibers also produces intense immunoreactivity in large piriform cells of the basolateral amygdaloid nucleus (McDonald *et al.*, 1989). Pyramidal neurons in the subiculum, which show similar intense glutamate immunoreactivity (McDonald *et al.*, 1989), also project to the cingulate cortex, but primarily to the posterior portions. Hence of the various potential sites of origin for the increased vertical fibers observed in the anterior cingulate cortex in schizophrenia, the amygdala seems to be most compelling.

Evidence for excitotoxicity in schizophrenia

Taking the above observations together with those of volume shrinkage and neuronal loss, an excitotoxic process has been postulated to play a role in the pathophysiology of schizophrenia (Benes, 1993c; Coyle and Puttfarcken, 1993; Olney and Farber, 1995). Neurochemical investigations of the cingulate cortex in which 'grind-and-bind' assays or low resolution autoradiography have been employed have reported no differences in high affinity binding to the phencyclidine (Weissman *et al.*, 1991), the sigma opiate (Weissman *et al.*, 1991; Shibuya *et al.*, 1992), or non-*N*-methyl-D-aspartate (NMDA) glutamate (Kurumaji *et al.*, 1992) receptors in schizophrenia. Increased phencyclidine receptor binding has, however, been reported in frontal cortex (Kornhuber *et al.*, 1989; Simpson *et al.*, 1992), and in the entorhinal region, hippocampus, and putamen (Kornhuber *et al.*, 1989). Since the phencyclidine site non-competitively blocks the NMDA receptor complex (Harrison and Simmonds, 1985), the increased binding in these regions could theoretically represent either an overall increase of NMDA-sensitive glutamate binding or a compensatory response of postsynaptic cells to limit the effect of glutamate on the receptor complex. A recent study has demonstrated an increase of the $NMDAR_{2D}$ subunit mRNA selectively in the prefrontal cortex of schizophrenics (Akbarian *et al.*, 1996b); no differences in other subunits were observed. These results are consistent with the possibility that there could be an over-expression of an anomalous form of the NMDA receptor complex. It is difficult to predict, however, whether such an anomaly would result in increased or decreased NMDA-mediated glutamatergic activity in cortical circuits. Another recent study found the mRNA for the $NMDAR_1$ subunit reduced in the superior temporal cortex in schizophrenia and to correlate with the degree of cognitive impairment (Humphries *et al.*, 1996).

Changes have also been reported for non-NMDA (AMPA and kainate) subtypes of glutamate receptor in schizophrenia, the nature of which differs between hippocampus and frontal cortex. In hippocampus, a reduction in the binding of ^{3}H-kainate was observed (Kerwin *et al.*, 1988, 1990), particularly in the area dentata, CA4, CA3, CA1, and parahippocampal gyrus. There is an accompanying loss of the mRNA transcripts encoding both AMPA and kainate receptor subunits (Harrison *et al.*, 1991; Eastwood *et al.*, 1995; Porter *et al.*, 1997), and decreased abundance of the AMPA receptor subunits $GluR_2$ and $GluR_3$ (Breese *et al.*, 1995; Eastwood *et al.*, 1997). Other data (Kostoulakos *et al.*, 1998; Benes *et al.*, 2001) also suggest immunoreactivity for the $GluR_{5,6,7}$ subunit of the kainate receptor in schizophrenia is decreased on apical dendrites of pyramidal neurons in the stratum radiatum and moleculare of CA1 to CA3, especially in CA2 where the decreased interneuron density was found (Benes *et al.*, 1998). In frontal lobe, elevated ^{3}H-kainate binding is seen, both in orbitofrontal cortex (Deakin *et al.*, 1989), medial frontal cortex, and frontal eye field (Nishikawa *et al.*, 1983; Toru *et al.*, 1988). While these findings might suggest a compensatory increase of receptor binding in response to diminished glutamatergic activity in frontal cortex, the concomitant increase of ^{3}H-aspartate receptor binding (a marker for glutamate reuptake) has led to the suggestion that glutamatergic innervation may be *increased* in these regions in schizophrenia (Deakin *et al.*, 1989).

It is clear that these findings do not lend themselves to straightforward conclusions as to whether excitotoxicity plays a role in schizophrenia. For example, do decreased kainate receptor indices in the hippocampus reflect (a) a compensatory down-regulation occurring in the setting of an increased action of glutamate on postsynaptic receptors; or (b) a drop-out of pyramidal neurons expressing this receptor on their dendrites? Both mechanisms imply that, at some point in the illness, there has been an increase of glutamate activity generated either within the hippocampus, or in other regions that project to it. As anterior cingulate cortex sends abundant projections to the hippocampus (Domesick, 1969; Beckstead, 1979), the latter possibility seems plausible, particularly given the reduction of non-pyramidal neurons in CA2 (Benes *et al.*, 1998); the excitatory input from the baso-lateral amygdala may also play a role (Benes and Berretta, 2000). A neuroleptic dose-related increase of GAD_{65}-IR terminals was also found in this sector, suggesting that a reduction of GABAergic terminals in drug-free schizophrenics may reflect the occurrence of oxida-tive stress (Todtenkopf and Benes, 1998). Thus, the evidence is consistent with the possibility that excitotoxicity may contribute to changes in the cortical volume and neuronal density found in schizophrenia. If such a mechanism is operative, the inconsistent findings of cell counting studies may reflect regional, or temporal, variation in the nature and extent of glutamatergic dysfunction.

The cortical dopamine system

Most studies of the dopamine system in schizophrenia have been targeted at subcortical regions. A variety of markers, including the levels of dopamine and parameters related to its synthesis, degradation, and reuptake, have not yielded any consistent pattern of changes (Davis *et al.*, 1991); increased D2 receptor binding in the striatum is well documented but is attributable largely to neuroleptic medication (Zakzanis and Hansen, 1998). Moving to the cortex, a recent study has explored the cytoarchitectonic distribution of D2 receptors in various subdivisions of the temporal lobe (Goldsmith *et al.*, 1997). The data indicate that this receptor may be decreased in superficial layers of the superior temporal gyrus in schizophrenia; this finding appears to be region-specific since a similar pattern was not noted in other portions of the temporal lobe.

A critical issue for our understanding of schizophrenia is whether there is any overt change in the distribution of dopaminergic fibers in the cortex. A commonly used marker for these fibers is the dopamine transporter. In one recent such study, no differences between controls and schizophrenics were detected (Hitri *et al.*, 1995). Alternatively, TH immuno-cytochemistry can be used as a marker for catecholaminergic neurons and fibers. While TH is not specific for the dopamine system, anti-TH antibodies yield a relatively selective visualization of dopamine fibers (Lewis *et al.*, 1987; Gaspar *et al.*, 1989; Williams and Goldman-Rakic, 1993). Consistent with the dopamine transporter data, no overall differ-ences in the distribution of TH-immunoreactive varicosities were seen in the anterior cingulate or prefrontal cortices in schizophrenia (Benes *et al.*, 1997*a*), though a decreased density of the varicosities was observed in the neuropil of layers V and VI in the anterior cingulate cortex in medicated (but not unmedicated) subjects (Benes *et al.*, 1997*a*). A decrease of TH-immnuoreactive fibers has also been reported in the entorhinal cortex in schizophrenia (Lewis and Akil, 1997).

More detailed studies of TH mmunoreactivity have provided additional information. The density of TH-immunoreactive varicosities in contact with non-pyramidal neurons in layer II was three times higher than that for pyramidal neurons in layer II in schizophrenia; this finding did not appear related to neuroleptic exposure (Benes *et al.*, 1997*a*). Interestingly, when the data are closely examined (Fig. 3.3), it is evident that there is a modest reduction in the number of the varicosities on pyramidal neurons, but an increase on non-pyramidal cells, in layer II of the schizophrenics when compared to the controls. This suggests the possibility that the increase of TH-immunoreactive varicosities on non-pyramidal neurons in schizophrenia may not necessarily be due to a loss of GABAergic neurons, but to a shift in location from pyramidal to non-pyramidal neurons (Fig. 3.4). In other words, schizophrenia could involve a miswiring of dopaminergic afferents in layer II of the anterior cingulate cortex, perhaps related to a disturbance of perinatal development (Benes, 1993*b*, 1995*b*). Since the cortical dopamine system shows selective increase of release during stress (Thierry *et al.*, 1976; Roth *et al.*, 1988), the normal ingrowth of these fibers which occurs until early adulthood (Benes *et al.*, 1996*c*) could serve as a trigger for the onset of schizophrenia during this period (Benes, 1995*a*).

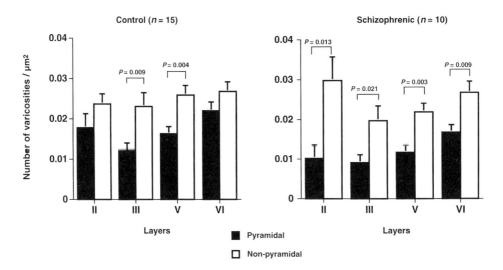

Fig. 3.3 A comparison of the density of tyrosine hydroxylase-immunoreactive (TH-IR) varicosities on pyramidal (PN) versus non-pyramidal (NP) neurons in the anterior cingulate cortex of normal controls (left panel) and schizophrenic subjects (right panel). The controls show a marked tendency for NPs to have a higher density of TH-IR varicosities forming appositions with their cell bodies, particularly in layers III and V. The schizophrenics show a similar pattern, except that it is more marked, particularly in layer II where the density of TH-IR varicosities is three times higher on NPs when compared to PNs. These data are consistent with a model in which there is a shift of dopaminergic varicosities from PNs to NPs in layer II of anterior cingulate cortex in schizophrenics. (Adapted from Benes *et al.*, 1996*a*.)

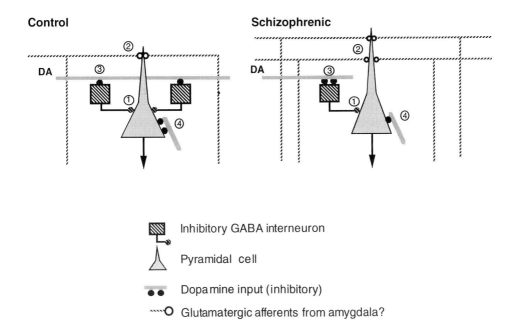

Control   **Schizophrenic**

DA   DA

▨   Inhibitory GABA interneuron

△   Pyramidal cell

●●   Dopamine input (inhibitory)

⟿O   Glutamatergic afferents from amygdala?

Fig. 3.4 A schematic diagram depicting a working model for alterations in layer II of the anterior cingulate cortex of schizophrenics. *Control circuit*: a pyramidal neuron (PN) receives (1) inhibitory inputs from two GABAergic cells, and (2) excitatory inputs from two incoming afferents. Both the PN (3) and the GABAergic (4) neuron receive inputs from dopaminergic (DA) varicosities and their relative number has been normalized with respect to the data in Fig. 3.3, and adjusted for the average size of the two cell types. Accordingly, each GABAergic neuron is depicted as receiving an input from one DA varicosity, while the PN has contact with two DA varicosities. *Schizophrenic circuit*: The diagram is similar to that for the control circuit, except that (1) one of the GABAergic cells is missing to indicate a reduction in either the number or activity of these cells, and (2) the PN is receiving excitatory inputs from four incoming afferents (Benes *et al.*, 1987, 1992*a*). The GABA cell (3) is receiving input from two DA varicosities, while the PN is receiving input from only one. There is an increase of vertical axons (Benes *et al.*, 1987) that appear to be glutamatergic afferents coursing toward layers I and II (Benes *et al.*, 1992*a*). If dopamine exerts an inhibitory influence on neurons, the model predicts that the schizophrenic circuit would have a decreased inhibitory modulation exerted on the PN as a result of two separate factors: a decrease of GABAergic activity and the increased DA input to GABA cells. The increase of $GABA_A$ receptor binding on the PN may be due either to (a) a compensatory up-regulation resulting from an inhibition of the GABAergic cell by DA inputs; (b) a primary defect in the genetic regulation of the GABA receptor complex; or (c) a glucocorticoid-mediated effect on the regulation of the $GABA_A$ receptor (see text for details). (Adapted from Benes, 1993*a*, 1998.)

Cortical pathology and the neurodevelopmental hypothesis

There has been intense interest in the idea that schizophrenia might be a neurodevelopmental disorder. The hypothesis originated with the finding of pyramidal cell disarray in the hippocampal formation which led to the suggestion by Kovelman and Scheibel (1984) that the disorder involves a disturbance in the early development of this region. Shortly thereafter, Jakob and Beckmann (1986) described cytoarchitectural anomalies in the pre-α layer (layer II) of the entorhinal cortex and suggested that there might be a disruption of normal neuronal migration during embryogenesis. Further support came the same year when a reduced density of neurons, without gliosis, in the prefrontal, anterior cingulate, and primary motor cortices of schizophrenics was shown, as detailed above (Benes *et al.*, 1986). In the latter study, it was suggested that an hypoxic insult during the perinatal period might potentially account for such a pattern. The fact that neuronal density was found to be lower leads to the the corollary suggestion that the surrounding neuropil has been increased (cf. Selemon and Goldman-Rakic, 1999). Other evidence in support of the neurodevelopmental hypothesis has come from the preponderance of anomalies observed in cortical layer II (see above) which has led to the suggestion that a disturbance of neuronal cell migration and/or maturation could be responsible for the changes (Benes, 1995*c*).

The neurodevelopmental hypothesis of schizophrenia is described in detail elsewhere in this volume, notably Chapter 8. Discussion here is limited to matters relevant to the neurochemical and circuitry issues outlined above. It was recently concluded from a study of the GABA$_A$ receptor in the hippocampus in schizophrenia that a very broad window of opportunity exists for inducing such changes (Benes *et al.*, 1996*a*; Benes, 1997*b*); it could be as early as the second trimester *in utero* (Jacobsen and Kinney, 1980), or perinatally when the maturation of neuronal processes is actively occurring, or perhaps even in late adolescence and early adulthood when the prodrome of the illness is beginning (Benes, 1988). It is very difficult to prove one way or another which of these developmental stages is a critical period for imparting the vulnerability to schizophrenia. Recent attempts at obtaining empirical evidence for such a hypothetical process in schizophrenics have included the study of the distribution of nicotinamide adenine dinucleotide phosphate-diaphorase (NADPH-D) containing neurons as markers for cell migration. In the first study, these cells showed a significantly higher density in the deeper portions of white matter in prefrontal cortex in schizophrenics (Akbarian *et al.*, 1993), interpreted as being consistent with disrupted neuronal migration. In a second study the authors noted a similar pattern, but only in 35 per cent of subjects (Akbarian *et al.*, 1996*a*; see also Chapter 13). A confound to the interpretation of these results is the fact that NADPH-D neurons, which are believed to be GABAergic, continue to migrate into the cortical mantle into the early postnatal period (Yan *et al.*, 1993). Accordingly, it is possible that any disturbance in schizophrenia has not occurred during the second trimester, but perinatally. Using antibodies against the neuronal marker microtubule associated protein 2 (MAP2), another group has explored the same issue, demonstrating no overall difference in schizophrenia, though there was a higher density compared to the controls at more superficial levels of the white matter (Andersen *et al.*, 1996). These data suggest that if a disturbance of cell migration and/or differentiation in the cortex does play a role in the pathophysiology of schizophrenia, it is a very subtle process, and one not readily accessible to empirical analysis.

An important issue regarding cortical pathology in schizophrenia is whether there are normal structural changes during adolescence that activate latent defects in corticolimbic circuitry. Most evidence suggests that people who develop schizophrenia are relatively 'normal' until adolescence or early adulthood, raising the possibility that a pathological process, possibly one involving excitotoxicity (see above), is not triggered until the second or third decade. This observation underscores the importance of learning more about the later postnatal development and maturation of the human brain (see Chapters 8 to 10). Thus far, increased myelination in the medial temporal lobe (Benes *et al.*, 1994) and synaptic pruning in the dorsolateral prefrontal cortex (Huttenlocher and Dabholkar, 1997) have been demonstrated to occur in adolescence; both of these changes could play a role in the onset of schizophrenia. In rat anterior cingulate cortex, other discrete changes in neural circuitry, such as the ingrowth of dopamine fibers (see Benes *et al.*, 1996*c*) and their increased interaction with intrinsic cortical elements such as GABAergic interneurons (Benes *et al.*, 1996*c*) have been detected. Are there similar changes occurring in human brain? If so, they might trigger the induction of wiring abnormalities in individuals vulnerable to schizophrenia. Some recent evidence in rodents suggests that such a change could be related, at least in part, to the combined effects of stress, not only during the perinatal period, but also during early adulthood (Benes, 1998). What specific cellular and molecular mechanisms contribute to such a process are unknown; however, a disturbance of neuroplasticity provides one potential source for inducing a trophic shift in cortical dopamine fibers (Taylor *et al.*, 1998; Benes *et al.*, 2000).

Conclusions

The above discussion has sought to demonstrate the approaches that are being used to study cortical pathology in a brain disorder in which there are no 'classic' histopathological features. As recently concluded by others, there are several different categories of findings that have emerged (Arnold and Trojanowski, 1996). Some of the findings are non-specific in nature (e.g. volume loss) but are nevertheless confirmatory of changes reported in structural *in vivo* imaging studies. Other findings, however, have pointed to a subtle degree of neuronal loss being found in some, though not all corticolimbic regions. These, together with other more discrete changes in specific neurotransmitter systems detected with cytochemical approaches have suggested that there are probably circumscribed changes in the microscopic connectivity of both extrinsic and intrinsic components of the corticolimbic system.

The findings of volume and neuronal loss are consistent with the idea that schizophrenia may involve a subtle and perhaps prolonged process of excitotoxicity. It seems likely that such an injury would vary in severity from one patient to another and probably also among various subtypes of schizophrenia. Indeed, the clinical severity of schizophrenia could, in part, be a reflection of the relative amount of excitotoxicity that has been present at some time during the subject's life and thence to the degree of neuronal loss. Such changes in the glutamate system could result either in neuronal death or in a less overt form of injury to distal branches of pyramidal cell dendrites, as has been suggested for dorsolateral prefrontal cortex (Selemon *et al.*, 1995). From a theoretical standpoint, there could be a loss of neurons in some brain regions in schizophrenia, while elsewhere there are only subtle atrophic changes (e.g. smaller neuronal somata; Rajkowska *et al.*, 1998) in an otherwise viable population of neurons.

Genetic factors in schizophrenia may also determine whether inappropriate interconnections or interactions occur between chemically normal components of the brain (Kety, 1959). Today, investigations are beginning to unravel the manner in which neural circuitry may be altered. With time, it may eventually be possible to define the constitutional vulnerability for schizophrenia by using a two-pronged strategy to characterize the alterations of neural circuitry associated with the schizophrenia phenotype: one directed at identifying the effect(s) of an abnormal gene and one directed at identifying the effects of an early disturbance of brain development. A genetic factor could act either alone or in combination with pre- and/or perinatal stress to alter normal brain development, either focally or in a generalized way, so that a change in 'wiring' is induced. Subsequent changes that normally occur during adolescence, such as the ingrowth of dopamine fibers, could then trigger the phenotypic expression of this altered constitution by inducing the formation of connections with a pre-existing network in which altered neural circuitry has been in a latent state (Benes *et al.*, 1996c). In the years to come, neuropathological studies of schizophrenia will be seeking to define precisely how the expression of an abnormal gene(s) may interplay with the effects of stress at critical periods when individuals at risk for the illness are apt to develop functional abnormalities.

An important question concerning the various microscopic changes seen in schizophrenia is whether the alterations appeared before, during, or after the onset of illness. The answer to this question may eventually help to define the pathophysiology of the disorder in terms of the development of precise neural circuits and lead to the evolution of novel therapeutic strategies, ones that may be applied early in the course of the illness. In this way, it may be eventually possible to offset the progressive deterioration in functioning that typically occurs during the first 5 to 10 years of illness and leads to the permanent impairments seen in many patients.

Acknowledgements

The author wishes to thank Mrs Maureen Medeiros for her help in preparing this manuscript. This work has been supported by grants from the National Institute of Mental Health (MH00423, MH42261, MH31862, MH311540), the Scottish Rite Foundation, and the Stanley Foundation.

References

Abercrombie, M. (1946) Estimation of nuclear population from microtomic sections. *Anatomic Review*, **94**, 239.

Akbarian, S., Bunney, W. E., Potkin, S. G. *et al.* (1993) Altered distribution of nicoti-namide-adenine dinucleotide phosphate-diaphorase cells in frontal lobe of schizophrenics implies disturbances of cortical development. *Archives of General Psychiatry*, **50**, 227–230.

Akbarian, S., Huntsman, M. M., Kim. J. J. *et al.* (1995*a*) GABA$_A$ receptor subunit gene expression in human prefrontal cortex: comparison of schizophrenics and controls. *Cerebral Cortex,* **6**, 550–560.

Akbarian, S., Kim, J.J., Potkin, S.G., *et al.* (1995*b*) Gene expression for glutamatic acid decarboxylase is reduced without loss of neurons in prefrontal cortex of schizophrenics. *Archives General Psychiatry,* **52**, 258–278.

Akbarian S., Kim, J. J., Potkin, S. G., Hetrick, W. P., Bunney, W. E., Jr, Jones, E. G. (1996*a*) Maldistribution of interstitial neurons in prefrontal white matter of the brains of schizophrenic patients. *Archives of General Psychiatry,* **53**, 425–436.

Akbarian, S., Sucher, N. J., Bradley, D. *et al.* (1996*b*) Selective alterations in gene expression for NMDA receptor subunits in prefrontal cortex of schizophrenics. *Journal of Neuroscience*, **16**, 19–30.

Amaral, D. G., Price, J. L., Pitkanen, A., Carmichael, S. T. (1992) Anatomical organization of the primate amygdaloid complex. In: J. P. Aggleton, (Ed.). *The amygdala.* Wiley-Liss, New York.

Anderson, S. A., Volk, D. W., Lewis, D. A. (1996) Increased density of microtubule associated protein 2-immunoreactive neurons in the prefrontal white matter of schizophrenic subjects. *Schizophrenia Research,* **19**, 111–119.

Arnold, S. E., Trojanowski, J. Q. (1996). Recent advances in defining the neuropathology of schizophrenia. *Acta Neuropathologica*, **92**, 217–231.

Arnold, S. E., Franz, B. R., Gur, R. C. *et al.* (1995) Smaller neuron size in schizophrenia in hippocampal subfields that mediate cortical-hippocampal interactions. *American Journal of Psychiatry*, **152**, 738–748.

Arnold, S. E., Franz, B. R., Trojanowski. J. Q., Moberg, P. J., Gur, R. E. (1996) Glial fibrillary acidic protein-immunoreactive astrocytosis in elderly patients with schizophrenia and dementia. *Acta Neuropathologica*, **91**, 269–277.

Beasley, C. L., Reynolds, G. P. (1996) Parvalbumin-immunoreactive neurons are reduced in the prefrontal cortex of schizophrenics. *Schizophrenia Research,* **24**, 349–355.

Beckstead, R. M. (1979). An autoradiographic examination of cortico-cortical and subcortical projections of the mediodorsal-projection (prefrontal) cortex in the rat. *Journal of Comparative Neurology*, **184**, 43–62.

Benes, F. M. (1988). Post-mortem structural analyses of schizophrenic brain. Study designs and the interpretation of data. *Psychiatric Developments*, **6**, 213–226.

Benes, F. M. (1993*a*). Post-mortem correlates of brain imaging findings in schizophrenia. *Harvard Review of Psychiatry*, **1**, 100–109.

Benes, F. M. (1993*b*) Development of the corticolimbic system. In: *Human behavior and the developing brain.* Guilford, New York.

Benes, F. M. (1993*c*) Cingulate cortex in schizophrenia and other psychiatric disorders. In: B. A. Vogt and M. Gabriel (Eds). *The neurobiology of cingulate cortex and limbic thalamus.* Birkhauser Inc, Boston, MA.

Benes, F. M. (1995a) Is there a neuroanatomic basis for schizophrenia? An old question revisited. *The Neuroscientist*, **1**, 104–115.

Benes, F. M. (1995b) Microscopic findings in the cortex and hippocampus of schizophrenic and schizoaffective patients. In: Marneros, A., Andreasen, N. C., Tsuang, M. T. (Eds). *Psychotic continuum,* pp. 127–136. Springer-Verlag, Berlin.

Benes, F. M. (1995c) A neurodevelopmental approach to the understanding of schizophrenia and other mental disorders. In: Cicchetti, D. and Cohen, D. J. (Eds). *Developmental psychopathology,* Volume 1. Wiley, Chichester.

Benes, F. M. (1996) The role of glutamate in the pathophysiology of schizophrenia. In: Conti, F., Hicks, T. P. (Eds). *Excitatory amino acids and the cerebral cortex*, pp. 361–374. MIT Press, Cambridge, MA.

Benes F. M. (1997a) Is there evidence for neuronal loss in schizophrenia? *International Review of Psychiatry*, **9**, 429–436.

Benes F. M. (1997b) The role of stress and dopamine-GABA interactions in the vulnerability for schizophrenia. *Journal of Psychiatric Research,* **31**, 257–275.

Benes, F. M. (1998) Model generation and testing in the study of postmortem schizophrenic brain. *Schizophrenia Bulletin*, **24**, 219–230.

Benes F. M., Bird E. D. (1987) An analysis of the arrangement of neurons in the cingulate cortex of schizophrenic patients. *Archives of General Psychiatry*, **44**, 608–616.

Benes, F.M., Davidson J., Bird, E. D. (1986) Quantitative cytoarchitectural studies of cerebral cortex of schizophrenics. *Archives of General Psychiatry*, **43**, 31–35.

Benes, F. M., Majocha, R., Bird, E. D., Marrotta, C. A. (1987). Increased vertical axon numbers in cingulate cortex of schizophrenics. *Archives of General Psychiatry*, **44**, 1017–1021.

Benes F. M., McSparren, J., Bird, E. D., Vincent, S. L., SanGiovanni, J. P. (1991a). Deficits in small interneurons in prefrontal and anterior cingulate cortex of schizophrenic and schizoaffective patients. *Archives of General Psychiat*ry, **48**, 996–1001.

Benes, F. M., Sorensen, I., Bird, E. D. (1991b) Morphometric analyses of the hippocampal formation in schizophrenic brain. *Schizophrenia Bulletin*, **17**, 597–608.

Benes, F. M., Sorensen, I., Vincent, S. L., Bird, E. D., Sathi, M. (1992a) Increased density of glutamate-immunoreactive vertical processes in superficial laminae in cingulate cortex of schizophrenic brain. *Cerebral Cortex*, **2**, 503–512.

Benes, F. M., Vincent, S. L., Alsterberg, G., Bird, E.D, San Giovanni, J. P. (1992b) Increased GABA-A receptor binding in superficial layers of cingulate cortex in schizophrenics. *Journal of Neuroscience*, **12**, 924–929.

Benes, F. M., Turtle, M., Khan, Y., Farol, P. (1994) Myelination of a key relay zone in the hippocampal formation occurs in the human brain during childhood, adolescence and adulthood. *Archives of General Psychiatry*, **51**, 477–484.

Benes, F. M., Khan, Y., Vincent, S. L., Wickramasinghe, R. (1996a) Differences in the subregional and cellular distribution of GABA-$_A$ receptor binding in the hippocampal formation of schizophrenic brain. *Synapse*, **22**, 338–349.

Benes, F. M., Vincent, S. L., Marie, A., Khan, Y. (1996b) Upregulation of GABA$_A$ receptor binding on neurons of prefrontal cortex in schizophrenic subjects. *Neuroscience*, **75**, 1021–1031.

Benes, F. M., Vincent, S. L., Molloy, R. (1996c) Increased interaction of dopamine-immunoreactive varicosities with GABA neurons of rat medial prefrontal cortex occurs during the post-weanling period. *Synapse, 23*, 237–245.

Benes, F. M, Todtenkopf, M. S., Taylor, J. B. (1997a) Differential distribution of tyrosine hydroxylase fibers on neuronal subtypes in layer II of anterior cingulate cortex of schizophrenic brain. *Synapse, 25*, 80–92.

Benes, F. M., Wickramasinghe, R., Vincent, S. L., Khan, Y., Todtenkopf, M. S. (1997b) Uncoupling of GABA$_A$ and benzodiazepine receptor binding activity in the hippocampal formation of schizophrenic brain. *Brain Research, 755*, 121–129.

Benes, F. M., Kwok, E., Vincent, S. L. (1998) Relative distribution of pyramidal (PN) and nonpyramidal (NP) neurons in the hippocampus of schizophrenic (SZ) and manic depressive (MD) brain. *Biological Psychiatry, 44*, 88–97.

Benes, F. M., Berretta, S. (2000) Amygdalo-entorhinal inputs to the hippocampal formation in relation to schizophrenia. *Annals of the New York Academy of Sciences* (in press).

Benes F. M., Taylor, J. B., Cunningham, M. C. (2000) Convergence and plasticity of monoaminergic system in medial prefrontal cortex during postnatal period: implications for the development of psychopathology. *Cerebral Cortex* (in press).

Benes, F. M., Todtenkopf, M. S., Kostoulakos, P. (2001) Decreased GluR$_{5, 6, 7}$ subunit immunoreactivity on apical dendrites in hippocampus of schizophrenics, but not manic depressives. *Hippocampus* (in press).

Bentoviglio, M., Kutlas-Ilinsky, K., Ilinsky, I. (1993) Limbic thalamus: structure, intrinsic organization, and connections, In: B. A. Vogt, M. Gabriel (Eds). *Neurobiology of cingulate cortex and limbic thalamus*, pp. 71–122. Birkhauser, Boston.

Bird, E. D., Spokes, E. G. S., Iversen, L. L. (1979) Increased dopamine concentrations in limbic areas of brain from patients dying with schizophrenia. *Brain, 102*, 347–360.

Breese, C. R., Freedman, R., Leonard, S. S. (1995) Glutamate receptor subtype expression in human postmortem brain tissue from schizophrenics and alcohol abusers. *Brain Research, 674*, 82–90.

Coggeshall, R. E., Lekan, H. A. (1996) Methods for determining numbers of cell and synbapses: A case for more uniform standards of review. *Journal of Comparative Neurology, 364*, 6–15.

Colon, E. J. (1972) Quantitative cytoarchitectonics of the human cerebral cortex. *Psychiatria, Neurologia, Neurochirurgia, 74*, 291–302.

Conde, F., Lund, J. S., Jacobowitz, D. M., Baimbridge, K. G., Lewis, D. A. (1994) Local circuit neurons immunoreactive for calretinin, calbindin D-28k or parvalbumin in monkey prefrontal cortex: distribution and morphology. *Journal of Comparative Neurology, 341*, 95–116.

Conti, F, Fabri, M., Manzoni, T. (1988) Glutamate-positive cortico-cortical neurons in the somatic sensory areas I and II of cats. *Journal of Neuroscience, 8*, 2948–2960.

Coyle, J. T., Puttfarcken, P. (1993) Oxidative stress, glutamate and neurodegenerative disorders. *Science, 262*, 689–695.

Davis, K. L., Kahn, R. S., Ko, G., Davidson, M. (1991) Dopamine in schizophrenia: a review and reconceptualization. *American Journal of Psychiatry, 148*, 1474–1486.

Daviss, S. R., Lewis, D. A. (1995) Local circuit neurons of the prefrontal cortex in schizophrenia: selective increase in the denisty of calbindin-immunoreactive neurons. *Psychiatry Research*, **59**, 81–96.

Deakin, J. F. W., Slater P., Simpson, M. D. *et al.* (1989) Frontal cortical and left temporal glutamatergic dysfunction in schizophrenia. *Journal of Neurochemistry*, **52**, 1781–1786.

Detre, T. P., Jarecki, H. G. (1971) *Modern psychiatric treatment*, pp. 108–116. J. B. Lippincott, Philadelphia.

Dom, R. (1976) Neostriatal and thalamic interneurons. Their role in the pathophysiology of Huntington's chorea, Parkinson's disease and catatonic schizophrenia. Doctoral dissertation, Karolinska Institute.

Dom, R., de Saedeler, J., Bogerts, B., Hopf, A. (1981) Quantitative cytometric analysis of basal ganglia in catatonic schizophrenics. In: Perris, C., Struwe, G., Jansson, B. (Eds). *Biological Psychiatry*. Elsevier, Amsterdam, pp. 723–726.

Domesick, V. B. (1969) Projections from the cingulate cortex in the rat. *Brain Research*, **12**, 296–230.

Eastwood S. L., McDonald, B., Burnet, P. W. J., Beckwith, J. P., Kerwin, R. W., Harrison, P. J. (1995) Decreased expression of mRNAs encoding non-NMDA glutamate receptors GluR1 and GluR2 in medial temporal lobe neurons in schizophrenia. *Molecular Brain Research*, **29**, 211–223.

Eastwood, S. L., Kerwin, R. W., Harrison, P. J. (1997) Immunoautoradiographic evidence for a loss of AMPA-preferring non-NMDA glutamate receptor subunits within the medial temporal lobe in schizophrenia. *Biological Psychiatry*, **41**, 636–643.

Fairen, A., DeFelipe, J., Regidor, J. (1982) Nonpyramidal neurons. In: Peters, A., Jones, E. G. (Eds). *Cerebral cortex*, Volume 1: *Cellular components of cerebral cortex*. Plenum Press, New York, pp. 201–253.

Gabriel, S. M., Haroutunian, V., Powchik, P. *et al.* (1997) Increased concentrations of presynaptic proteins in the cingulate cortex of subjects with schizophrenia. *Archives of General Psychiatry*, **54**, 559–566.

Gaspar, P., Berger, B., Febvret, A., Vigny, A., Henry, J. P. (1989) Catecholamine innervation of the human cerebral cortex as revealed by comparative immunohistochemistry of tyrosine hydroxylase and dopamine beta-hydroxylase. *Journal of Comparative Neurology*, **279**, 249–271.

Glantz, L.A., Lewis, D. A. (1997) Reduction of synaptophysin immunoreactivity in the prefrontal cortex of subjects with schizophrenia. *Archives of General Psychiatry*, **54**, 943–952.

Goldsmith, S. K., Shapiro, R. M., Joyce, J. N. (1997) Disrupted pattern of D$_2$ dopamine receptors in the temporal lobe in schizophrenia. *Archives of General Psychiatry*, **54**, 649–658.

Gundersen, H. J. G., Bagger, P., Bendtsen, T. F. *et al.* (1988) The new stereological tools: Disector, fractionator, nucleator and point sampled intercepts and their use in pathological research and diagnosis. *Acta Pathologica Methodol Immunol Sci*, **96**, 857–881.

Hanada, S., Mita, T., Nishinok, N., Tankaka, C. (1987) ^{3}H-Muscimol binding sites increased in autopsied brains of chronic schizophrenics. *Life Sciences*, **40**, 259–266.

Harrison, N. L., Simmonds, M. A. (1985) Quantitative studies on some antagonists of *N*-methyl-D-aspartate in slices of rat cerebral cortex. *British Journal of Pharmacology*, **84**, 381–391.

Harrison, P. J., McLaughlin, D., Kerwin, R. W. (1991) Decreased hippocampal expression of a glutamate receptor gene in schizophrenia. *Lancet,* **337***,* 450–452.

Heckers, S., Heinsen, H., Geiger, B., Beckmann, H. (1991) Hippocampal neuron number in schizophrenia. *Archives of General Psychiatry*, **48**, 1002–1008.

Hitri, A., Casanova, M. F., *et al.* (1995) Age-related changes in [^{3}H]GBR 12935 binding site density in the prefrontal cortex of controls and schizophrenics. *Biological Psychiatry,* **37**, 175–182.

Humphries, C., Mortimer, A., *et al.* (1996) NMDA receptor mRNA correlation with ante-mortem cognitive impairment in schizophrenia. *Neuroreport,* **7**, 2051–2055.

Huttenlocher, P. R., Dabholkar, A. S. (1997) Regional differences in synaptogenesis in human cerebral cortex. *Journal of Comparative Neurology*, **387**, 167–178.

Jacobsen, B., Kinney, D. K. (1980) Perinatal complications in adopted and non-adopted schizophrenics and their controls: Preliminary results. *Acta Psychiatrica Scandinavica*, **238**, 103–123.

Jakob, H., Beckman, H. (1986) Prenatal developmental disturbances in the limbic allo-cortex in schizophrenics. *Journal of Neural Transmission,* **65**, 303–326.

Jones, E. G. (1984) Laminar distribution of cortical efferent cells. In: Peters, A., Jones, E. G. (Eds). *Cerebral Cortex* Volume 1. *Cellular components of the cerebral cortex*, pp. 521–554. Plenum Press, New York.

Kerwin, R. W., Patel, S., Meldrum, B. S., Czudek, C., Reynolds, G. P. (1988) Asymmetrical loss of glutamate receptor subtype in left hippocampus in schizophrenia. *Lancet,* **1**, 583–584.

Kerwin R. W., Patel, S. Meldrum, B. (1990) Quantitative autoradiographic analysis of gluta-mate binding sites in the hippocampal formation in normal and schizophrenic brain post mortem. *Neuroscience*, **39**, 25–32.

Kety, S. (1959) Biochemical theories of schizophrenia. Part I of a two-part critical review of current theories and of the evidence used to support them. *Science*, **129**, 1528–1596.

Kornhuber, J., Mack-Burkhardt, F., Riederer, P. *et al.* (1989) [^{3}H]MK-801 binding sites in postmortem brain regions of schizophrenic patients. *Journal of Neural Transmission*, **77**, 231–236.

Kostoulakos, P. M., Todtenkopf, M. S., Benes, F. M. (1998) Down-regulation of GluR5,6,7 subunit expression on apical dendrites of pyramidal cells in schizophrenic hippocampus. *Society for Neuroscience Abstracts*, **24**, 1275.

Kovelman, J. A., Scheibel, A. B. (1984) A neurohistological correlate of schizophrenia. *Biological Psychiatry*, **19**, 1601–1621.

Kurumaji, A., Ishimaru, T., Toru, M. (1992) Alpha-[^{3}H]amino-3-hydroxy-5-methylisoxa-zole-4-propionic acid binding to human cerebral cortical membranes: minimal changes in postmortem brains of chronic schizophrenics. *Journal of Neurochemistry,* **59**, 829–837.

Lewis, D. A., Akil, M. (1997) Cortical dopamine in schizophrenia: strategies for post-mortem studies. *Journal of Psychiatric Research*, **31**, 175–195.

Lewis, D. A., Campbell, M. J., Foote, S., Goldstein, M., Morrison, J. H. (1987) The distri-bution of tyrosine hydroxylase immmunoreactive fibers in primate neocortex is widespread but regionally specific. *Journal of Neuroscience,* **7**, 279–290.

Longson, D., Deakin, J. W. F., Benes, F. M. (1996) Increased density of entorhinal gluta-mate-immunoreactive vertical fibers in schizophrenia. *Journal of Neural Transmission,* **103**, 503–507.

Luntz-Leybman, V., Rotter, A., Zdilar, D., Frostholm, A. (1995) Uncoupling of GABA$_A$/benzodiazepine receptor α1, ß2, and γ2 subunit mRNA expression in cerebellar Purkinje cells of staggerer mutant mice. *Journal of Neuroscience,* **15**, 8121–8130.

McDonald, A. J., Beitz, A. J., Larson, A. A., Kuriyama, R., Sellitto, C., Madi, J. E. (1989) Co-localization of glutamate and tubulin in putative excitatory neurons of the hippocampus and amygdala: an immunohistochemical study using monoclonal antibodies. *Neuroscience,* **30**, 405–421.

Majocha, R., Marotta, C., Benes, F. M. (1985) Immunostaining of neurofilament protein in human post-mortem cortex. A sensitive and specific approach to the pattern analysis of human cortical cytoarchitecture. *Canadian Journal of Biochemistry,* **63**, 577–584.

Martin, K. A. C. (1984) Neuronal circuits in cat striate cortex. In: Jones E. G., Peters, A. (Eds). *Cerebral cortex* Volume 2. *Functional properties of cortical cells.* Plenum Press, New York, pp. 241–284.

Monaghan, D. T., Cotman, C. W. (1985) Distribution of *N*-methyl-D-aspartate-sensitive L-^{3}H-glutamate-binding sites in the rat brain. *Journal of Neuroscience,* **5**, 2905–2919.

Nishikawa, T., Takashima, M., Toru, M. (1983) Inceased [^{3}H]kainic acid binding in the prefrontal cortex in schizophrenia. *Neuroscience Letters,* **40**, 245–250.

Olney, J. W., Farber, N. B. (1995) Glutamate receptor dysfunction and schizophrenia. *Archives of General Psychiatry,* **52**, 998–1007.

Pakkenberg, B. (1990) Pronounced reduction of total neuron number in mediodorsal thal-amic nucleus and nucleus accumbens in schizophrenic. *Archives of General Psychiatry,* **47**, 1023–1028.

Pakkenberg, B. (1993) Total nerve cell numbers in neocortex in chronic schizophrenics and controls estimated using optical dissectors. *Biological Psychiatry,* **34**, 768–772.

Perrone-Bizzozero, N. I., Sower, A. C. *et al.* (1996) Levels of growth-associated GAP-43 are selectively increased in association cortices in schizophrenia. *Proceedings of the National Academy of Sciences USA,* **93**, 14182–14187.

Porter, R. H. P., Eastwood, S. L., Harrison, P. J. (1997) Distribution of kainate receptor subunit mRNAs in human hippocampus, neocortex and cerebellum, and bilateral reduc-tions of hippocampal GluR6 and KA2 transcripts in schizophrenia. *Brain Research,* **751**, 217–231.

Rabow, L. E., Russek, S. J., Farb, D. H. (1995) From ion currents to genomic analysis: Recent advances in GABA$_A$ receptor research. *Synapse,* **21**, 189–274.

Rajkowska, G., Selemon, L. D., Goldman-Rakic, P. S. (1998) Neuronal and glial somal size in the prefrontal cortex: a postmortem morphometric study of schizophrenia and Huntington's disease. *Archives of General Psychiatry,* **55**, 215–224.

Reynolds, G. P., Czudek, C., Andrews, H. (1990) Deficit and hemispheric asymmetry of GABA uptake sites in the hippocampus in schizophrenia. *Biological Psychiatry,* **27**, 1038–1044.

Roberts, E. (1972) An hypothesis suggesting that there is a defect in the GABA system in schizophrenia. *Neurosciences Research Program Bulletin,* **10**, 468–482.

Roth, R. H., Tam, S. Y., Ida, Y., Yang, J. X., Deutch, A. Y. (1988) Stress and the meso-corticolimbic dopamine systems. *Annals of the New York Academy of Sciences*, **537**, 138–147.

Selemon, L. D., Goldman-Rakic, P. S. (1999) The reduced neuropil hypothesis. A circuit-based model of schizophrenia. *Biological Psychiatry*, **45**, 17–25.

Selemon, L. D., Rajkowska, G., Goldman-Rakic, P. S. (1995) Abnormally high neuronal density in the schizophrenic cortex. A morphometric analysis of prefrontal area 9 and occipital area 17. *Archives of General Psychiatry*, **52**, 805–818

Selemon, L. D., Rajkowska, G., Goldman-Rakic, P. S. (1998) Elevated neuronal density in prefrontal area 46 in brains from schizophrenic patients. *Journal of Comparative Neurology*, **392**, 402–412.

Shibuya, H., Mori, H., Toru, M. (1992) Sigma receptors in schizophrenic cerebral cortices. *Neurochemistry Research*, **17**, 983–990.

Simpson, M. D., Slater, P., Deakin, J. F., Royston, M. C., Skan, W. J. (1989) Reduced GABA uptake sites in the temporal lobe in schizophrenia. *Neuroscience Letters*, **107**, 211–215.

Simpson, M. D., Slater, P., Royston, M. C., Deakin, J. F. W. (1992) Alterations in phen-cyclidine and sigma binding sites in schizophrenic brains. *Schizophrenia Research*, **6**, 41–48

Squires, R. F., Lajtha, A., Saederup, E., Palkovits, M. (1993) Reduced [^{3}H]-Flunitrazepam binding in cingulate cortex and hippocampus of postmortem schizophrenic brains. *Neurochemistry Research*, **18**, 219–223.

Stevens, J. R. (1992) Abnormal reinnervation as a basis for schizophrenia: a hypothesis. *Archives of General Psychiatry*, **49**, 238–243.

Tamminga, C. (1998) Schizophrenia and glutamatergic transmission. *Critical Reviews in Neurobiology*, **12**, 21–36.

Taylor, J. B., Cunningham, M. C., Benes, F. M. (1998) Neonatal raphe lesions increase dopamine fibers in prefrontal cortex of adult rats. *Neuroreport*, **9**, 1811–1815.

Thierry, A. M., Tassin, J. P., Blanc, G., Glowinski, J. (1976) Selective activation of the mesocortical DA system by stress. *Nature*, **263**, 242–244.

Todtenkopf, M. S., Benes, F. M. (1998) Distribution of GAD$_{65}$-immunoreactive puncta on pyramidal and non-pyramidal neurons in the hippocampus of schizophrenic brain. *Synapse*, **29**, 323–332.

Toru, M., Watanbe, S., Shibuyam H. *et al.* (1988) Neurotransmitters, receptors and neuropep-tides in post-mortem brains of chronic schizophrenic patients. *Acta Psychiatrica Scandinavica*, **78**, 121–137.

Van Hoesen, G. W., Morecraft, R. J., Vogt, B. A. (1993) Connections of the monkey cingu-late cortex. In: Vogt, B. A., Gabriel, M. (Eds). *Neurobiology of cingulate cortex and limbic thalamus*. Birkhauser, Boston, pp. 249–284.

Vincent, S. L., Todtenkopf, M. S., Benes, F. M. (1997) A comparison of pyramidal and nonpyramidal neurons in the anterior cingulate cortex of schizophrenics and manic depres-sives. *Society for Neuroscience Abstracts*, **23**, 2199

Weibel, E. R. (1979) Elementary introduction to stereological principles. *Stereological methods*, Volume 1. *Practical methods for biological morphometry*. Academic Press, New York, pp. 46–57.

Weissman, A. D., Casanova, M. F., Kleinman, J. E., London, E. D., DeZouza, E. B. (1991) Selective loss of cerebral cortical sigma, but not PCP binding sites in schizophrenia. *Biological Psychiatry,* **29**, 41–54.

Williams, R. W., Rakic, P. (1988) Three-dimensional counting: An accurate and direct method to estimate numbers of cells in sectioned material. *Journal of Comparative Neurology,* **278**, 344–352.

Williams, S. M., Goldman-Rakic, P. S. (1993) Characterization of the dopaminergic innervation of the primate frontal cortex using a dopamine-specific antibody. *Cerebral Cortex,* **3**, 199–222.

Wisden, W., Laurie, D. J., Monyer, H., Seeburg, P. H. (1992) The distribution of 13 GABA$_A$ receptor subunit mRNAs in the rat brain. 1. Telencephalon, diencephalon, mesencephalon. *Journal of Neuroscience,* **12**, 1040–1062.

Yan, X. X., Garey, L. J., Jen, L. S. (1993) Development of NADPH-diaphorase activity in the rat neocortex. *Developmental Brain Research,* **79**, 29–38.

Zakzanis, K. K., Hansen, K. T. (1998) Dopamine D2 receptor densities and the schizophrenic brain. *Schizophrenia Research* **32**, 201–206.

4 Synaptic Pathology

William G. Honer, Clint Young, and Peter Falkai

Assessment of synapses
  Golgi technique
  Ultrastructural characteristics
  Synaptic proteins
Models of synaptic abnormalities in schizophrenia
Studies of synapses in schizophrenia
  Golgi studies and postsynaptic MAPs
  Ultrastructural studies
  Synaptic proteins
Discussion and conclusions
  Overall conclusions: relationship to models of Feinberg and Stevens
  Animal models of abnormal neural connectivity
  Synaptic pathology in dementia

Synapses are a defining characteristic of neurons, and pathology at these sites is proposed to be a mechanism for psychiatric disorders. Studies of neurotransmitters and receptors provide one perspective on synaptic pathophysiology in schizophrenia, however there are other equally informative, complementary approaches to investigate synaptic abnormalities in the disorder. In the past decade, molecular elements of the synaptic complex, both pre- and postsynaptic, have been defined in considerable detail. The aims of this chapter are to assess critically the techniques available to study synapses in the human brain, and evaluate the evidence for synaptic pathology in schizophrenia from morphological and molecular vantage points. We conclude with a brief discussion of its potential origins and functional implications.

Assessment of synapses

The classical neurodegenerative disorders involve cellular pathology, manifested as accumulations of abnormal proteins and neuronal loss (Chapter 11). Schizophrenia and other 'functional' psychiatric disorders do not share these characteristics, and increasingly the focus of research is on the integrity of neuronal connections rather than neurons themselves (Goodman, 1989; McGuire and Frith, 1996; Lewis, 1997). In contrast to the situation in experimental animals, there are few methods available to assess connectivity in humans in terms of tract tracing (Crick and Jones, 1993). However, synapses represent the final common pathway of neural connections, and several techniques now allow study of synapses in human postmortem tissue.

Golgi technique

Although synapses are comprised of pre- and postsynaptic elements, several of the techniques to be discussed visualize or assess only one component. The Golgi technique is one of these, a classical method to stain neurons and their processes (Golgi, 1894). This method of silver impregnation forms a visible complex on neurons, as well as glia and some vessels. The technique has many variations, with the 'rapid Golgi' staining most widely used. This technique stains only a small subset of neurons in a section; the reasons why certain neurons stain and not others are not clear. The method seems to work very well with embryonal tissue or tissue from young animals. While the exquisite detail of postsynaptic spines and dendrites which can be observed is unquestioned, the variability of the technique makes comparing results between studies challenging. In a study comparing techniques (Buell, 1982), the Golgi–Cox method resulted in impregnation of many neurons with a rich dendritic plexus and normal overall appearance. Occasional cells appeared grossly atrophic with irregular somata and apparent loss of apical and basilar dendritic segments. In contrast, with the rapid Golgi method the vast majority of impregnated neurons exhibited a grossly atrophic appearances, while few if any impregnated neurons had rich dendritic plexuses or otherwise appeared normal. The rapid Golgi method appeared highly sensitive to postmortem delay or other factors affecting human brain tissues obtained at autopsy (Chapter 14).

Ultrastructural characteristics

With the advent of electron microscopy in the early 1950s, details of synaptic structure were revealed. The morphological counterpart of a chemical synapse is the synaptic organelle or synaptic complex formed by the presynaptic element, the postsynaptic component, and the synaptic cleft or intracellular space separating them. The structural characteristics of these elements allowed a classification of synapses and an attempt to correlate structure with inhibitory or excitatory function. Several different synaptic taxonomies have been elaborated.

Type I and type II synapses

The first attempt to classify synaptic contacts in the cerebral cortex was made by Gray (1959), who described two types on the basis of their junctional features. In type I synapses, pre- and postsynaptic membranes bear noticeable cytoplasmic densities, particularly a very prominent postsynaptic differentiation, and possess a widened synaptic cleft of 20 to 30 nm. Type I synapses are formed with dendritic spines and some shafts. In type II synapses, the synaptic cleft is about 15 nm, and the postsynaptic differentiation is much less pronounced. Type II synapses are formed with dendritic shafts and the soma. It is now clear that type I and II synapses are the extreme cases of a continuum of differentiation, and that intermediate forms can be encountered. Type I and II synapses were renamed by Colonnier (1968) based upon configuration: type I were termed asymmetrical synapses, and type II symmetrical synapses. Despite the inappropriateness of this nomenclature (the functional polarity of the synapses implies structural asymmetry), it has been commonly used.

Classification according to synaptic vesicle shape

The most commonly found vesicles in central axon terminals are small synaptic vesicles (SSV), which appear as either rounded or flattened structures in aldehyde-fixed material. This artefactual change in shape caused by aldehyde fixation is useful, because it permits identification of precise populations of axon terminals (Peters and Palay, 1996). Moreover, in cortical structures, correlation between the electrophysiological properties (excitation or inhibition) of axon terminals and their ultrastructural identification can be made. As a generalization, excitatory synapses are formed by boutons containing rounded vesicles whilst inhibitory ones are filled with pleomorphic (rounded as well as flattened) vesicles. Most asymmetrical synapses contain rounded vesicles carrying excitatory neurotransmitters such as glutamate, whereas most symmetrical ones are filled with flattened vesicles containing inhibitory neurotransmitters such as GABA or glycine. However, this correlation may not apply in all brain regions.

Other approaches to classifying synapses are based on the types of neuronal elements involved (e.g. axoaxonal synapses) or according to the complexity of the arrangement of synaptic partners (e.g. synaptic ribbons in the outer plexiform layer of the retina).

Synaptic proteins

The application of immunological and molecular techniques has allowed individual protein components of synapses to be isolated and defined in detail. At present, well over 30 families of molecules are described as being enriched at synapses (Südhof, 1995). As well as being involved in neurotransmission, certain of these proteins are differentially expressed during brain development. Individual isoforms of proteins from these families of molecules are expressed in subsets of synapses. The relationship between this differential regional expression and the distribution of classical neurotransmitters and receptors is generally unclear. Deciding which synaptic proteins to include here (Table 4.1) was guided by the principle of avoiding inclusion of enzymes and receptor proteins regularly discussed in neurochemical reviews.

SNARE proteins

There are several families of proteins which are expressed at high levels in synapses and contribute to the unique properties of these structures. Neurotransmitters are packaged and stored in vesicles in presynaptic terminals, and there are specific proteins which form the vesicles. Other synaptic proteins are involved in docking and fusion of vesicles to the presynaptic membrane, in determining when these events should occur, and in recycling the vesicle proteins following fusion. A group of proteins participating in this process of synaptic vesicle cycling and recycling are called SNARE proteins, and are found

Table 4.1 Distribution of presynaptic terminal proteins

Protein	Molecular weight (kDa)	Chromosome	Terminal type	Protein levels in hippocampal layers				mRNA levels in hippocampal regions		
				or	rad	mol	mf	CA1	CA3	CA4
Synaptophysin	38	Xp11.22–23	All nerve terminals	++	++	++	+++	+++	+++	+++
Syntaxin			Asymmetric terminals							
1A	35	7q11.2		++	++	++	+	++		
1B		16q11.2		+++	+++	++	++++		+++	
SNAP-25	25	20p11–12	Subpopulation of terminals	+++	+++	++	++++	++	++++	++++
Rab3	24		Most terminals	+++	+++	++	++++	++	++++	+++
GAP-43	43	3	Most terminals	+++	++++	++	+	+	++	+++
Complexin										
I	18		Axosomatic (mostly inhibitory)	++	++	+++	++	+	++	++
II	19	5	Axospinous and axodendritic (mostly excitatory)	+++	+++	+++	++++	+++	++++	+++
NCAM	105–180	11q23		+++	+++	++	++	++++	++++	+++
Synapsin	86	Xp11.2	All nerve terminals	++	++	++	+++			
la	86									
lb	80									
lla	74	3p	Not in GABAergic							
llb	55	3p	Cholinergic and others							

Immunoreactivity and *in situ* hybridisation signal strength are shown for hippocampus as an example region to demonstrate differences between proteins, and between brain subregions. Most information is derived from rat.

Hippocampal layers: or, oriens; rad, radiatum; mol, moleculare; mf, mossy fibre pathway.

Signal density: ++++ intense, +++ strong, ++ moderate, + slight.

Synaptophysin: Jahn et al, 1985; Wiedenmann and Franke, 1985; Navone et al, 1986; Ozcelik et al, 1990; Fykse et al, 1993; Mahata et al, 1993; Eastwood et al, 1994.

Syntaxin: Sesak and Snyder, 1995; Ruiz-Montasell et al, 1996; Smirnova et al, 1996; Nakayama et al, 1997.

SNAP-25: Branks and Wilson, 1986; Boschert et al, 1996; Hess et al, 1995; Oyler et al, 1989; Geddes et al, 1990; Duc and Catsicas, 1995.

Rab3: Fischer von Molard et al, 1990; Mizoguchi et al, 1990; Stettler et al, 1995.

GAP-43: Gispen et al, 1985; Oestreicher and Gispen, 1986; Kosik et al, 1988; van Lookeren Campagne et al, 1990; Eastwood and Harrison, 1998.

Complexins: McMahon et al, 1995; Takahashi et al, 1995; Harrison and Eastwood, 1998; Ono et al, 1998; Young and Honer, unpublished.

NCAM: Miller et al, 1993; Telatar et al, 1995.

Synapsin: De Camilli et al, 1983; Südhof et al, 1989; Kirchgessner et al, 1991; Melloni et al, 1993; Li et al, 1995ab.

NCAM: Neural cell adhesion molecule; GAP, growth associated protein.

on the synaptic vesicle (v-SNAREs), in the cytosol of the presynaptic terminal, and in the target areas of the presynaptic membrane (t-SNAREs) (Söllner *et al.*, 1993; Südhof, 1995). The v-SNARE called VAMP (vesicle associated membrane protein or synaptobrevin) and the t-SNAREs named SNAP-25 and syntaxin form a stable complex during the process of vesicle fusion to the presynaptic membrane (Fig. 4.1; Söllner *et al.*, 1993). Other molecules interact with the complex at different time points during neurotransmitter release.

Syntaxin   The syntaxins are a family of proteins which form a component of the presynaptic membrane (Bennett *et al.*, 1992). The syntaxins bind to SNAP-25 and to the α_{1a}/α_{1b} subunits of the voltage gated calcium channel (also part of the presynaptic membrane), and to VAMP which is part of the vesicle membrane (Rettig *et al.*, 1996; Woodman, 1997). These interactions implicate syntaxin as part of the vesicle docking/fusion complex, and indicate a potential role in coupling the sequence of events forming the docking/fusion complex to the calcium flux across the presynaptic membrane. Syntaxin expression in rat hippocampus is increased during induction of long-term potentiation and kindling (Smirnova *et al.*, 1993; Kamphuis *et al.*, 1995). Several studies indicate syntaxin is not limited to the presynaptic membrane, but is also found in preterminal axons (Koh *et al.*, 1993; Sesack and Snyder, 1995); although its function in axons is unclear, it may play a role in active modification of

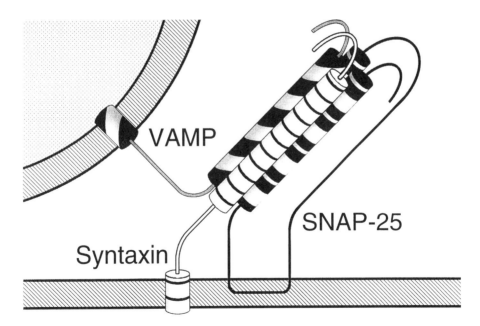

Fig. 4.1 SNARE mechanism: illustration of the proposed structure of interactions between the t-SNARE proteins SNAP-25 and syntaxin, with the v-SNARE VAMP (according to the model of Sutton *et al.*, 1998). Other proteins such as synaptophysin, complexin, and rab3 are important in modulating vesicular neurotransmission.

the axonal membrane. Of interest, in the presynaptic terminal, syntaxin appears restricted to those terminals showing an asymmetric profile (see above), possibly implying a role for certain isoforms of the molecule in excitatory but not inhibitory transmission (Sesack and Snyder, 1995). A role for syntaxin in development is suggested by the finding that in *Drosophila*, its deletion results in embryonic lethality (Schulz *et al.*, 1995). Of further interest, the syntaxin 1A gene in humans is located in the region of chromosome 7 which exhibits a microdeletion in Williams' syndrome, a neurodevelopmental disorder associated with mental handicap and behavioural abnormalities (Osborne *et al.*, 1997).

SNAP-25   SNAP-25 (synaptosomal associated protein) is a presynaptic protein which also participates in the synaptic vesicle docking/fusion complex (Oyler *et al.*, 1989). Like syntaxin, SNAP-25 binds to VAMP and to the α_{1a}/α_{1b} subunits of the voltage gated calcium channel (Rettig *et al.*, 1996; Woodman, 1997). SNAP-25 may be involved in neurite formation (Osen-Sand *et al.*, 1993), and an alternatively spliced isoform is increased during development as well as transiently following brain lesions (Oyler *et al.*, 1991; Boschert *et al.*, 1996; Patanow *et al.*, 1997). SNAP-25 is present in most, but apparently not all, synapses (Oyler *et al.*, 1989; Geddes *et al.*, 1990; Duc and Catsicas, 1995). The distribution of SNAP-25 in hippocampus changes during development (Oyler *et al.*, 1991; Boschert *et al.*, 1996), presumably reflecting maturation of a subgroup of synapses.

Hemizygous coloboma mice (*Cm/+*) have a chromosomal deletion which encompasses the encoding gene, *Snap* (Hess *et al.*, 1992). These animals exhibit significant behavioral deviations including hyperactivity, maternal neglect of offspring, and delayed developmental milestones (Hess *et al.*, 1992, 1996; Heyser *et al.*, 1995). Although gross morphological deviations were not observed, abnormalities of neurotransmission were described, including decreased glutamate release, region-specific impairment in dopamine and serotonin release, and reduced synaptosomal glutamate as well as altered electrophysiological responses to hippocampal stimulation including long-term potentiation (Steffensen *et al.*, 1996; Raber *et al.*, 1997). Although this mouse mutant was originally proposed as a model of attention deficit disorder, the phenotypic associations with reduced SNAP-25 may also have interesting parallels to abnormalities of behavioral development, cognition, and neurotransmission in schizophrenia.

Rab3   The rab family of proteins are GTP-binding proteins involved in membrane trafficking, and exist in cytosolic and synaptic vesicle membrane-bound forms (Südhof, 1995). Stimulation of rab3 results in hydrolysis of the associated GTP to GDP. Rab proteins contribute to regulation of vesicle fusion, by acting as a throttle to alter the kinetic control of SNARE complex assembly, or by modifying the complex stability (Geppert *et al.*, 1997; Rothman and Söllner, 1997).

Complexins   Complexins I and II are small proteins thought to be similar to rab3 in functioning as modulators of the SNARE complex (Ishizuka *et al.*, 1995; McMahon *et al.*, 1995; Takahashi *et al.*, 1995). Each isoform may be differentially localized to subpopulations of presynaptic terminals, and play different modulatory roles in neurotransmitter release (Takahashi *et al.*, 1995; Ono *et al.*, 1998).

Other synaptic proteins

A host of molecules in addition to SNARE proteins are enriched at synapses. These proteins may play roles in synaptic development and maturation, and possibly contribute to neurotransmission.

Synapsin Synapsin was one of the first synaptic vesicle proteins to be characterized (De Camilli *et al.*, 1983; Huttner *et al.*, 1983). The synapsins form a family of phosphorylated proteins associated with the surface of the synaptic vesicle, rather than spanning the synaptic vesicle membrane (Greengard *et al.*, 1993). The role of these molecules is not entirely clear. They can form complexes with cytoskeletal proteins, which may stabilize synaptic vesicles in the cytoplasm prior to the arrival of a stimulus for release of neurotransmitter (Südhof, 1995). Although mice lacking synapsin genes do not have obvious neurodevelopmental abnormalities, various forms of synaptic plasticity are impaired and they are prone to seizures. The synapsins are expressed during neuronal development prior to the period of extensive synapse formation, suggesting that these proteins may have different roles in the fetal and adult nervous systems (Chun and Shatz, 1988).

Synaptophysin Synaptophysin is an integral part of the synaptic vesicle membrane (Jahn *et al.*, 1985; Wiedenmann and Franke, 1985). Synaptophysin may be part of a larger family of proteins which includes the related protein synaptoporin (Knaus *et al.*, 1990). The function of synaptophysin is not entirely clear, although this protein does interact with the v-SNARE called VAMP-2 (Woodman, 1997). All nerve terminals appear to contain synaptophysin, and this marker is largely absent from axons (Navone *et al.*, 1986). Synaptophysin levels alter during brain development, and increased expression of synaptophysin occurs as synapses are formed in the immature nervous system (Leclerc *et al.*, 1989). This protein is also present in nerve growth cones, presumably in a non-vesicle associated form (Devoto and Barnstable, 1987).

GAP-43 Growth associated protein (GAP-43) is a membrane phosphoprotein which is involved in neural development, response to injury, and synaptic plasticity (Benowitz and Perrone-Bizzozero, 1991). There is evidence for a calcium-dependent interaction between GAP-43 and the SNARE complex proteins syntaxin, SNAP-25 and VAMP (Haruta *et al.*, 1997).

NCAM Neural cell adhesion molecule (NCAM) was initially characterized as a protein involved in cell–cell adhesion during brain development (Edelman, 1984). Subsequent studies indicated NCAM is highly expressed in synaptic terminals (Persohn *et al.*, 1989). NCAM is expressed as several isoforms, and during development is modified by the addition of complex side chains (polysialyation) (Rutishauser *et al.*, 1988; Jørgensen, 1995*a*). Dynamic changes in NCAM expression occur during hippocampal long-term potentiation suggesting a role for NCAM regulation in the synaptic processes involved in learning and memory (Cremer *et al.*, 1994; Lüthl *et al.*, 1994; Rose, 1995). The effects of NCAM gene disruptions on brain development range from subtle to severe, depending on which isoforms are targeted (Tomasiewicz *et al.*, 1993; Rabinowitz *et al.*, 1996).

MAPs   Microtubule associated proteins (MAPs) are proteins which regulate the dynamic properties of neuronal microtubules through promotion of assembly and stabilization of these organelles (Sheetz *et al.*, 1998). MAPs are large, complex proteins, which exhibit variable phosphorylation and isoform expression that can change during development (Sheetz *et al.*, 1998). MAPs are localized to the somatodendritic compartment of neurons (De Camilli *et al.*, 1984). Glutamate can influence MAP organization, leading to a hypothesis that primary abnormalities of glutamate receptors in schizophrenia could result in neurodevelopmental disturbances mediated through MAP changes in cellular structure (Kerwin, 1993). Studies of human immunodeficiency virus (HIV) infections indicate that MAP immunocytochemistry may be an indicator of severity of dendritic damage (Masliah *et al.*, 1997).

Technical aspects of studying synaptic proteins

Investigations of synaptic proteins use a range of immunological techniques to study the proteins directly, or molecular approaches to assess the encoding mRNA. Protein-based methods rely on the availability of suitable antibodies, which may be polyclonal (reactive with a range of antibody binding sites or epitopes on the target protein) or monoclonal (reactive with a single epitope). Many antibodies are now available commercially. Since these are derived from different sources, each antibody may have individual properties, including degree of specificity to selected isoforms of a particular synaptic protein, as well as differences in epitopes detected on the same isoform. Proteins are malleable molecules, and individual epitopes (therefore individual antibodies) may show differential sensitivity to factors such as postmortem interval and tissue fixation which generally decrease antibody binding. The most frequently used techniques are described here; many of the caveats and limitations apply to less commonly used and older techniques as well.

ELISA/immunoblotting   Antibodies can be used in a wide range of assay formats, each with advantages and limitations. Solid phase assays such as enzyme-linked immunoadsorbent assay (ELISA) and immunoblotting have largely replaced the radioimmunoassay (RIA). In the ELISA, minute amounts (micro- to nanograms) of brain protein or extracts are applied to a clear plastic plate and incubated with antibody, following blocking of non-specific binding. The amount of antibody bound is determined by the amount of antigen present, and is quantified with a chromogen reaction and a spectrophotometer. ELISA studies can be quantitated over a wide range of sample dilution (more than 10-fold), allowing a linear range of response to be defined for accurate comparisons. ELISAs are well characterized and reliable (Hamilton and Adkinson, 1988). Disadvantages include the need for large volumes of antibody, unfixed tissue samples, and the loss of anatomical detail following tissue homogenization. Adhesion of protein to the ELISA plate also likely involves a component of denaturation, which can distort epitopes. Finally, since no information about the specificity of antibody binding is obtained from an ELISA, antibodies and their targets must be characterized in advance using immunoblotting and other techniques with the assumption that the same target is being detected in the ELISA.

   Immunoblotting techniques first use protein electrophoresis through polyacrylamide gel to sort proteins according to molecular weight. The proteins are then transferred from the gel to nitrocellulose or other membrane which permanently binds protein and can be exposed to antibodies, then used for colorimetric or radiometric assays. Immunoblotting has the advantage of separating proteins according to molecular weight, allowing increased certainty of interpreting antibody binding data. Frequently, less antibody is required for these assays compared to ELISA. The limitations include lower sensitivity, and a more limited linear range of response (sometimes only three- to fourfold) (Peretti-Renucci *et al.*, 1991; Sze *et al.*, 1997). Serial dilutions of samples are necessary for accuracy of quantification, and this is quite time consuming.

Immunocytochemistry   This technique involves applying the antibodies directly to tissue sections, detecting the amount and distribution of bound antibody using a chromogen or radio-label, and performing one of several image analysis techniques for quantification (Calhoun *et al.*, 1996). The great advantage is preservation of anatomical detail, which can be resolved to the subcellular level with chromogen-based techniques (Fig. 4.2). The main disadvantage is that, as currently applied, immunocytochemistry is at best semi-quantitative, since serial dilutions of a sample cannot be performed and a linear relationship between the amount of antigen and signal cannot be defined. This is a considerable limitation, particularly with chromogen-based techniques, as signal amplification occurs which may not be linear over all concentrations of antigen. Tissue samples for immunocytochemistry are generally fixed with aldehydes or other agents which often disrupt epitopes and limit antibody binding. Embedding tissue in paraffin for sectioning, followed by deparaffinization with solvents further limits the range of antibodies which will still exhibit useful binding. Also, reliability data on immunocytochemical approaches is fairly sparse. Despite these problems, technical studies have demonstrated reasonably good correlations between synaptic immunocytochemical assays and quantification using immunoblotting or other solid phase assays (Masliah *et al.*, 1989, 1990, 1991*b*; Alford *et al.*, 1994).

Interpreting results: animal models and lesions   Once proteins enriched in synapses could be assayed, animal studies using lesions were used to determine if these proteins, used as synaptic markers, accurately reflected synaptic pathology. Chemical lesions to limbic brain areas were associated with losses of synaptophysin and increases of glial fibrillary acidic protein, a marker of injury (Brock and O'Callaghan, 1987). As well as direct effects, lesions to one brain region have predictable consequences on the axons and terminals in the projection fields. Cortical lesions in rodents were associated with the expected reductions in synaptic protein markers in the target regions (Walaas *et al.*, 1988; Geddes *et al.*, 1990; Masliah *et al.*, 1991*a*; Cabalka *et al.*, 1992; Poltorak *et al.*, 1993; Patanow *et al.*, 1997). Of interest, while markers such as synaptophysin, synapsin, and SNAP-25 are reduced following lesions, other proteins such as NCAM show increased expression, at least transiently, perhaps as part of a plasticity response (Jørgensen and Stein, 1992; Poltorak *et al.*, 1993; Jørgensen, 1995*a*, 1997). These observations led Jørgensen (1995*a*) to propose that an elevated NCAM to synaptophysin (or SNAP-25) ratio might be suggestive of increased synaptic turnover or remodelling. While still speculative, this idea reinforces the notion that individual components of the synaptic apparatus may be differentially regulated, and have a spectrum of consequences for mechanism of illness.

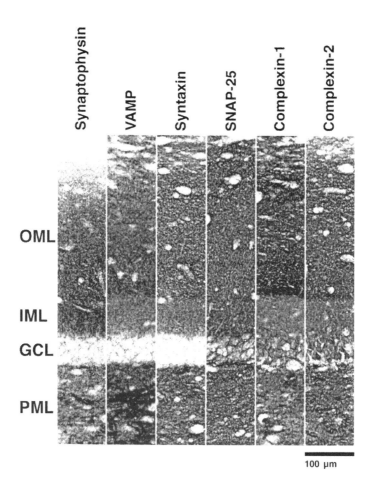

Fig. 4.2 Immunocytochemical distribution of presynaptic terminal proteins in dentate gyrus of the hippocampus. Different patterns of immunoreactivity are observed in individual layers. GCL, granule cell layer; IML, inner molecular layer; OML, outer molecular layer; PML, polymorph layer.

Models of synaptic abnormalities in schizophrenia

Even prior to the development of techniques permitting analysis of synaptic proteins, synaptic pathology was proposed to be a mechanism of illness in schizophrenia. Two possible routes to synaptic pathology were proposed, the first relating to abnormalities of development and maturation, the second relating to aberrant reinnervation following lesions.

The developmental profile of synapses was established in rodent and primate studies using electron microscopic counting techniques, supplemented by a few human studies (Cragg, 1975; Rakic *et al.*, 1986; Bourgeois *et al.*, 1994; Huttenlocher and Dabholkar, 1997). Synapse formation begins *in utero*, and continues to increase during the first postnatal months, reaching a peak number of synapses at approximately 3 months of age in auditory cortex, and 15 months of age in middle frontal gyrus. Following this, synaptic number declines in late childhood and early adolescence, again at a slightly earlier age in auditory cortex compared to middle frontal gyrus. It is likely that both genetic and experiential factors influence these patterns of synaptic formation and selective elimination (Rakic *et al.*, 1986; Bourgeois *et al.*, 1994; Huttenlocher and Dabholkar, 1997).

Golgi studies of dendritic spines also demonstrate changes associated with brain maturation. Dendritic length increases largely in parallel with increases in synaptic number (reviewed in Huttenlocher and Dabholkar, 1997). A pronounced loss of frontal pyramidal cell spines was reported to occur during the third and fourth decades of life, with numbers and density stabilizing thereafter (Jacobs *et al.*, 1997). These changes appear to be occurring somewhat later than the loss of synaptic profiles, however since the studies of dendritic spines lack data obtained during infancy and childhood, the relative reduction in spine number may not be as large as it appears. Feinberg (1982–83; 1990) related the pattern of synaptic development to profiles of brain metabolism and patterns of EEG activity, and proposed that schizophrenia might be associated with either too much or too little remodelling ('pruning') of synapses following the peak in early childhood. More recent elaborations of this hypothesis have focused on the maturation of prefrontal cortical circuitry during adolescence (Lewis, 1997; Chapter 10). Other studies have used computer modelling with neural networks to support the possibility of fewer synapses in schizophrenia, perhaps on a developmental basis (Hoffman and Dobscha, 1989; Hoffman and McGlashan, 1993, 1997).

The alternative hypothesis for synaptic pathology in schizophrenia is aberrant synaptic plasticity (Haracz, 1984; Stevens, 1992). Following brain lesions, dynamic changes occur in connected brain regions. Synapses are lost from the afferent fibres originating in the lesioned region, but proliferation or sprouting of connections from viable terminals in the same projection field occurs. These new connections are argued by some to be responsible for improvement in function, however, aberrant connections may also be responsible for new symptomatology, such as seizures. Stevens (1992) proposed a model of reduced hippocampal efferent fibres secondary to a lesion such as viral infection, followed by aberrant reinnervation and misfunctioning connections in the target regions. The strength of this model is the focus on regional connectivity in brain, rather than considering all synaptic populations changing in unison in a disease state. However, the precise nature of the lesion responsible for the stimulus to reinnervation remains unclear.

Studies of synapses in schizophrenia

Golgi studies and postsynaptic MAPs

Early neuropathological studies of schizophrenia sometimes included silver staining techniques, and while there were several descriptions of dendritic abnormalities, no specific information was available concerning dendritic spines or other components of synapses (David, 1957; Tatetsu, 1964). The available studies of schizophrenia using the Golgi technique are summarized in Table 4.2. Several of these studies are only available in preliminary form, and appear to contradict the findings of earlier investigations. It is likely that careful

Table 4.2 Dendrites in schizophrenia: studies using Golgi staining and microtubule associated protein (MAP) immunostaining

Study	Assay method	Samples	Results
Frontal cortex			
(Senitz and Winkelmann, 1981	Golgi-Kopsch	10 sch	Increased density of pyramidal cell spines, irregularly positioned triangular cells in lamina VI with thickened dendrites and increased spine density (BA 10, 11)
(Senitz and Winkelmann, 1991)	Golgi-Bubenaite	20 sch 'many' con	Increased spine number, a small group of layer III pyramidal cells observed with atypical long spines and splitting of spine heads (BA 11)
(Lewis and Glantz, 1997)	Rapid Golgi	10 sch 10 con 10 oth	Decreased spine density in layer III (BA 46 and visual cortex, BA 17). Sample too small for statistical significance
(Garey et al, 1998)	Rapid Golgi	4 sch 5 con 1 oth	Decreased density of spines in layer III (BA 10, 11, 45 mixed)
Temporal cortex			
(Garey et al, 1998)	Rapid Golgi	13 sch 9 con	Decreased density of spines in layer III (BA 22, 38 mixed)
Hippocampus			
(Arnold et al, 1991)	MAP2 and MAP5 ICC	6 sch 6 con	Decreased somatodendritic MAP2 and MAP5 in subiculum in sch (5/6 cases) and entorhinal cortex (4/6)
(Rosoklija et al, 1995)	MAP2 ICC	15 sch 6 con 14 oth	Decreased MAP2 immunoreactivity in schizophrenia, in subiculum and CA4
(Cotter et al, 1997)	MAP2 ICC, phosphorylated (P) and non-phosphorylated (NP) forms	8 sch 11 con	No overall difference in MAP2-NP densitometry, leftsided decrease in subiculum and CA1 in schizophrenia. No difference in MAP2-P counts

sch, schizophrenia; con, control; oth, other psychiatric disorder controls; ICC, peroxidase immunocytochemistry; MAP, microtubule associated protein; BA, Brodmann area.

interpretation in the context of age, regional and lateralized (Chapter 6) variation in the dynamics of spine formation, and remodelling will be necessary for this work, and may resolve apparent contradictions (Anderson and Rutledge, 1996; Jacobs *et al.*, 1997).

Immunocytochemical studies of MAPs provide a complementary technique for investigating dendrites in schizophrenia (Table 4.2). Studies of the amount of immunostaining in hippocampal neurons are relevant to understanding synaptic pathology, but are contradictory (Arnold *et al.*, 1991; Cotter *et al.*, 1997). (Other investigations used MAP2 immunostaining as a marker for persisting cortical subplate neurons, and are not directly relevant here; Chapters 3 and 10).

Ultrastructural studies

The electron microscopic studies of synapses in schizophrenia (including preliminary studies) are described in Table 4.3. Although the technical challenges to performing these studies are considerable, significant findings have been made. Most consistent are the reports of qualitative and quantitative synaptic pathology in the basal ganglia. However, these results need to be interpreted with considerable caution since of all brain regions, the basal ganglia appear to be most likely to show structural change in relation to antipsychotic drug treatment (Chapter 15).

Synaptic proteins

Studies of synaptic proteins in schizophrenia are summarized in Table 4.4 and the overall conclusions discussed below.

Firstly, synaptic terminals do not appear to be affected equally in all brain regions. In frontal cortex, and probably in hippocampus, most evidence indicates reduced synaptophysin and reduced SNAP-25, suggesting terminals are decreased overall. This interpretation would be consistent with the preliminary Golgi study reports of reduced dendritic spines (Glantz and Lewis, 2000; Garey *et al.*, 1998), and with suggestions of reduced in frontal cortex neuropil in schizophrenia (Selemon *et al.*, 1995; Chapter 3). One study reporting unchanged frontal synaptophysin and SNAP-25 comprised elderly individuals with schizophrenia, many of whom were demented (Gabriel *et al.*, 1997). As discussed in Chapter 2, further studies may clarify whether elderly demented individuals with schizophrenia represent a distinct subgroup, and how the mechanism of schizophrenic dementia differs from that of degenerative diseases (in which synaptic proteins are decreased). In contrast to the prefrontal cortex, cingulate cortex synaptic proteins (in particular the t-SNARE components) appear to be increased. Of interest, unlike most cortical regions, cingulate cortex is not reduced in volume in schizophrenia, and neuronal density may be slightly reduced, possibly indicating an expanded neuropil compartment (Benes *et al.*, 1986; Young *et al.*, 1991; Noga *et al.*, 1995; Chapter 3). The findings of increased syntaxin are consistent with the reported increase in axospinous synapses observed in electron microscopy (Agranova and Uranova, 1992), and the increase in ascending, glutamatergic axons (Benes *et al.*, 1987, 1992). Finally, even with a single region such as hippocampus, different subfields may show differing alterations (Harrison and Eastwood, 1998; Young *et al.*, 1998).

Table 4.3 Synapses in schizophrenia: studies using electron microscopy

Study	Assay method	Samples	Results
Frontal cortex (Miyakawa et al, 1972)	Qualitative examination of biopsies	5 sch 4 oth	Many synapses in schizophrenia were normal. Abnormalities such as membrane-bound debris, filaments forming whorls, dense granules in postsynaptic elements, and synapses without vesicles were also observed (BA 10)
(Senitz and Winklemann, 1981)	Qualitative	10 sch	Artefacts related to postmortem effects were thought to be responsible for any deviations in the schizophrenia group (BA 10, BA 11)
(Uranova et al, 1997)	Quantitative	21 sch 20 con	Increased volume density of postsynaptic density overall, and decreased mitochondria per axon terminal in a subset of cases with predominant negative symptoms (BA 10, layer VI)
Cingulate cortex (Agranova and Uranova, 1992)	Morphometry and counting	5 sch 7 con 2 bi	Increased axospinous synapses in schizophrenia, as well as in bipolar disorder (although attenuated). Decreased axodendritic synapses in schizophrenia only. An increase in convex, and a decrease in imperforate, synapses in schizophrenia was also seen (BA 24)
Temporal cortex (Ong and Garey, 1993)	Qualitative, biopsy	1 sch	Unusual morphology of asymmetric synapses (temporal pole, BA 38)
Basal ganglia (Uranova et al, 1997)	Quantitative	21 sch 20 con	Fewer mitochondria per axon terminal, and decreased mitochondrial area in substantia nigra in a subgroup of cases with predominant negative symptoms. Decreased spine area in caudate.
(Uranova et al, 1996)	Qualitative, (subset quantitative)	25 (7) sch 25 (7) con	Polymorphous changes in some synapses in schizophrenia including swelling of terminals, swollen mitochondria, poverty of vesicles, shrinkage of boutons, concentric lamellar bodies and dark Wallerian degeneration of boutons. Axospinous synapses in caudate had a significant increase of postsynaptic density volume (both length and width).

Table 4.3 continued

Study	Assay method	Samples	Results
(Kolomeets et al, 1996)	Qualitative	25 sch 25 con	Polymorphous changes in axodendritic synapses in schizophrenia including dystrophy, shrinkage and atrophy, particularly of asymmetric terminals, as well as hypertrophy and swelling of others.
(Roberts et al, 1996)	Morphometry and counting	6 sch 6 con	Reduced spine size in schizophrenia. Morphological characteristics of spines unchanged (striatum).
(Kung et al, 1998)	Morphometry and counting	6 sch, 7 con 3 oth	Schizophrenics: decreased ratio of caudate : putamen synaptic density (specifically symmetric profiles and symmetric axospinous synapses); decreased density of perforated striatal synapses. Some additional differences were observed in a subset of schizophrenics.
Cortex (Soustek, 1989)	Qualitative examination	8 sch, 5 con	Relative reduction in synapses in layer 1 of cortex relative to deeper layers in schizophrenia. Vesicles described as being aggregated.

sch, Schizophrenia; con, control; bi, bipolar; oth, other; BA; Brodmann area.

Table 4.4 Synapses in schizophrenia: studies of presynaptic proteins

Study	Assay method	Samples	Results
Prefrontal cortex			
(Glantz and Lewis 1993, 1997)	ICC synaptophysin ICC rab 3A	10 sch 10 con	Synaptophysin decreased in schizophrenia, unchanged in other psychiatric illness (BA 9, BA 46). Rab3A unchanged.
(Stefan et al, 1995)	ICC SNAP-25	15 sch 4 con 5 oth	SNAP-25 decreased in schizophrenia (BA 47).
(Barbeau et al, 1995)	IB NCAM	10 sch 9 con	NCAM 180, 140, 120 isoforms unchanged in schizophrenia.
(Perrone-Bizzozero et al, 1996)	IB synaptosomal membranes: GAP-43, synaptophysin	5–6 sch 4–6 con	Synaptophysin decreased, GAP-43 increased in schizophrenia (BA 9 and BA 10).
(Gabriel et al, 1997)	ELISA: synaptophysin, SNAP-25, syntaxin	19 sch 16 con	Synaptophysin, SNAP-25 and syntaxin unchanged in frontal cortex (BA 8) in schizophrenia.
(Thompson et al, 1998)	IB synaptosomal membranes: SNAP-25	5–10 sch 5–6 con 6 oth	SNAP-25 decreased in schizophrenia (BA 10), increased in BA 9.
(Vawter et al, 1998)	IB extracts for NCAM	10 sch 10 con 10 oth (suicide)	105–155 *kDa* isoform NCAM increased in schizophrenia, no differences in 140 *kDa* NCAM isoform or in L1 protein.
(Eastwood and Harrison, 1998)	*In situ* hybridisation of GAP-43 mRNA	11 sch 11 con	Unchanged in schizophrenia (BA 46).
(Honer et al, 1999)	ELISA: synaptophysin and GAP-43	13 sch (6 suicide) 10 con 11 dep (suicide)	Synaptophysin decreased in schizophrenia (death of natural causes) unchanged in both suicide groups. GAP-43 unchanged in schizophrenia (anterior frontal).
(Karson et al, 1999)	IB homogenates for synaptophysin and SNAP-25; Northern blotting for mRNAs	14 sch 12 con	Synaptophysin and SNAP-25 proteins decreased in schizophrenia, neither mRNA different from controls (BA 10).

Table 4.4 continued

Study	Assay method	Samples	Results
Cingulate cortex			
(Honer et al, 1997)	ELISA: synaptophysin, SNAP-25, syntaxin, NCAM	18 sch 24 con	Syntaxin and NCAM elevated in schizophrenia, synaptophysin and SNAP-25 unchanged.
(Powchik et al, 1998)	ELISA: synaptophysin, SNAP-25, syntaxin	28 sch	Significant correlation of PANSS negative symptom score with synaptophysin.
(Gabriel et al, 1997)	ELISA: synaptophysin, SNAP-25, syntaxin	19 sch 16 con	Synaptophysin, SNAP-25, and syntaxin all elevated in schizophrenia (BA 24).
(Eastwood and Harrison, 1998)	*In situ* hybridisation of GAP-43 mRNA	11 sch 11 con	Decreased in schizophrenia (BA 24).
Temporal cortex			
(Powchik et al, 1998)	ELISA: synaptophysin, SNAP-25, syntaxin	28 sch	Significant correlation of positive symptom score with synaptophysin (BA 36).
(Tcherepanov and Sokolov, 1997)	Reverse transcription-polymerase chain reaction	24 sch 10 con	Synaptophysin, synapsin 1A and synapsin 1B mRNA inversely correlated with age in schizophrenia, no correlation in controls (BA 21 and BA 22).
(Gabriel et al, 1997)	ELISA: synaptophysin, SNAP-25, syntaxin	19 sch 16 con	Synaptophysin, SNAP-25 and syntaxin unchanged in schizophrenia (BA 20).
(Perrone Bizzozero et al, 1996)	IB synaptosomal membranes: GAP-43, synaptophysin	6 sch 4 con 2 oth	Synaptophysin decreased, GAP-43 increased in schizophrenia (BA 20).

Table 4.4 continued

Study	Assay method	Samples	Results
(Thompson et al, 1998)	IB synaptosomal membranes: SNAP-25	4 sch 7 con 2 oth	SNAP-25 decreased in schizophrenia (BA 20), no difference in other neuroleptic treated illnesses.
(Eastwood and Harrison, 1998)	In situ hybridisation of GAP-43 mRNA	11 sch 11 con	Unchanged in schizophrenia (BA 22).
Parietal cortex (Gabriel et al, 1997)	ELISA: synaptophysin, SNAP-25, syntaxin	19 sch 16 cor	All unchanged in schizophrenia (BA 7).
Occipital cortex (Perrone-Bizzozero et al, 1996)	IB synaptosomal membranes: GAP-43, synaptophysin	10 sch 6 con 4 oth	Both unchanged in schizophrenia (BA 17).
(Glantz and Lewis, 1993, 1997)	ICC synaptophysin ICC rab3A	10 sch 10 cor 5 oth	Unchanged in schizophrenia (BA 17).
(Thompson et al, 1998)	IB synaptosomal membranes SNAP-25	9 sch 10 cor 4 oth	SNAP-25 unchanged in schizophrenia (BA 17).
(Eastwood and Harrison, 1998)	In situ hybridisation of GAP-43 mRNA	11 sch 11 con	GAP-43 mRNA decreased in schizophrenia (BA 17).
Hippocampus (Browning et al, 1993)	IB: synaptophysin, synapsin	7 sch 7 con	Synapsin I and synapsin IIb reduced, synaptophysin unchanged.
(Barbeau et al, 1995)	IB NCAM ICC PSA-NCAM	10 sch 9 con	NCAM 180, 140, 120 isoforms unchanged in schizophrenia. Reduced expression of polysialylated (embryonic) NCAM in hilar cells.

Table 4.4 continued

Study	Assay method	Samples	Results
(Eastwood et al, 1995)	In situ hybridisation of synaptophysin mRNA: ICC for synaptophysin	7 sch 13 con	mRNA reduced in CA4, CA3, subiculum, parahippocampal gyrus, no difference in CA1 or dentate gyrus. No differences detected by ICC.
(Eastwood and Harrison, 1995)	Immuno-autoradiography of synaptophysin	11 sch 14 con	Synaptophysin reduced in right dentate gyrus molecular layer, subiculum and parahippocampal gyrus, unchanged in CA4, CA3, CA1, all regions on left.
(Harrison and Eastwood, 1998)	In situ hybridisation of complexin I and II mRNA; immuno-autoradiography of complexin I and II	11 sch 11 con	Complexin I mRNA decreased overall, complexin II mRNA decreased in CA4, CA1, granule cell layer, subiculum, and parahippocampal gyrus. Complexin I protein unchanged, complexin II protein decreased in CA3 and parahippocampal gyrus.
(Vawter et al, 1998)	IB extracts for NCAM and L1	16 sch 13 con 6 bipolar 7 oth (suicide)	105–155 kDa isoform NCAM increased in schizophrenia, no differences in 140 kDa NCAM isoform or in L1 protein.
(Eastwood and Harrison, 1998)	In situ hybridisation of GAP-43 mRNA	11 sch 11 con	GAP-43 mRNA overall lower in schizophrenia, particularly CA3, CA4, subiculum, parahippocampal gyrus, perirhinal gyrus.
(Young et al, 1998)	ELISA/ICC: synaptophysin and SNAP-25	12–13 sch 12–13 con	ELISA: no differences. ICC: SNAP-25 reduced in schizophrenia in perforant pathway termination zone, synaptophysin increased in dentate granule cell layer.
Cortex (Grebb and Greengard, 1990)	Phosphorylation assay of immunoprecipitated synapsin	16 sch 26 con	Frequency of synapsin variants unchanged in schizophrenia.

ICC, peroxidase immunocytochemistry; ELISA, enzyme-linked immunoadsorbent assay; IB, immunoblotting; sch, schizophrenia; con, control; oth, other psychiatric illness; dep, depression; BA, Brodmann area; GAP, growth associated protein; NCAM, neural cell adhesion molecule.

Secondly, different synaptic proteins may not be equally affected. In frontal, cingulate, and occipital cortices, changes have been observed in at least one synaptic marker, while in the same studies other markers were changed in the opposite direction, or were not significantly affected (Table 4.4). Just as impairments in any part of a neuronal circuit may lead to the same functional consequences, the molecular mechanism of neurotransmission may have multiple vulnerabilities with similar functional implications.

Thirdly, there is some evidence of diagnostic specificity to the findings. The pattern of changes in frontal cortex in schizophrenia differed from a small group of mixed diagnosis psychiatric controls (Glantz and Lewis, 1997), and the cingulate cortex findings in elderly subjects with schizophrenia differed from Alzheimer's disease (Gabriel *et al.*, 1997). Also, SNAP-25 is decreased in the hippocampus in schizophrenia (Young *et al.*, 1998), whereas a small study of endogenous depression indicated an increase in the D3 protein (subsequently identified as SNAP-25) (Jørgensen and Riederer, 1985; Jørgensen, 1995*b*). As well as these differences, similarities across diagnoses may be important. In a recent study, several synaptic and plasticity related proteins were similar in schizophrenics and depressed individuals who died of suicide, but differed from schizophrenics who died of natural causes (Honer *et al.*, 1999).

Synaptic proteins as candidate genes

Another strategy to investigate the potential aetiological contribution of synaptic proteins to schizophrenia is to consider the genes which code for these proteins as candidates for linkage or association studies. A precedent is provided by α-synuclein, a synaptic protein gene which causes familial Parkinson's disease (Polymeropoulos *et al.*, 1997). To date, few synaptic protein genes have yet been tested in schizophrenia; there are negative results for NCAM and synaptic vesicular monoamine transporter genes (Persico *et al.*, 1995; Vincente *et al.*, 1997).

Discussion and conclusions

Overall conclusions: relationship to models of Feinberg and Stevens

Research on synaptic terminals has established that abnormalities are present in schizophrenia (Tables 4.3 and 4.4). However the early stage of investigations limits the extent to which conclusions can be used to support either the Feinberg developmental model or the Stevens reinnervation model. At present, the observations of reduced synaptic terminal markers in frontal cortex appear to be most relevant to *in vivo* studies of schizophrenia (Goldman-Rakic and Selemon, 1997). New research studies investigating synaptic pathology in parallel with anatomical markers of neurodevelopmental abnormality, or molecular markers of injury and plasticity, may help resolve the relative contributions of development and dynamic changes. Augmenting further direct studies of this kind, the relationship of developmental disorders and synaptic connectivity can be investigated in animal models, and the implications of altered synaptic connectivity in schizophrenia can be considered in the context of clinicopathological correlations in dementia.

Animal models of abnormal neural connectivity

Mouse strains can be developed in which individual genes coding for synaptic proteins are deleted or 'knocked out', as described above. Another experimental approach is to investigate connectivity in animals selected for developmental disability. The mutant mouse *reeler* is a consequence of a mutation in the gene encoding reelin, a protein involved in addressing neurons to appropriate sites during development. In *reeler* mice, the normal inside-out pattern of organization of the six cortical layers is lost. The abnormal position of cortical neurons is associated with abnormalities of cortical microconnections and behavior (Rakic and Caviness, 1995). In a mutant called *barrelless* the normal barrel-shaped clusters of neurons in somatosensory cortex do not form properly, thalamocortical inputs to these areas are not distributed in the expected fashion, and sensory processing is abnormal (Welker *et al.*, 1996). A final animal model includes microgyri and ectopic positioned neurons, which can be induced following a microfreezing lesion of cortex, or which is observed spontaneously in autoimmune mice (Sherman *et al.*, 1987; Humphreys *et al.*, 1991). Neurofilament staining in these animals demonstrates abnormal connections and disruption of cortical layers in the vicinity of heterotopic clusters of neurons (Sherman *et al.*, 1990). Other animal models of schizphrenia are discussed in Chapter 12.

Synaptic pathology in dementia

Studies indicate reductions of multiple synaptic proteins in dementia, both in brain regions directly affected by pathological changes, and in the terminal fields of neurons which project from these regions (Masliah *et al.*, 1989, 1990, 1991*b*). These studies are corroborated by direct electron microscopic demonstration of synaptic pathology (DeKosky *et al.*, 1996), confirming that synaptic protein studies provide meaningful correlates of *in vivo* dysfunction, and supporting their application in schizophrenia. For example, the severity of cognitive impairment has been shown to be related to the magnitude of loss of presynaptic proteins. For example, immunocytochemical and immunoblotting studies of neocortex and hippocampus in Alzheimer's disease demonstrate significant correlations between cognitive impairment and loss of synaptophysin or syntaxin (Terry *et al.*, 1991; Lassmann *et al.*, 1992; Wakabayashi *et al.*, 1994; Sze *et al.*, 1997). An ELISA study of synaptophysin also observed significant correlations with antemortem cognitive function (Dickson *et al.*, 1995), as did an *in situ* hybridization study of synaptophysin mRNA in temporal cortex (Heffernan *et al.*, 1998).

In summary, studying neural connectivity in schizophrenia is a promising approach. At the cellular and molecular level, synaptic mechanisms are the final common pathway of connectivity, and it is noteworthy that both anatomical and functional abnormalities of synapses appear to be present in the disorder. Continued postmortem investigation of synapses will be an important complement to evolving *in vivo* neuroimaging studies of connectivity in schizophrenia.

References

Agranova, É. A., Uranova, N. A. (1992) Morphometric analysis of synaptic contacts in the anterior limbic cortex in the endogenous psychoses. *Neuroscience and Behavioural Physiology*, **22**, 59–65.

Alford, M. F., Masliah, E., Hansen, L. A., Terry, R. D. (1994) A simple dot-immunobinding assay for quantification of synaptopysin-like immunoreactivity in human brain. *Journal of Histochemistry and Cytochemistry*, **42**, 283–287.

Anderson, B., Rutledge, V. (1996) Age and hemisphere effects on dendritic structure. *Brain*, **119**, 1983–1990.

Arnold, S. E., Lee, V. M.-Y., Gur, R. E., Trojanowski, J. Q. (1991) Abnormal expression of two microtubule-associated proteins (MAP2 and MAP5) in specific subfields of the hippocampal formation in schizophrenia. *Proceedings of the National Academy of Sciences USA*, **88**, 10850–10854.

Barbeau, D., Liang, J. J., Robitaille, Y., Quirion, R., Srivastava, L. K. (1995) Decreased expression of the embyronic form of the nerve cell adhesion molecule in schizophrenic brains. *Proceedings of the National Academy of Sciences USA*, **92**, 2785–2789.

Benes, F. M., Davidson, J., Bird, E. D. (1986) Quantitative cytoarchitectural studies of cerebral cortex of schizophrenics. *Archives of General Psychiatry*, **43**, 31–35.

Benes, F. M., Majocha, R., Bird, E. D., Marotta, C. A. (1987) Increased vertical axon numbers in cingulate cortex of schizophrenics. *Archives of General Psychiatry*, **44**, 1017–1021.

Benes, F. M., Sorensen, I., Vincent, S. L., Bird, E. D. Sathi, M. (1992) Increased density of glutamate-immunoreactive vertical processes in superficial laminae in cingulate cortex of schizophrenic brain. *Cerebral Cortex*, **2**, 503–512.

Bennett, M. K., Calakos, N., Scheller, R. H. (1992) Syntaxin: a synaptic protein implicated in docking of synaptic vesicles at presynaptic active zones. *Science*, **257**, 255–259.

Benowitz, L. I., Perrone Bizzozero, N. I. (1991) The expression of GAP 43 in relation to neuronal growth and plasticity: when, where, how, and why? *Progress in Brain Research*, **89**, 69–87.

Boschert, U., O'Shaughnessy, C., Dickinson, R. *et al.* (1996) Developmental and plasticity-related differential expression of two SNAP-25 isoforms in rat brain. *Journal of Comparative Neurology*, **367**, 177–193.

Bourgeois, J. P., Goldman-Rakic, P. S., Rakic, P. (1994) Synaptogenesis in the prefrontal cortex of rhesus monkeys. *Cerebral Cortex*, **4**, 78–96.

Branks, P. L., Wilson, M. C. (1986) Patterns of gene expression in the murine brain revealed by in situ hybridization of brain-specific mRNAs. *Molecular Brain Research*, **1**, 1–16.

Brock, T., O'Callaghan, J. (1987) Quantitative changes in the synaptic vesicle proteins synapsin I and p38 and the astrocyte-specific protein glial fibrillary acidic protein are associated with chemical-induced injury to the rat central nervous system. *Journal of Neuroscience*, **7**, 931–942.

Browning, M. D., Dudek, E. M., Rapier, J. L., Leonard, S., Freedman, R. (1993) Significant reductions in synapsin but not synaptophysin specific activity in the brains of some schizophrenics. *Biological Psychiatry*, **34**, 529–535.

Buell, S. J. (1982) Golgi-Cox and rapid Golgi methods as applied to autopsied human brain tissue: widely disparate results. *Journal of Neuropathology and Experimental Neurology*, **41**, 500–507.

Cabalka, L., Hyman, B., Goodlett, C., Ritchie, T., van Hoesen, G. (1992) Alteration in the pattern of nerve terminal protein immunoreactivity in the perforant pathway in Alzheimer's disease and in rats after entorhinal lesions. *Neurobiology of Aging*, **13**, 283–291.

Calhoun, M. E., Jucker, M., Martin, L. J., Thinakaran, G., Price, D. L., Mouton, P. R. (1996) Comparative evaluation of synaptophysin-based methods for quantification of synapses. *Journal of Neurocytology*, **25**, 821–828.

Chun, J. J. M., Shatz, C. J. (1988) Redistribution of synaptic vesicle antigens is correlated with the disappearance of a transient synaptic zone in the developing cerebral cortex. *Neuron*, **1**, 297–310.

Colonnier, M. (1968) Synaptic patterns on different cell types in the different laminae of the cat visual cortex. An electron microscope study. *Brain Research*, **9**, 268–287.

Cotter, D., Kerwin, R., Doshi, B., Martin, C. S., Everall, I. P. (1997) Alterations in hippocampal non-phosphorylated MAP2 protein expression in schizophrenia. *Brain Research*, **765**, 238–246.

Cragg, B. (1975) The density of synapses and neurons in normal, mentally defective and ageing human brains. *Brain*, **98**, 81–90.

Cremer, H., Lange, R., Cristoph, A. *et al.* (1994) Inactivation of the N-CAM gene in mice results in size reduction of the olfactory bulb and deficits in spatial learning. *Nature*, **367**, 455–459.

Crick, F. and Jones, E. (1993) Backwardness of human neuroanatomy. *Nature*, **361**, 109–110.

David, G. B. (1957). The pathological anatomy of the schizophrenias. In Richter D. (Ed.). *Schizophrenia: somatic aspects.* Pergamon Press, London, pp. 93–130.

De Camilli, P., Cameron, R., Greengard, P. (1983) Synapsin I (protein I), a nerve terminal-specific phosphoprotein. I. Its general distribution in synapses of the central and peripheral nervous system demonstrated by immunofluorescence in frozen and plastic sections. *Journal of Cell Biology*, **96**, 1337–1354.

De Camilli, P., Miller, P. E., Navone, F., Theurkauf, W. E. and Vallee, R. B. (1984) Distribution of microtubule-associated protein 2 in the nervous system of the rat studied by immunofluorescence. *Neuroscience*, **11**, 819–846.

DeKosky, S. T., Scheff, S. W., Styren, S. D. (1996) Structural correlates of cognition in dementia: Quantification and assessment of synapse change. *Neurodegeneration*, **5**, 417–421.

Devoto, S., Barnstable, C. (1987) SVP38: a synaptic vesicle protein whose appearance correlates closely with synaptogenesis in the rat central nervous system. *Annals of the New York Academy of Sciences*, **493**, 493–496.

Dickson, D. W., Crystal, H. A., Bevona, C., Honer, W., Vincent, I., Davies, P. (1995) Correlations of synaptic and pathological markers with cognition in the elderly. *Neurobiology of Aging*, **16**, 285–304.

Duc, C., Catsicas, S. (1995) Ultrastructural localization of SNAP-25 within the rat spinal cord and peripheral nervous system. *Journal of Comparative Neurology*, **356**, 152–163.

Eastwood, S. L., Harrison, P. J. (1995) Decreased synaptophysin in the medial temporal lobe in schizophrenia demonstrated using immunoautoradiography. *Neuroscience*, **69**, 339–343.

Eastwood, S. L., Harrison, P. J. (1998) Hippocampal and cortical growth-associated protein-43 messenger RNA in schizophrenia. *Neuroscience*, **86**, 437–448.

Eastwood, S. L., Burnet, P. W. J., McDonald, B., Clinton, J., Harrison, P. J. (1994) Synaptophysin gene expression in human brain: a quantitative in situ hybridization and immunocytochemical study. *Neuroscience*, **59**, 881–892.

Eastwood, S. L., Burnet, P. W. J., Harrison, P. J. (1995) Altered synaptophysin expression as a marker of synaptic pathology in schizophrenia. *Neuroscience*, **66**, 309–319.

Edelman, G. M. (1984) Modulation of cell adhesion during induction, histogenesis, and perinatal development of the nervous system. *Annual Review of Neuroscience*, **7**, 339–377.

Feinberg, I. (1982–83) Schizophrenia: caused by a fault in programmed synaptic elimination during adolescence? *Journal of Psychiatric Research*, **17**, 319–334.

Feinberg, I. (1990) Cortical pruning and the development of schizophrenia. *Schizophrenia Bulletin*, **16**, 567–568.

Fischer von Molard, G., Mignery, G. A., Baumert, M. *et al.* (1990) rab3 ia a small GTP-binding protein exclusively localized to synaptic vesicles. *Proceedings of the National Academy of Sciences USA*, **87**, 1988–1992.

Fykse, E. M., Takei, K., Walch-Solimena, C. *et al.* (1993) Relative properties and localizations of synaptic vesicle protein isoforms: the case of the synaptophysins. *Journal of Neuroscience*, **13**, 4997–5007.

Gabriel, S. M., Haroutunian, V., Powchik, P. *et al.* (1997) Increased concentrations of presynaptic proteins in the cingulate cortex of schizophrenics. *Archives of General Psychiatry*, **54**, 559–566.

Garey, L. J., Ong, W. Y., Patel, T. S. *et al.* (1998) Reduced dendritic spine density on cerebral cortical pyramidal neurons in schizophrenia. *Journal of Neurology, Neurosurgery and Psychiatry*, **65**, 446–453.

Geddes, J. W., Hess, E. J., Hart, R. A., Kesslak, J. P., Cotman, C. W., Wilson, M. C. (1990) Lesions of hippocampal circuitry define synaptosomal-associated protein-25 (SNAP-25) as a novel presynaptic marker. *Neuroscience*, **38**, 515–525.

Geppert, M., Goda, Y., Stevens, C. F., Südhof, T. C. (1997) The small GTP-binding protein Rab3A regulates a late step in synaptic vesicle fusion. *Nature*, **387**, 810–814.

Gispen, W. H., Leunissen, J. L., Oestreicher, A. B., Verkleij, A., Zwiers, H. (1985) Presynaptic localization of B-50 phosphoprotein: the (ACTH)-sensitive protein kinase substrate involved in rat brain polyphosphoinositide metabolism. *Brain Research*, **328**, 381–385.

Glantz, L. A., Lewis, D. A. (1993) Synaptophysin and not rab3A is specifically reduced in the prefrontal cortex of schizophrenic subjects. *Society for Neuroscience Abstracts*, **20**, 622.

Glantz, L. A., Lewis, D. A. (1997) Reduction of synaptophysin immunoreactivity in the prefrontal cortex of subjects with schizophrenia: regional and diagnostic specificity. *Archives of General Psychiatry*, **54**, 943–952.

Glantz, L. A., Lewis, D. A. (2000) Decreased dendritic spine density on prefrontal cortical pyramidal neurons in schizophrenia. *Archives of General Psychiatry*, **57**, 65–73.

Goldman-Rakic, P. S., Selemon, L. D. (1997) Functional and anatomical aspects of prefrontal pathology in schizophrenia. *Schizophrenia Bulletin*, **23**, 437–458.

Golgi, C. (1894) *Untersuchungen über den feineren Bau des zentralen und peripheren Nervensystems.* G Fischer, Jena.

Goodman, R. (1989) Neuronal misconnections and psychiatric disorder: is there a link? *British Journal of Psychiatry*, **154**, 292–299.

Gray, E. G. (1959) Axo-somatic and axo-dendritic synapses of the cerebral cortex: an electron-microscope study. *Journal of Anatomy*, **93**, 420–433.

Grebb, J. A., Greengard, P. (1990) An analysis of synapsin II, a neuronal phosphoprotein, in postmortem brain tissue from alcoholic and neuropsychiatrically ill adults and medically ill children and young adults. *Archives of General Psychiatry*, **47**, 1149–1156.

Greengard, P., Valtorta, F., Czernik, A. J., Benfenati, F. (1993) Synaptic vesicle phosphoproteins and regulation of synaptic function. *Science*, **259**, 780–785.

Hamilton, R. G., Adkinson, N. F. (1988) Quantitative aspects of solid phase immunoassays. In Kemeny D. M., Challacombe S.J. (Eds). *ELISA and other solid phase immunoassays: theoretical and practical aspects.* John Wiley, Chichester, pp. 57–84.

Haracz, J. L. (1984) A neural plasticity hypothesis of schizophrenia. *Neuroscience and Biobehavioural Reviews*, **8**, 55–71.

Harrison, P. J., Eastwood, S. L. (1998) Preferential involvement of excitatory neurons in medial temporal lobe in schizophrenia. *Lancet*, **352**, 1669–1673.

Haruta, T., Takami, N., Ohmura, M., Misumi, Y., Ikehara, Y. (1997) Ca^{2+}-dependent interaction of the growth-associated protein GAP-43 with the synaptic core complex. *Biochemical Journal*, **325**, 455–463.

Heffernan, J. M., Eastwood, S. L., Nagy, Z., Sanders, M. W., McDonald, B., Harrison, P. J. (1998) Temporal cortex synaptophysin mRNA is reduced in Alzheimer's disease and is negatively correlated with the severity of dementia. *Experimental Neurology*, **150**, 235–239.

Hess, E. J., Jinnah, H. A., Kozak, C. A., Wilson, M. C. (1992) Spontaneous locomotor hyperactivity in a mouse mutant with a deletion including the Snap gene on chromosome 2. *Journal of Neuroscience*, **12**, 2865–2874.

Hess, E. J., Rogan, P. K., Domoto, M., Tinker, D. E., Ladda, R. L., Ramer, J. C. (1995) Absence of linkage of apparently single gene mediated ADHD with the human syntenic region of the mouse mutant coloboma. *American Journal of Medical Genetics (Neuropsychiatric Genetics)*, **60**, 573–579.

Hess, E. J., Collins, K. A. and Wilson, M. C. (1996) Mouse model of hyperkinesis implicates SNAP-25 in behavioral regulation. *Journal of Neuroscience*, **16**, 3104–3111.

Heyser, C. J., Wilson, M. C., Gold, L. (1995) Coloboma hyperactive mutant exhibits delayed neurobehavioral developmental milestones. *Developmental Brain Research*, **89**, 264–269.

Hoffman, R. E., Dobsha, S. K. (1989) Cortical pruning and the development of schizophrenia: a computer model. *Schizophrenia Bulletin*, **15**, 477–490.

Hoffman, R. E., McGlashan, T. H. (1993) Parallel distributed processing and the emergence of schizophrenic symptoms. *Schizophrenia Bulletin*, **19**, 119–140.

Hoffman, R. E., McGlashan, T. H. (1997) Synaptic elimination, neurodevelopment, and the mechanisms of hallucinated 'voices' in schizophrenia. *American Journal of Psychiatry*, **154**, 1683–1689.

Honer, W. G., Falkai, P., Young, C. *et al.* (1997) Cingulate cortex synaptic terminal proteins and neural cell adhesion molecule in schizophrenia. *Neuroscience*, **78**, 99–110.

Honer, W. G., Falkai, P., Chen, C., Arango, V., Mann, J. J., Dwork, A. J. (1999) Synaptic and plasticity associated proteins in anterior frontal cortex in severe mental illness. *Neuroscience*, **91**, 1247–1255.

Humphreys, P., Rosen, G. D., Press, D. M., Sherman, G. F., Galaburda, A. M. (1991) Freezing lesions of the newborn rat brain: a model for cerebrocortical microgyria. *Journal of Neuropathology and Experimental Neurology*, **50**, 145–160.

Huttenlocher, P. R., Dabholkar, A. S. (1997) Regional differences in synaptogenesis in human cerebral cortex. *Journal of Comparative Neurology*, **387**, 167–178.

Huttner, W. B., Schiebler, W., Greengard, P., De Camilli, P. (1983) Synapsin I (protein I), a nerve terminal-specific phosphoprotein. III. Its association with synaptic vesicles studied in a highly purified synaptic vesicle preparation. *Journal of Cell Biology*, **96**, 1374–1388.

Ishizuka, T., Saisu, H., Odani, S., Abe, T. (1995) Synaphin: a protein associated with the docking/fusion complex in presynaptic terminals. *Biochemical and Biophysical Research Communications*, **213**, 1107–1114.

Jacobs, B., Driscoll, L., Schall, M. (1997) Life-span dendritic and spine changes in areas 10 and 18 of human cortex: a quantitative Golgi study. *Journal of Comparative Neurology*, **386**, 661–680.

Jahn, R., Schiebler, W., Ouimet, C., Greengard, P. (1985) A 38,000-dalton membrane protein (p38) present in synaptic vesicles. *Proceedings of the National Academy of Sciences USA*, **82**, 4137–4141.

Jørgensen, O. S. (1995*a*) Nerve cell adhesion molecule (NCAM) as a quantitative marker in synaptic remodelling. *Neurochemistry Research*, **20**, 533–547.

Jørgensen, O. S. (1995*b*) SNAP-25 is the major immunoreactive component of the brain-specific D3 protein. *NeuroReport*, **7**, 73–76.

Jørgensen, O. S., Riederer, P. (1985) Increased synaptic markers in hippocampus of depressed patients. *Journal of Neural Transmission*, **64**, 55–66.

Jørgensen, O. S., Stein, D. G. (1992) Transplant and ganglioside G1 mediated neuronal recovery in rats with brain lesions. *Restorative Neurology and Neuroscience*, **3**, 311–320.

Jørgensen, O. S., Hansen, L. I., Hoffman, S. W., Fülöp, Z., Stein, D. G. (1997) Synaptic remodelling and free radical formation after brain contusion injury in the rat. *Experimental Neurology*, **144**, 326–338.

Kamphuis, W., Smirnova, T., Hicks, A., Hendriksen, H., Mallet, J., Lopes da Silva, F. H. (1995) The expression of syntaxin 1B/GR33 mRNA is enhanced in the hippocampal kindling model of epileptogenesis. *Journal of Neurochemistry*, **65**, 1974–1980.

Karson, C. N., Mrak, R. E., Schluterman, K. O., Stumer, W. Q., Sheng, J. G., Griffin, W. S. T. (1999) Alterations in synaptic proteins and their encoding mRNAs in prefrontal cortex in schizophrenia: a possible neurochemical basis for 'hypofrontality'. *Molecular Psychiatry*, **4**, 39–45.

Kerwin, R. (1993) Glutamate receptors, microtubule associated protins and developmental anomaly in schizophrenia: an hypothesis. *Psychological Medicine*, **23**, 547–551.

Kirchgessner, C. U., Trofatter, J. A., Mahtani, M. M., Willard, H. F., DeGennaro, L. J. (1991) A highly polymorphic dinucleotide repeat on the proximal short arm of the human X chromosome: linkage mapping of the synapsis 1/A-raf-1 genes. *American Journal of Human Genetics*, **49**, 184–191.

Knaus, P., Marquéze-Pouey, B., Scherer, H., Betz, H. (1990) Synaptoporin, a novel putative channel protein of synaptic vesicles. *Neuron*, **5**, 453–462.

Koh, S., Yamamoto, A., Inoue, A. *et al.* (1993) Immunoelectron microscopic localization of the HPC-1 antigen in rat cerebellum. *Journal of Neurocytology*, **22**, 995–1005.

Kolomeets, N. S., Uranova, N. A., Orlovskaya, D. D. (1996) The ultrastructure of the synaptic contacts on the dopaminergic neurons in postmortem substantia nigra of schizophrenics. *Schizophrenia Research*, **18**, 180–181.

Kosik, K. S., Orecchio, L. D., Bruns, G. A. *et al.* (1988) Human GAP-43: its deduced amino acid sequence and chromosomal localization in mouse and human. *Neuron*, **1**, 127–132.

Kung, L., Conley, R., Chute, D. J., Smialek, J., Roberts, R. C. (1998) Synaptic changes in the striatum of schizophrenic cases: A controlled postmortem ultrastructural study. *Synapse*, **28**, 125–139.

Lassmann, H., Weiler, R., Fischer, P. *et al.* (1992) Synaptic pathology in Alzheimer's disease: immunological data for markers of synaptic and large dense-core vesicles. *Neuroscience*, **46**, 1–8.

Leclerc, N., Beesley, P. W., Brown, I. *et al.* (1989) Synaptophysin expression during synaptogenesis in the rat cerebellar cortex. *Journal of Comparative Neurology*, **280**, 197–212.

Lewis, D. A. (1997) Development of the prefrontal cortex during adolescence: insights into vulnerable neural circuits in schizophrenia. *Neuropsychopharmacology*, **16**, 385–398.

Lewis, D. A., Glantz, L. A. (1997) Specificity of decreased spine density on layer III pyramidal cells in schizophrenia. *Schizophrenia Research*, **24**, 39.

Li, L., Chin, L.-S., Greengard, P., Copeland, N. G., Gilbert, D. J., Jenkins, N. A. (1995a) Localization of the synapsin II (SYN2) gene to human chromosome 3 and mouse chromosome 6. *Genomics*, **28**, 365–366.

Li, X., Rosahl, T. W., Südhof, T. C., Francke, U. (1995b) Mapping of synapsin II (SYN2) genes to human chromosome 3p and mouse chromosome 6 band F. *Cytogenetics and Cell Genetics*, **71**, 301–305.

Lüthl, A., Laurent, J. P., Figurov, A., Muller, D., Schachner, M. (1994) Hippocampal long-term potentiation and neural cell adhesion molecules L1 and NCAM. *Nature*, **372**, 777–779.

McGuire, P. K., Frith, C. D. (1996) Disordered functional connectivity in schizophrenia. *Psychological Medicine*, **26**, 663–667.

McMahon, H. T., Missler, M., Li, C., Südhof, T. C. (1995) Complexins: cytosolic proteins that regulate SNAP receptor function. *Cell*, **83**, 111–119.

Mahata, M., Mahata, S. K., Fischer-Colbrie, R., Winkler, H. (1993) Ontogenic development and distribution of mRNAs of chromogranin A and B, secretogranin II, p65 and synaptin/synaptophysin. *Developmental Brain Research*, **76**, 43–58.

Masliah, E., Terry, R. D., DeTeresa, R. M., Hansen, L. A. (1989) Immunohistochemical quantification of the synapse-related protein synaptophysin in Alzheimer disease. *Neuroscience Letters*, **103**, 234–239.

Masliah, E., Terry, R. D., Alford, M., DeTeresa, R. (1990) Quantitative immunohistochemistry of synaptophysin in human neocortex: an alternative method to estimate density of presynaptic terminals in paraffin sections. *Journal of Histochemistry and Cytochemistry*, **38**, 837–844.

Masliah, E., Fagan, A. M., Terry, R. D., DeTeresa, R., Mallory, M., Gage, F. H. (1991*a*) Reactive synaptogenesis assessed by synaptophysin immunoreactivity is associated with GAP-43 in the dentate gyrus of the adult rat. *Experimental Neurology*, **113**, 131–142.

Masliah, E., Terry, R. D., Alford, M., DeTeresa, R., Hansen, L. A. (1991*b*) Cortical and subcortical patterns of synaptophysin-like immunoreactivity in Alzheimer's disease. *American Journal of Pathology*, **138**, 235–246.

Masliah, E., Heaton, R. K., Marcotte, T. D. *et al.* (1997) Dendritic injury is a pathological substrate for human immunodeficiency virus-related cognitive disorders. *Annals of Neurology*, **42**, 963–972.

Melloni, R. H., Hemmendinger, L. M., Hamos, J. E., DeGennaro, L. J. (1993) Synapsin I gene expression in the adult rat brain with comparative analysis of mRNA and protein in the hippocampus. *Journal of Comparative Neurology*, **327**, 507–520.

Miller, P. D., Chung, W. W., Lagenaur, C. F., DeKosky, S. T. (1993) Regional distribution of neural cell adhesion molecule (N-CAM) and L1 in human and rodent hippocampus. *Journal of Comparative Neurology*, **327**, 341–349.

Miyakawa, T., Sumiyoshi, S., Deshimaru, M. *et al.* (1972) Electron microscopic study on schizophrenia: mechanisms of pathological changes. *Acta Neuropathologica*, **20**, 67–77.

Mizoguchi, A., Kim, S., Ueda, T. *et al.* (1990) Localization and subcellular distribution of smg p25A, a ras p21-like GTP-binding protein, in rat brain. *Journal of Biological Chemistry*, **265**, 11872–11879.

Nakayama, T., Fujiwara, T., Miyazawa, A. *et al.* (1997) Mapping of the human HPC-1/syntaxin 1A gene (STX1A) to chromosome 7 band q11.2. *Genomics*, **42**, 173–176.

Navone, F., Jahn, R., Di Gioia, G., Stukenbrok, H., Greengard, P., De Camilli, P. (1986) Protein p38: an integral membrane protein specific for small vesicles of neurons and neuroendocrine cells. *Journal of Cell Biology*, **103**, 2511–2527.

Noga, J. T., Aylward, E., Barta, P. , Pearlson, G. D. (1995) Cingulate gyrus in schizophrenic patients and normal volunteers. *Psychiatry Research: Neuroimaging*, **61**, 201–208.

Oestreicher, A. B., Gispen, W. H. (1986) Comparison of the immunocytochemical distribution of the phosphoprotein B-50 in the cerebellum and hippocampus of immature and adult rat brain. *Brain Research*, **375**, 267–279.

Ong, W. Y., Garey, L. J. (1993) Ultrastructural features of biopsied temporopolar cortex (area 38) in a case of schizophrenia. *Schizophrenia Research*, **10**, 15–27.

Ono, S., Baux, G., Sekiguchi, M. *et al.* (1998) Regulatory roles of complexins in neuro-transmitter release from mature presynaptic nerve terminals. *European Journal of Neuroscience*, **10**, 2143–2152.

Osborne, L. R., Soder, S., Shi, X.-M. *et al.* (1997) Hemizygous deletion of the syntaxin 1A gene in individuals with Williams syndrome. *American Journal of Human Genetics*, **61**, 449–452.

Osen-Sand, A., Catsicas, M., Staple, J. K. *et al.* (1993) Inhibition of axonal growth by SNAP-25 antisense oligonucleotides in vitro and in vivo. *Nature*, **364**, 445–447.

Oyler, G. A., Higgins, G. A., Hart, R. A. *et al.* (1989) The identification of a novel synaptosomal-associated protein, SNAP-25, differentially expressed by neuronal subpopulations. *Journal of Cell Biology*, **109**, 3039–3052.

Oyler, G. A., Polli, J. W., Wilson, M. C., Billingsley, M. L. (1991) Developmental expression of the 25-kDa synaptosomal-associated protein (SNAP-25) in rat brain. *Proceedings of the National Academy of Sciences USA*, **88**, 5247–5251.

Ozcelik, T., Lafreniere, R. G., Archer, B. T. I. *et al.* (1990) Synaptophysin: structure of the human gene and assignment to the X chromosome in man and mouse. *American Journal of Human Genetics*, **47**, 551–561.

Patanow, C. M., Day, J. R., Billingsley, M. L. (1997) Alterations in hippocampal expression of SNAP-25, GAP-43, stannin and glial fibrillary acidic protein following mechanical and trimethyltin-induced injury in the rat. *Neuroscience*, **76**, 187–202.

Peretti-Renucci, R., Feuerstein, C., Manier, M. *et al.* (1991) Quantitative image analysis with densitometry for immunohistochemistry and autoradiography of receptor binding sites: methodological considerations. *Journal of Neuroscience Research*, **28**, 583–600.

Perrone-Bizzozero, N. I., Sower, A. C., Bird, E. D., Benowitz, L. I., Ivins, K. J., Neve, R. L. (1996) Levels of the growth-associated protein GAP-43 are selectively increased in association cortices in schizophrenia. *Proceedings of the National Academy of Sciences USA*, **93**, 14182–14187.

Persico, A. M., Wang, Z. W., Black, D. W., Andreasen, N. C., Uhl, G. R., Crowe, R. R. (1995) Exclusion of close linkage between the synaptic vesicular monoamine transporter locus and schizophrenia spectrum disorders. *American Journal of Medical Genetics (Neuropsychiatric Genetics)*, **60**, 563–565.

Persohn, E., Pollerberg, G. E., Schachner, M. (1989) Immunoelectron-microscopic localization of the 180 kD component of the neural cell adhesion molecule N-CAM in postsynaptic membranes. *Journal of Comparative Neurology*, **288**, 92–100.

Peters, A., Palay, S. L. (1996) The morphology of synapses. *Journal of Neurocytology*, **25**, 687–700.

Poltorak, M., Herranz, A. S., Williams, J., Lauretti, L., Freed, W. J. (1993) Effects of frontal cortical lesions on mouse striatum: reorganization of cell recognition molecule, glial fiber, and synaptic protein expression in the dorsomedial striatum. *Journal of Neuroscience*, **13**, 2217–2223.

Polymeropoulos, M. H., Lavedan, C., Leroy, E. *et al.* (1997) Mutation in the a-synuclein gene identified in families with Parkinson's disease. *Science*, **276**, 2045–2047.

Powchik, P., Davidson, M., Haroutunian, V. *et al.* (1998) Postmortem studies in schizophrenia. *Schizophrenia Bulletin*, **24**, 325–341.

Raber, J., Mehta, P. P., Kreifeldt, M. *et al.* (1997) Coloboma hyperactive mutant mice exhibit regional and transmitter-specific deficits in neurotransmission. *Journal of Neurochemistry*, **68**, 176–188.

Rabinowitz, J. E., Rutishauser, U., Magnuson, T. (1996) Targeted mutation of NCAM to produce a secreted molecule results in a dominant embryonic lethality. *Proceedings of the National Academy of Sciences USA*, **93**, 6421–6424.

Rakic, P., Caviness, V. S. (1995) Cortical development: view from neurological mutants two decades later. *Neuron*, **14**, 1101–1104.

Rakic, P., Bourgeois, J.-P., Eckenhoff, M. F., Zecevic, N., Goldman-Rakic, P. S. (1986) Concurrent overproduction of synapses in diverse regions of the primate cerebral cortex. *Science*, **232**, 232–235.

Rettig, J., Sheng, Z.-H., Kim, D. K., Hodson, C. D., Snutch, T. P., Catterall, W. A. (1996) Isoform-specific interaction of the (1A subunits of brain Ca^{2+} channels with the presynaptic proteins syntaxin and SNAP-25. *Proceedings of the National Academy of Sciences USA*, **93**, 7363–7368.

Roberts, R. C., Conley, R., Kung, L., Peretti, F. J., Chute, D. J. (1996) Reduced striatal spine size in schizophrenia: a postmortem ultrastructural study. *NeuroReport*, **7**, 1214–1218.

Rose, S. P. R. (1995) Cell-adhesion molecules, glucocorticoids and long-term-memory formation. *Trends in Neurosciences*, **18**, 502–506.

Rosoklija, G., Kaufman, M. A., Liu, D. *et al.* (1995) Subicular MAP-2 immunoreactivity in schizophrenia. *Society for Neuroscience Abstracts*, **21**, 835.10.

Rothman, J. E., Söllner, T. H. (1997) Throttles and dampers: controlling the engine of membrane fusion. *Science*, **276**, 1212–1213.

Ruiz-Montasell, B., Aguado, F., Majó, G. *et al.* (1996) Differential distribution of syntaxin isoforms 1A and 1B in the rat central nervous system. *European Journal of Neuroscience*, **8**, 2544–2552.

Rutishauser, U., Acheson, A., Hall, A. K., Mann, D. M., Sunshine, J. (1988) The neural cell adhesion molecule (NCAM) as a regulator of cell-cell interactions. *Science*, **240**, 53–57.

Schulz, K. L., Broadie, K., Perin, M. S., Bellen, H. J. (1995) Genetic and electrophysiological studies of *Drosophila* syntaxin-1A demonstrate its role in nonneuronal secretion and neurotransmission. *Cell*, **80**, 311–320.

Selemon, L. D., Rajkowska, G., Goldman-Rakic, P. S. (1995) Abnormally high neuronal density in the schizophrenic cortex: a morphometric analysis of prefrontal area 9 and occipital area 17. *Archives of General Psychiatry*, **52**, 805–818.

Senitz, D., Winkelmann, E. (1981) Über morphologische Befunde in der orbitofrontalen Rinde bei Menschen mit schizophrenen Psychosen. *Psychiatrie, Neurologie und Medizinische Psychologie*, **1**, 1–9.

Senitz, D., Winkelmann, E. (1991) Neuronale Strukturanormalität im orbito-frontalen Cortex bei Schizophrenien. *Journal fur Hirnforschung*, **32**, 149–158.

Sesack, S. R., Snyder, C. L. (1995) Cellular and subcellular localization of syntaxin-like immunoreactivity in the rat striatum and cortex. *Neuroscience*, **67**, 993–1007.

Sheetz, M. P., Pfister, K. K., Bulinski, J. C., Cotman, C. W. (1998) Mechanisms of trafficking in axons and dendrites: implications for development and neurodegeneration. *Progress in Neurobiology*, **55**, 577–594.

Sherman, G. F., Galaburda, A. M., Behan, P. O., Rosen, G. D. (1987) Neuroanatomical anomalies in autoimmune mice. *Acta Neuropathologica*, **74**, 239–242.

Sherman, G. F., Stone, J. S., Press, D. M., Rosen, G. D., Galaburda, A. M. (1990) Abnormal architecture and connections disclosed by neurofilament staining in the cerebral cortex of autoimmune mice. *Brain Research*, **529**, 202–207.

Smirnova, T., Laroche, S., Errington, M. L., Hicks, A. A., Bliss, T. V. P., Mallet, J. (1993) Transsynaptic expression of a presyaptic glutamate receptor during hippocampal long-term potentiation. *Science*, **262**, 433–436.

Smirnova, T., Miniou, P., Viegas-Pequignot, E., Mallet, J. (1996) Assignment of the human syntaxin 1B gene (STX) to chromosome 16p11.2 by fluorescence in situ hybridization. *Genomics*, **36**, 551–553.

Söllner, T., Whiteheart, S. W., Brunner, M. *et al.* (1993) SNAP receptors implicated in vesicle targeting and fusion. Nature, **362**, 318–324.

Soustek, Z. (1989) Ultrastructure of cortical synapses in the brain of schizophrenics. *Zentralblatt Allgemeine Pathologie und Pathologische Anatomie*, **135**, 25–32.

Stefan, M. D., Horton, K., Johnston, P., Bruton, C. J., Roberts, G. W., Royston, M. C. (1995) Synaptic pathology in schizophrenia: abnormalities of the prefrontal cortex. *Schizophrenia Research*, **15**, 32.

Steffensen, S. C., Wilson, M. C., Hendriksen, S. J. (1996) Coloboma contiguous gene deletion encompassing Snap alters hippocampal plasticity. *Synapse*, **22**, 281–289.

Stettler, O., Nothias, F., Tavitian, B., Vernier, P. (1995) Double in situ hybridization reveals overlapping neuronal populations expressing the low molecular weight GTPases Rab3a and Rab3b in rat brain. *European Journal of Neuroscience*, **7**, 702–713.

Stevens, J. (1992) Abnormal reinnervation as a basis for schizophrenia: a hypothesis. *Archives of General Psychiatry*, **49**, 238–243.

Südhof, T. C. (1995) The synaptic vesicle cycle: a cascade of protein–protein interactions. *Nature*, **375**, 645–653.

Südhof, T., Czernik, A., Kao, H.-T. *et al.* (1989) Synapsins: mosaics of shared and individual domains in a family of synaptic vesicle phosphoproteins. *Science*, **245**, 1474–1480.

Sutton, R. B., Fasshauer, D., Jahn, R., Brunger, A. (1998) Crystal structure of a SNARE complex involved in synaptic exocytosis at 2.4 Å resolution. *Nature*, **395**, 347–353.

Sze, C.-I., Troncoso, J. C., Kawas, C., Mouton, P., Price, D. L., Martin, L. J. (1997) Loss of the presynaptic vesicle protein synaptophysin in hippocampus correlates with cognitive decline in Alzheimer disease. *Journal of Neuropathology and Experimental Neurology*, **56**, 933–944.

Takahashi, S., Yamamoto, H., Matsuda, Z. *et al.* (1995) Identification of two highly homologous presynaptic proteins distinctly localized at the dendritic and somatic synapses. *FEBS Letters*, **368**, 455–460.

Tatetsu, S. (1964) A contribution to the morphological background of schizophrenia. *Acta Neuropathologica*, **3**, 558–571.

Tcherepanov, A. A., Sokolov, B. P. (1997) Age-related abnormalities in expression of mRNAs encoding synapsin 1A, synapsin 1B, and synaptophysin in temporal cortex of schizophrenics. *Journal of Neuroscience Research*, **49**, 639–644.

Telatar, M., Lange, E., Uhrhammer, N., Gatti, R. A. (1995) New localization of NCAM, proximal to DRD2 at chromosome 11q23. *Mammalian Genome*, **6**, 59–60.

Terry, R. D., Masliah, E., Salmon, D. P. *et al.* (1991) Physical basis of cognitive alterations in Alzheimer's disease: synapse loss is the major correlate of cognitive impairment. *Annals of Neurology*, **30**, 572–580.

Thompson, P. M., Sower, A. C.., Perrone-Bizzozero, N. I. (1998) Altered levels of the synaptosomal associated protein SNAP-25 in schizophrenia. *Biological Psychiatry*, **43**, 239–243.

Tomasiewicz, H., Ono, K., Yee, D., Thompson, C., Goridis, C., Rutishauser, U., Magnuson, T. (1993) Genetic deletion of a neural cell adhesion molecule variant (N-CAM-180) produces distinct defects in the central nervous system. *Neuron*, **11**, 1163–1174.

Uranova, N. A., Casanova, M. F., DeVaughn, N. M., Orlovskaya, D. D., Denisov, D. V. (1996) Ultrastructural alterations of synaptic contacts and astrocytes in postmortem caudate nucleus of schizophrenic patients. *Schizophrenia Research*, **22**, 81–83.

Uranova, N. A., Orlovskaya, D. D., Kolomeets, N. S., Vikchreva, O. V., Zimina, I. S., Denisov, D. V. (1997) Morphometric study of synaptic size in autopsied prefrontal cortex, caudate nucleus and substantia nigra of schizophrenics. *Schizophrenia Research*, **24**, 41–42.

van Lookeren Campagne, M., Oestreicher, A. B., van Bergen en Henegouwen, P. M. P., Gispen, W. H. (1990) Ultrastructural double localization of B-50/GAP43 and synaptophysin (p38) in the neonatal and adult rat hippocampus. *Journal of Neurocytology*, **19**, 948–961.

Vawter, M. P., Cannon-Spoor, H. E., Hemperly, J. J. *et al.* (1998) Abnormal expression of cell recognition molecules in schizophrenia. *Experimental Neurology*, **149**, 424–432.

Vincente, A. M., Macciardi, F., Verga, M. *et al.* (1997) NCAM and schizophrenia: genetic studies. *Molecular Psychiatry*, **2**, 65–69.

Wakabayashi, K., Honer, W. G., Masliah, E. (1994) Synapse alterations in the hippocampal-entorhinal formation In Alzheimer's disease with and without Lewy body disease. *Brain Research*, **667**, 24–32.

Walaas, S. I., Jahn, R., Greengard, P. (1988) Quantitation of nerve terminal populations: synaptic vesicle-asociated proteins as markers for synaptic density in the rat neostriatum. *Synapse*, **2**, 516–520.

Welker, E., Armstrong-Jones, M., Bronchti, G. *et al.* (1996) Altered sensory processing in the somatosensory cortex of the mouse mutant barrelless. *Nature*, **271**, 1864–1867.

Wiedenmann, B., Franke, W. (1985) Identification and localization of synaptophysin, an integral membrane glycoprotein of Mr 38,000 characteristic of synaptic vesicles. *Cell*, **41**, 1017–1028.

Woodman, P. G. (1997) The roles of NSF, SNAPs and SNAREs during membrane fusion. *Biochimica et Biophysica Acta*, **1357**, 155–172.

Young, A. H., Blackwood, D. H. R., Roxborough, H., McQueen, J. K., Martin, M. J., Kean, D. (1991) A magnetic resonance imaging study of schizophrenia: brain structure and clinical symptoms. *British Journal of Psychiatry*, **158**, 158–164.

Young, C. E., Arima, K., Xie, J. *et al.* (1998) SNAP-25 deficit and hippocampal connectivity in schizophrenia. *Cerebral Cortex*, **8**, 261–268.

5 Gliosis and its Implications for the Disease Process

Gareth W. Roberts and Paul J. Harrison

In a disorder notable for its neuropathological complexity and obscurity, gliosis has been called the 'most inscrutable lesion' (Bruton *et al.*, 1990). Establishing if gliosis is present in schizophrenia has been one of the key questions addressed in contemporary studies, because of the significant implications which it has for understanding the nature of the disorder. Put simply, gliosis would equate with a progressive, neurodegenerative process, as Kraepelin believed was the case. Conversely, an absence of gliosis, in the presence of macroscopic (Chapter 1) and cytoarchitectural (Chapters 2 to 4) alterations, can be construed as supportive of a neurodevelopmental disease process (Chapter 8). This chapter reviews the evidence and concludes that gliosis is indeed not a feature of the brain in schizophrenia. The caveats to, and interpretation of, this important negative result are then discussed.

Glia and gliosis

Glial subtypes

There are three major glial cell types in the brain: astrocytes, oligodendrocytes, and microglia (Ellison *et al.*, 1998). Astrocytes play several roles, including contributions to neuronal migration, synaptic neurotransmission, and maintenance and plasticity of neuronal circuits (Liedtke *et al.*, 1996; Kreutzberg *et al.*, 1997; Porter and McCarthy, 1997). Of most relevance here, astrocytes are also central to the response to neural injury and scar formation in the brain. They are subdivided into protoplasmic astrocytes (in grey matter) and fibrous astrocytes (in white matter). Numerically, they outnumber neurons 10 to 1, and occupy a third of cortical volume (Norenberg, 1994). Oligodendrocytes are involved in myelination, whilst microglia are mainly responsible for phagocytosis of cell debris and secretion of cytokines (Kreutzberg *et al.*, 1997).

Astrocytes and gliosis

In neuropathological parlance, the term gliosis is often used as shorthand for, and is implicitly synonymous with, astrocytic gliosis (also called reactive gliosis or astrogliosis). This brevity has been the convention in schizophrenia research and it is adopted here. (Nevertheless, it risks overlooking the contribution of microglia to gliosis which is increasingly recognised (Streit *et al.*, 1999) and the possibility of microglial involvement in schizophrenia; for example, Pakkenberg (1990) reported a loss of microglia as well as of astrocytes in the thalamus, and Bayer *et al.* (1999) have provided evidence of microglial activation in the frontal cortex.)

Gliosis consists of several types of alterations in astrocytes, including initial swelling, hypertrophy, activation, elongation of cellular processes, proliferation, and formation of fibrils. Neurochemically, the most prominent, though still functionally mysterious, astrocytic protein is glial fibrillary acidic protein (GFAP). GFAP is detectable in most resting astrocytes, depending on how the tissue is processed, and its expression increases rapidly and massively during the gliotic response (Norton *et al.*, 1992; Eng and Ghirnikar, 1994). There are many astrocytic markers apart from GFAP, including vimentin and S-100β (Eddleston and Mucke, 1993).

Detection of gliosis

Gliosis can be detected in two main ways: by traditional stains, notably the Holzer technique, and by immunochemical methods which take advantage of the selectivity, robustness, and quantifiability of GFAP (Table 5.1). In recent years, GFAP-based methods have become the more widely used, and in schizophrenia research they are now the standard approach.

Although GFAP detection has become the standard marker of gliosis, it is not without limitations. The abundance of GFAP is not an invariable correlate of, or directly proportional to, the degree of gliosis. GFAP expression can be increased by stimuli (e.g. seizures) without any evidence of tissue damage; conversely, elevated GFAP is not always detectable despite independent evidence that gliosis is present (Eng and Ghirnikar, 1994; Norenberg, 1994). In particular, a decline of GFAP towards normal levels sometimes occurs weeks or months after experimental lesions, especially at distant sites; the magnitude of the initial response is also affected by the location and nature of the lesion (Anezaki *et al.*, 1992; Kalman *et al.*, 1993; Dell'Anna *et al.*, 1995; Berman *et al.*, 1998). In human brain, it has been suggested that chronic gliosis is more readily detected by the Holzer stain than by GFAP immunohistochemistry, perhaps because of the relatively weak GFAP staining of astrocytic fibrils (J.R. Stevens *et al.*, 1988; Stevens *et al.*, 1992). Furthermore, different GFAP antisera

Table 5.1 Methods for detecting gliosis

Traditional stains
  Holzer
  Lithium carbonate
  Phosphotungstic acid haematoxylin
  Nissl

Glial fibrillary acidic protein (GFAP)[1]
  Immunocytochemistry
    number, density, or size of immunoreactive cells
  Immunohistochemistry
    tissue densitometry
  Western or dot blotting
  Hybridization methods for GFAP mRNA

[1] the same range of methods can in principle be applied to other molecules selectively expressed by astrocytes, such as vimentin.

can give markedly different results (Halliday *et al.*, 1996) and, like all immunological methods, GFAP detection may be affected by perimortem factors (Chapter 14).

Despite these considerations, there are good reasons why GFAP detection has largely replaced conventional stains for detecting gliosis. Firstly, GFAP has advantages because of its specificity for astrocytes, ease and safety of use, and the more readily quantifiable and less capricious nature of molecular methods. Secondly, the Holzer stain has its own problems, including a failure to detect reliably the marked gliosis seen in Huntington's disease (Nieto and Escobar, 1972) or in the early stages of a gliotic response (Stevens *et al.*, 1992). Although Nissl stains are simple and are used widely (mainly because they are required anyway to assess neurons), they have inherent limitations in this context because astrocytes cannot be distinguished clearly from small neurons and other glia.

In addition to these methodological complications, there is uncertainty as to what parameter is most important in the diagnosis of gliosis—is it astrocyte size, density, number, fibrils, etc? For instance, in the presence of atrophy, gliosis in terms of increased glial density may be profound, yet glial number is not increased (Miyake *et al.*, 1988). In a systematic study, da Cunha *et al.* (1993) compared different GFAP indices (cell size, cell density, and intensity of staining, in both white matter and grey matter) with a 'gliosis index' which was based upon the raters' impressions of routine staining. Only the size of white matter astrocytes correlated with the gliosis index; other parameters did not. There was also variation between the four raters. As well as highlighting the subjective element and lack of uniformity in the assessment of gliosis, the data question the assumption that increased astrocytic density, however identified, is largely synonymous with gliosis (da Cunha *et al.*, 1993).

In summary, the definition, detection, and quantification of gliosis are not straightforward. These somewhat arcane matters are mentioned because they have contributed to the controversy about gliosis in schizophrenia; in particular, whether, as discussed below, the lack of gliosis is real or apparent.

Gliosis in schizophrenia

The key studies

The landmark report by Stevens (1982*a*) was the first significant contemporary neuropathological study of schizophrenia. Using the Holzer technique, and in keeping with observations going back as far as Alzheimer (reviewed in Nieto and Escobar, 1972; Stevens 1982*b*), she found that gliosis was present in 70 per cent of her cases of schizophrenia. Only one of 18 control subjects showed any evidence of gliosis. The gliosis was usually located in periventricular and subependymal regions of the diencephalon or in adjacent basal forebrain structures. In keeping with the standard interpretation of gliosis mentioned above, the findings were taken as evidence not only of pathology *per se* in schizophrenia (thus helping to resurrect interest in this field), but also that it was suggestive of an inflammatory process, perhaps viral in origin (thus stimulating interest in the biological aetiology of the disorder).

Since 1982 there have been a large number of studies investigating gliosis in schizophrenia. As shown in Table 5.2, the overwhelming majority of reports have not confirmed the presence of gliosis in schizophrenia; indeed, they have largely ruled out the possibility. Although each study has limitations, it is noteworthy that the negative conclusions are seen in many brain areas, using different methods, and measuring different parameters of gliosis. These factors together make it unlikely that the lack of gliosis is due to the limitations of GFAP-based methods mentioned above (for debate see Roberts *et al.*, 1988; Stevens *et al.*, 1992). The recent study by Falkai *et al.* (1999) is important, being the largest series to date and because it included analysis of the periventricular region identified by Stevens (1982*a*) as a key site of gliosis, whereas many of the intervening studies had focused on cortical regions and therefore were unable to replicate or refute her original findings.

Gliosis in schizophrenia: coincidental pathologies

As shown in Table 5.1, the weight of evidence is firmly against gliosis as being present in schizophrenia, and this appears to be a true negative rather than a false negative result. A further issue which has complicated matters concerns the prevalence and meaning of other disorders with which schizophrenia coexists or is mistaken for, and which may themselves be associated with gliosis.

A higher proportion (~50 per cent) of brains from patients with schizophrenia than from age-matched controls contain non-specific focal degenerative abnormalities, such as small infarcts and white matter changes (Jellinger, 1985; Bruton *et al.*, 1990; Riederer *et al.*, 1995). These are presumably coincidental, in that they are variable in distribution and nature, do not affect the clinical picture (Johnstone *et al.*, 1994), and in some instances are documented as having occurred long after the onset of symptoms of schizophrenia. Their occurrence raises two points. One is whether the frequency of lesions is a sign that the brain in schizophrenia is more vulnerable to neurodegenerative and vascular impairment, perhaps in conjunction with chronic antipsychotic treatment (Chapter 15), or whether the finding is merely a collection artefact (Harrison, 1995). (The related question as to the

Table 5.2 Studies of gliosis in schizophrenia[1]

Author	Region	Number of cases/controls	Parameter measured	Technique	Finding in schizophrenia
(a) Studies without neuropathological purification					
Stevens, 1982a	Multiple areas	25/20	Gliosis	Holzer stain	Increased
Bogerts et al., 1983	Substantia nigra	6/6	Glial number	Nissl stain	Unchanged
Benes et al., 1986	Frontal and cingulate cortex (areas 4, 10, 24)	7–10/5–9	Glial density	Nissl stain	Unchanged/decreased
Falkai and Bogerts, 1986[a]	Hippocampus	15/9	Glial number	Nissl stain	Unchanged/decreased
Owen et al., 1987	Frontal and temporal cortex; hippocampus; amygdala; putamen; hypothalamus	39/44	MAO-B activity[2]	Enzyme assay	Unchanged/decreased
Falkai et al., 1988[a]	Entorhinal cortex	15/9	Glial number	Nissl stain	Unchanged
Bruton et al., 1990[b]	Cortex; periventricular region	48/56	Gliosis rating	Holzer stain	Increased
Casanova et al., 1990	Dentate gyrus	6/7	Glial number	Holzer stain	Unchanged
Pakkenberg, 1990	Mediodorsal thalamus; ventral striatum; basolateral amygdala	12/12	Absolute glial number	Nissl stain; physical disector	Unchanged/decreased
Karson et al., 1993	Frontal, temporal, and occipital cortex; thalamus; cerebellum; pontine tegmentum	4–12/3–10	GFAP abundance	Western blot	Unchanged
Arnold et al., 1996	Hippocampus, frontal and visual cortex	21/12	GFAP-positive astrocyte density; GFAP IR[3]; vimentin-positive astrocyte density	Immunocytochemistry	Unchanged[4]
Jonsson et al., 1997	Hippocampus	4/8	Glial density	Nissl stain	Unchanged
Falkai et al., 1999	Entorhinal cortex, subiculum, several white matter regions	33/26	GFAP-positive astrocyte density	Immunocytochemistry	Unchanged

Table 5.2 Continued

(b) Studies with neuropathological purification

Author	Region	Number of cases/controls	Parameter measured	Technique	Finding in schizophrenia
Roberts et al., 1986[c]	Multiple areas	5/7	Gliosis	GFAP IR[3]	Unchanged
Roberts et al., 1987	Multiple temporal lobe areas	18/12	Gliosis	GFAP IR[3]	Unchanged
C. D. Stevens et al., 1988[c]	Caudate, cingulate white matter, periventricular nuclei	5/7	GFAP-positive cell counts	Immunocyto-chemistry	Unchanged
Crow et al., 1989[b]	Temporal, frontal, and parietal cortex; hippocampus, amygdala and caudate	18/20	Gliosis	DBI IR[5], Holzer stain	Unchanged
Benes et al., 1991	Frontal and cingulate cortex (areas 10, 24)	15–18/9–12	Glial density	Nissl stain	Unchanged
Selemon et al., 1995[d]	Frontal and occipital cortex (areas 9, 17)	16/19	Glial density	Nissl stain	Unchanged
Perrone-Bizzozero et al., 1996	Frontal, temporal and occipital cortex (areas 9, 10, 17, 20)	5–10/4–6	GFAP abundance	Western blot	Unchanged
Öngur et al., 1998	Cingulate and parietal cortex (areas 24, 3b)	11/11	Glial density and number	Nissl stain	Unchanged
Rajkowska et al., 1998[d]	Frontal and occipital cortex (areas 9,17)	9/10	Glial size	Nissl stain	Unchanged
Karson et al., 1999	Frontal cortex (area 10)	14/12	GFAP and GFAP mRNA abundance	Western and northern blots	Unchanged

[1]Table adapted and updated from Harrison (1997). Studies in part (a) included all schizophrenics, or had clinical criteria for exclusion (e.g. a history of dementia). Studies in part (b) excluded brains with neuropathological abnormalities (e.g. presence of infarcts, trauma).
[2]MAO, monoamine oxidase. The B form of the enzyme is mainly glial.
[3]GFAP IR, glial fibrillary acidic protein; IR, immunoreactivity.
[4]Though schizophrenics with dementia (n = 14) had higher GFAP-positive astrocyte densities than those without (n = 7).
[5]DBI IR: diazepam-binding inhibitor immunoreactivity, measured densitometrically. DBI is a selective glial marker.
[a-d]Studies sharing the same superscript were carried out on the same brains.

frequency of Alzheimer's disease in schizophrenia is discussed in Chapter 2.) The second issue, which is directly relevant to this chapter, is that gliosis is to be expected as an accompaniment to these coincidental pathologies, and hence its frequency will be increased in schizophrenia unless brains with such changes are excluded. The pros and cons of this strategy have been discussed elsewhere (Harrison, 1995; Arnold and Trojanowski, 1996).

As a further complication, about 3 to 5 per cent of cases clinically diagnosed as schizophrenia turn out to be a known neurological disorder, such as temporal lobe epilepsy, syphilis, Wilson's disease, metachromatic leukodystrophy, and so on (Davison, 1983; Johnstone *et al.*, 1987). Some of these diseases may exhibit gliosis as part of the pathological process (as in the non-schizophrenic psychiatric control group in Stevens, 1982*a*) and hence confound the matter if they are unknowingly or knowingly included in brain series. Of the disorders listed above, the relationship between epilepsy and schizophrenia is particularly noteworthy in this regard (Roberts *et al.*, 1990; Bruton *et al.*, 1994; see Chapter 11).

Given these considerations, it is of note in Table 5.2b that no gliosis has ever been seen in schizophrenia in brain series which 'purified' their cases (i.e. rigorously excluded those where other neuropathological abnormalities were present). The study of Bruton *et al.* (1990) is illuminating, since the apparent excess of gliosis in their schizophrenia group was due to an increased frequency of the concurrent neuropathological abnormalities compared to the controls mentioned above. Once these brains were excluded, no gliosis was seen in the schizophrenics, but the other findings of decreased brain size (Bruton *et al.*, 1990) and ventricular enlargement (Crow *et al.*, 1989) were still observed. In other words, there is a pathology in schizophrenia which is more fundamental than, and can be dissociated from, gliosis. Hence the latter appears to be primarily a sign of coincidental or superimposed pathological changes.

The meaning of an absence of gliosis

Because gliosis is an invariable correlate of neural injury, its absence is taken to exclude any form of degenerative or progressive pathology, including classical neurodegenerative disorders, also inflammatory, ischaemic, infective, postinfective, or autoimmune processes, as occurring in schizophrenia. Implicit in this formulation is that schizophrenia is neuropathologically static, during its clinical course. In this respect, the lack of gliosis provides independent support for the same view which has emerged from structural brain imaging which finds changes present at first presentation with little good evidence for progression thereafter (Chapter 1).

The lack of gliosis has more significance attached to it than merely a pathology which is non-progressive with regard to the clinical disease: it is taken as prima-facie evidence that the changes must have originated before the onset of the glial response, which is said to begin during the second trimester *in utero* (i.e. between about 14 and 28 weeks; Friede, 1989). Hence, the lack of gliosis is taken as strong evidence to support a neurodevelopmental pathogenesis for schizophrenia which predates this time (Roberts, 1991; Bloom, 1993; see Chapter 8). This view is strengthened if it is considered in parallel with the heterotopias and other putative neuronal migrational abnormalities reported in some cyto-architectural studies (Chapters 2 and 3), since these processes are also ongoing at the same ontogenic stage. Parenthetically, such a timing renders birth complications as epiphenomena, being a sign of an already compromised brain rather than having a direct causal role in schizophrenia (as is also the case in cerebral palsy; MacLennan, 1999; see Chapter 8); this is also consistent with the evidence that true perinatal brain damage produces a different pathology (such as periventricular haemmorhage and leucomalacia), which is often accompanied by gliosis (Marin-Padilla, 1996, 1997).

Limitations of the assumptions

The second trimester inference

Despite the often-quoted statement that the gliotic response begins in the second trimester, it remains far from unequivocally established, let alone timed more accurately within the trimester as sometimes stated. Certainly, GFAP (Aquino et al., 1996) and GFAP-positive astrocytes (Roessmann and Gambetti, 1986) are detectable by about 20 weeks gestation, and there are case reports of gliosis after fetal lesions timed at 13 to 18 weeks (Cohen and Roessmann, 1994; Squier et al., 2000). However, we are not aware of good data showing when the phenomenon of reactive gliosis is *first* observed. As well as being a difficult question to answer, it may well be an oversimplistic one, since it assumes that there is such a time point before which gliosis is not demonstrable. It is also constrained by the the process of gliogenesis itself; unequivocal recognition of astrocytes in the cerebral cortex is not possible until 15 weeks gestation (Marin-Padilla, 1995), though detection of GFAP-positive fibrous astrocytes in cultures of 8 to 10 week fetal brain tissue has been reported (Elder and Major, 1988). Moreover, the emergence of GFAP expression is regionally variable in the human cerebral cortex (Aquino et al., 1996) as is the onset of experimental gliosis (Ajtai et al., 1997). When the glial response is first seen might also depend upon many other variables, such as genetic factors (cf. Overmyer et al., 1999) and the nature of the stimulus. Given these uncertainties, one should draw with great caution the inference that a lack of gliosis means that a pathological process must predate the third trimester; it would be prudent merely to argue that it is consistent with such a timing (Roberts et al., 1997).

Progressive disease process without gliosis?

The possibility that gliosis might not be present despite a disease which is progressive and continues well after the second trimester must be considered. A 'false negative' gliosis result of this kind could emerge for several reasons. Firstly, as noted above, detection of gliosis is not as straightforward as might be imagined, being influenced by many factors. In other words, it is difficult to rule out the possibility that there has been gliosis at some stage, or in some brain areas, in subjects with schizophrenia, but that all evidence of it has disappeared by the time of death. Secondly, if schizophrenia involves aberrant formation or refinement of neuronal and synaptic connections, as many data reviewed in this book suggest, it may be a form or subtlety of pathology which does not elicit a gliotic response, perhaps because it is just a minor quantitative deviation from normal maturational processes.

One such example could be an alteration in neuronal apoptosis, as has been advocated in schizophrenia, for which no accompanying gliosis would be expected.

Pathological heterogeneity

A final consideration is that gliosis might be present in a subset of schizophrenia, and that overemphasis on group averages overlooks informative cases or subgroups (Stevens, 1997). The finding of elevated GFAP-positive astrocyte densities in demented compared to non-demented elderly schizophrenics, despite an absence of any concurrent degenerative disorder, might be one indication of this (Arnold *et al.*, 1996). The possibility of neuropathological heterogeneity gains indirect support from recent imaging data suggesting there may be progression of structural changes in a subgroup of cases with poor outcome and poor treatment response (Woods, 1998; Chapter 1). Returning to the Stevens (1982*a*) study, it is noteworthy that most of the cases had presented as catatonic schizophrenia, a subtype also common in other earlier reports in which gliosis was observed (Stevens 1982*a,b*). Perhaps the increasing rarity of this form of schizophrenia—and of other catatonic syndromes such as von Economo's encephalitis which might have been mistaken for schizophrenia—contributes to the apparent 'declining incidence' of gliosis in schizophrenia.

Conversely, we should not lose sight of the fact that, to date, there has been no convincing evidence of a pathological heterogeneity of schizophrenia (with the exceptions, mentioned above, of cases which exhibit other pathologies underlying, or coincidental to, the schizophrenia phenotype). As such, the parsimonious view remains that schizophrenia has a single pathology, including the absence of gliosis, which varies only in severity (Roberts and Bruton, 1990).

Conclusions

There is little doubt that gliosis is not a core feature of the neuropathology of schizophrenia. This is a crucial negative conclusion, since it makes conventional neurodegenerative processes unlikely to be occurring in the disease. By default, neurodevelopmental abnormalities are therefore favoured.

Several outstanding issues remain. Firstly, clarification of whether there are circumstances in which gliosis does occur in schizophrenia. Secondly, to take into account the increasing appreciation of the molecular complexities of astrocytes and the heterogeneity of the glial response (Ridet *et al.*, 1997), and the corresponding need for more rigorous approaches to its definition, characterisation, and detection. Thirdly, a more critical and empirically grounded interpretation of what an absence of gliosis can and cannot reveal about the pathogenesis of the disorder. These topics are discussed further in Chapters 8 and 11.

Acknowledgement

We thank Janice Stevens for many stimulating discussions and for comments on an early draft of this chapter.

References

Ajtai BM, Kallai L, Kalman M (1997) Capability for reactive gliosis develops prenatally in the diencephalon but not in the cortex of rats. *Experimental Neurology* **146**, 151–158.

Anezaki T, Yanagisawa K, Takahashi H *et al.* (1992) Remote astrocytic response of prefrontal cortex is caused by the lesions in the nucleus basalis of Meynert, but not in the ventral tegmental area. *Brain Research* **574**, 63–69.

Aquino DA, Padin C, Perez JM, Peng D, Lyman WD, Chiu F-C (1996) Analysis of glial fibrillary acidic protein, neurofilament protein, actin and heat shock proteins in human fetal brain during the second trimester. *Developmental Brain Research* **91**, 1–10.

Arnold SE, Trojanowski JQ (1996) Recent advances in defining the neuropathology of schizophrenia. *Acta Neuropathologica* **92**, 217–231.

Arnold SE, Franz BR, Trojanowski JQ, Moberg PJ, Gur RE (1996) Glial fibrillary acidic protein-immunoreactive astrocytosis in elderly patients with schizophrenia and dementia. *Acta Neuropathologica* **91**, 269–277.

Bayer TA, Buslei R, Havas L, Falkai P (1999) Evidence for activation of microglia in patients with psychiatric illnesses. *Neuroscience Letters* **271**, 126–128.

Benes FM, Davidson J, Bird ED (1986) Quantitative cytoarchitectural studies of the cerebral cortex of schizophrenics. *Archives of General Psychiatry* **43**, 31–35.

Benes FM, McSparren J, Bird ED, SanGiovanni JP, Vincent SL (1991) Deficits in small interneurons in prefrontal and cingulate cortices of schizophrenic and schizoaffective patients. *Archives of General Psychiatry* **48**, 996–1001.

Berman NEJ, Raymond LA, Warren KA *et al.* (1998) Fractionator analysis shows loss of neurons in the lateral geniculate nucleus of macaques infected with neurovirulent simian immunodeficiency virus. *Neuropathology and Applied Neurobiology* **24**, 44–52.

Bloom FE (1993) Advancing a neurodevelopmental origin for schizophrenia. *Archives of General Psychiatry* **50**, 224–227.

Bogerts B, Häntsch J, Herzer M (1983) A morphometric study of dopamine-containing cell groups in the mesencephalon of normals, Parkinson patients and schizophrenics. *Biological Psychiatry* **18**, 951–969.

Bruton CJ, Crow TJ, Frith CD, Johnstone EC, Owens DGC, Roberts GW (1990) Schizophrenia and the brain: a prospective clinico-neuropathological study. *Psychological Medicine* **20**, 285–304.

Bruton CJ, Stevens J, Frith CD (1994) Epilepsy, psychosis and schizophrenia. Clinical and neuropathological considerations. *Neurology* **44**, 34–42.

Casanova MF, Stevens JR, Kleinman JE (1990) Astrocytosis in the molecular layer of the dentate gyrus, a study in Alzheimer's disease and schizophrenia. *Psychiatry Research, Neuromaging* **35**, 149–166.

Cohen M, Roessmann U (1994) *In utero* brain damage: relationship of gestational age to pathological consequences. *Developmental Medicine and Child Neurology* **36**, 263–268.

Crow TJ, Ball J, Bloom SR *et al.* (1989) Schizophrenia as an anomaly of development of cerebral asymmetry. *Archives of General Psychiatry* **46**, 1145–1150.

Da Cunha A, Jefferson JJ, Tyor WR, Glass JD, Jannotta F, Vitkovic L (1993) Gliosis in human brain: relationship to size but not other properties of astrocytes. *Brain Research* **600**, 161–165.

Davison K (1983) Schizophrenia-like psychoses associated with organic cerebral disorders: a review. *Psychiatric Developments* **1**, 1–34.

Dell'Anna ME, Geloso MC, Draisci G, Luthman J (1995) Transient changes in fos and GFAP immunoreactivity precede neuronal loss in the rat hippocampus following neonatal anoxia. *Experimental Neurology* **131**, 144–156.

Eddleston M, Mucke L (1993) Molecular profile of reactive astrocytes—implications for their role in neurologic disease. *Neuroscience* **54**, 15–36.

Elder GA, Major EO (1988) Early appearance of type II astrocytes in developing human fetal brain. *Developmental Brain Research* **42**, 146–150.

Ellison D, Love S, Cimelli L *et al.* (1998) *Neuropathology*. Mosby, St Louis.

Eng LF, Ghirnikar RS (1994) GFAP and astrogliosis. *Brain Pathology* **4**, 229–237.

Falkai P, Bogerts B (1986) Cell loss in the hippocampus of schizophrenics. *European Archives of Psychiatry and Neurological Science* **236**, 154–161.

Falkai P, Bogerts B, Rozumek M (1988) Limbic pathology in schizophrenia: the entorhinal region—a morphometric study. *Biological Psychiatry* **24**, 515–521.

Falkai P, Honer WG, David S, Bogerts B, Majtenyi C, Bayer TA (1999) No evidence for astrogliosis in brains of schizophrenic patients. A post-mortem study. *Neuropathology and Applied Neurobiology* **25**, 48–53.

Friede RL (1989) *Developmental neuropathology*, 2nd edn. Springer, Berlin, p. 577.

Halliday GM, Cullen KM, Kril JJ, Harding AJ, Harasty J (1996) Glial fibrillary acidic protein (GFAP) immunohistochemistry in human cortex: A quantitative study using different antisera. *Neuroscience Letters* **209**, 29–32.

Harrison PJ (1995) On the neuropathology of schizophrenia and its dementia: neurodevelopmental, neurodegenerative, or both? *Neurodegeneration* **4**, 1–12.

Harrison PJ (1997) Schizophrenia and its dementia. In: Esiri MM, Morris JH (eds). *The neuropathology of dementia*. Cambridge, Cambridge University Press, pp. 385–397.

Jellinger K (1985) Neuromorphological background of pathochemical studies in major psychoses. In: Beckmann H, Riederer P (eds). *Pathochemical markers in major psychoses*. Berlin, Springer, pp. 1–23.

Johnstone EC, McMillan JF, Crow TJ (1987) The occurrence of organic disease of possible or probable aetiological significance in a population of 268 cases of first episode schizophrenia. *Psychological Medicine* **17**, 371–379.

Johnstone EC, Bruton CJ, Crow TJ, Frith CD, Owens DGC (1994) Clinical correlates of postmortem brain changes in schizophrenia: decreased brain weight and length correlate with indices of early impairment. *Journal of Neurology, Neurosurgery and Psychiatry* **57**, 474–479.

Jonsson SAT, Luts A, Guidberg-Kjaer N, Brun A (1997) Hippocampal pyramidal cell disarray corelates negatively to cell number: implications for the pathogenesis of schizophrenia. *European Archives of Psychiatry and Neurological Science* **247**, 120–127.

Kalman M, Csillag A, Schleicher A, Rind C, Hajós F, Zilles K (1993) Long-term effects of anterograde degeneration on astroglial reaction in the rat geniculo-cortical system as revealed by computerized image analysis. *Anatomy and Embryology* **187**, 1–7.

Karson CN, Casanova MF, Kleinman JE, Griffin WST (1993) Choline acetyltransferase in schizophrenia. *American Journal of Psychiatry* **150**, 454–459.

Karson CN, Mrak RC, Schluterman KO, Sturner WQ, Sheng JG, Griffin WST (1999) Alterations in synaptic proteins and their encoding mRNAs in prefrontal cortex in schizophrenia: a possible neurochemical basis for 'hypofrontality'. *Molecular Psychiatry* **4**, 39–45.

Kreutzberg GW, Blakemore WF, Graeber MB (1997) Cellular pathology of the central nervous system. In: Graham DI, Lantos PE (eds). *Greenfield's neuropathology*, 6th edition. Edward Arnold, London, pp. 85–156.

Liedtke W, Edelmann W, Bieri PL *et al.* (1996) GFAP is necessary for the integrity of CNS white matter architecture and long-term maintenance of myelination. *Neuron* **17**, 607–615.

MacLennan A (1999) A template for defining a causal relation between acute intrapartum events and cerebral palsy: international consensus statement. *British Medical Journal* **319**, 1054–1059.

Marin-Padilla M (1995) Prenatal development of fibrous (white matter), protoplasmic (grey matter), and layer 1 astrocytes in the human cerebral cortex: a Golgi study. *Journal of Comparative Neurology* **357**, 554–572.

Marin-Padilla M (1996) Developmental neuropathology and impact of perinatal brain damage. I. Hemorrhagic lesions of neocortex. *Journal of Neuropathology and Experimental Neurology* **55**, 758–773.

Marin-Padilla M (1997) Developmental neuropathology and impact of perinatal brain damage. II. White matter lesions of the neocortex. *Journal of Neuropathology and Experimental Neurology* **56**, 219–235.

Miyake T, Kitamura T, Takamatsu T, Fujita S (1988) A quantitative analysis of human astrocytosis. *Acta Neuropathologica* **75**, 535–537.

Nieto D, Escobar A (1972) Major psychoses. In: Minkler J (ed.). *Pathology of the nervous system*, Volume 3. McGraw Hill, New York, pp. 2654–2665.

Norenberg MD (1994) Astrocyte responses to CNS injury. *Journal of Neuropathology and Experimental Neurology* **53**, 213–220.

Norton WT, Aquino DA, Hozumi I, Chui F-C, Brosnan CF (1992) Quantitative aspects of reactive gliosis: a review. *Neurochemistry Research* **17**, 877–885.

Öngur D, Drevets WC, Price JL (1998) Glial reduction in the subgenual prefrontal cortex in mood disorders. *Proceedings of the National Academy of Science USA* **95**, 13290–13295.

Overmyer M, Seppo H, Hilkka S, Markku L, Reikkenen P Sr, Alafuzoff I (1999) Astrogliosis and the ApoE genotype. *Dementia* **10**, 252–257.

Owen F, Crow TJ, Frith CD *et al.* (1987) Selective decreases in MAO-B activity in post-mortem brains from schizophrenic patients with type II syndrome. *British Journal of Psychiatry* **151**, 744–752.

Pakkenberg B (1990) Pronounced reduction of total neuron number in mediodorsal thalamic nucleus and nucleus accumbens in schizophrenics. *Archives of General Psychiatry* **47**, 1023–1028.

Perrone-Bizzozero NI, Sower AC, Bird ED, Benowitz LI, Ivins KJ, Neve RL (1996) Levels of the growth-associated protein GAP-43 are selectively increased in association cortices in schizophrenia. *Proceedings of the National Academy of Science USA* **93**, 14182–14187.

Porter JT, McCarthy KD (1997) Astrocytic neurotransmitter receptors *in situ* and *in vivo*. *Progress in Neurobiology* **51**, 439–455.

Rajkowska G, Selemon LD, Goldman-Rakic PS (1998) Neuronal and glial somal size in the prefrontal cortex—A post-mortem morphometric study of schizophrenia and Huntington disease *Archives of General Psychiatry* **55**, 215–224.

Ridet JL, Malhotra SK, Privat A, Gage FH (1997) Reactive astrocytes: cellular and molecular clues to biological function. *Trends in Neuroscience* **20**, 570–577.

Riederer P, Gsell W, Calza L, Franzek E, Jungkunz G, Jellinger K (1995) Consensus on minimal criteria of clinical and neuropathological diagnosis of schizophrenia and affective disorders for post mortem research. *Journal of Neural Transmission* **102**, 255–264.

Roberts GW (1991) Schizophrenia: a neuropathological perspective. *British Journal of Psychiatry* **158**, 8–17.

Roberts GW, Bruton CJ (1990) Notes from the graveyard: neuropathology and schizophrenia. *Neuropathology and Applied Neurobiology* **16**, 3–16.

Roberts GW, Colter N, Lofthouse R, Bogerts B, Zech N, Crow TJ (1986) Gliosis in schizophrenia. *Biological Psychiatry* **21**, 1043–1050.

Roberts GW, Colter N, Lofthouse R, Johnstone EC, Crow TJ (1987) Is there gliosis in schizophrenia? Investigation of the temporal lobe. *Biological Psychiatry* **22**, 1459–1468.

Roberts GW, Bruton CJ, Crow TJ (1988) Gliosis in schizophrenia. *Biological Psychiatry* **24**, 729–731.

Roberts GW, Done DJ, Bruton C, Crow TJ (1990) A 'mock-up' of schizophrenia: temporal lobe epilepsy and schizophrenia-like psychosis. *Biological Psychiatry* **28**, 127–143.

Roberts GW, Royston MC, Weinberger DR (1997) Schizophrenia. In: Graham DI, Lantos PE (eds). *Greenfield's neuropathology*, 6th edition. Edward Arnold, London, pp. 897–929.

Roessmann U, Gambetti P (1986) Pathological reaction of astrocytes in perinantal brain injury. Immunohistochemical study. *Acta Neuropathologica* **70**, 302–307.

Selemon LD, Rajkowska G, Goldman-Rakic PS (1995) Abnormally high neuronal density in the schizophrenic cortex. *Archives of General Psychiatry* **52**, 805–818.

Squier MV, Chamberlain P, Zaiwalla Z *et al.* (2000) Five cases of brain injury following mid-term amniocentesis. *Developmental Medicine and Child Neurology*.

Stevens CD, Altshuler LL, Bogerts B, Falkai P (1988) Quantitative study of gliosis in schizophrenia and Huntington's chorea. *Biological Psychiatry* **24**, 697–700.

Stevens JR (1982a) Neuropathology of schizophrenia. *Archives of General Psychiatry* **39**, 1131–1139.

Stevens JR (1982b) The neuropathology of schizophrenia. *Psychological Medicine* **12**, 695–700.

Stevens JR (1997) Anatomy of schizophrenia revisited. *Schizophrenia Bulletin* **23**, 373–383.

Stevens JR, Casanova M, Bigelow L (1988) Gliosis and schizophrenia. *Biological Psychiatry* **24**, 727–729.

Stevens JR, Casanova M, Poltorak M, Germain L, Buchan GC (1992) Comparison of immunocytochemical and Holzer's methods for detection of acute and chronic gliosis in human postmortem material. *Journal of Neuropsychiatry and Clinical Neuroscience* **4**, 168–173.

Streit WJ, Walter SA, Pennell NA (1999) Reactive microgliosis. *Progress in Neurobiology* **57**, 563–581.

Woods BT (1998) Is schizophrenia a progressive neurodevelopmental disorder? Toward a unitary pathogenetic mechanism. *American Journal of Psychiatry* **155**, 1661–1670.

6 Cerebral Asymmetry

Dorothy P. Holinger, Albert M. Galaburda, and Paul J. Harrison

Investigation of human brain lateralization began in earnest following Broca's (1861) report of language disturbance resulting from injury to the left hemisphere (see Harris (1999) for historical review). Proposals that cerebral asymmetry is relevant to insanity can be traced back to Wigan (1844), Crichton Browne (1879), and, more explicitly, to the neuropathologist Southard (1915) who stated 'the atrophies and aplasias [of schizophrenia], when focal, show a tendency to occur in the left cerebral hemisphere.' Despite these prescient statements, and the stimulus provided by Flor-Henry's (1969) report that schizophrenia was associated with left-sided foci in temporal lobe epilepsy, it is only in the past 20 years or so that the question has been investigated in any detail. Although no unequivocal answer can be yet given, this chapter reviews a range of evidence which suggests that the neuropathology of schizophrenia is asymmetrical, and considers the implications this has for the nature of the disorder. First, however, we discuss the normal anatomical cerebral asymmetries, since it need not be schizophrenia *per se* which is lateralized, but rather that the disorder affects these asymmetries.

Structural cerebral asymmetries

The frontal lobe is wider on the right than the left, with the occipital lobe showing the reverse pattern, a combination sometimes called (Yakovlevian) torque (LeMay, 1976; Le May and Kido, 1978; Weinberger *et al.*, 1982; Falkai *et al.*, 1995*b*). The right cerebral hemisphere is slightly larger than the left (von Bonin, 1962; Weis *et al.*, 1989; Kertesz *et al.*, 1990). In the context of these overall asymmetries, there are a number of localized left–right differences in cerebral structure and cytoarchitecture.

Planum temporale and superior temporal gyrus

The most robust cerebral asymmetry concerns the planum temporale (PT), a language-related region located on the upper surface of the posterior superior temporal gyrus (STG; Fig. 6.1; Harrison, 1995). The asymmetry was reported by Pfeiffer (1936) and expanded by Geschwind and Levitsky (1968) who showed that the length of the lateral border of the PT was longer on the left than the right in 65 of 100 adult brains. The asymmetry has been replicated in other autopsy series (Wada *et al.*, 1975; Galaburda *et al.*, 1987; Falkai *et al.*, 1995*a*) and *in vivo* with MRI (Steinmetz *et al.*, 1989, 1991; Foundas *et al.*, 1994; Barta *et al.*, 1997). Although some studies have failed to demonstrate left–right PT asymmetry (Steinmetz *et al.*, 1990; Witelson, 1991; Loftus *et al.*, 1993), its existence was confirmed in a recent systematic review which showed leftward asymmetry of the PT in

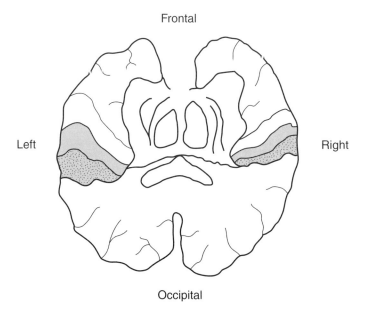

Fig. 6.1 Stylized horizontal section of the exposed upper surface of the temporal lobes, showing that the planum temporale (shaded) and the cytoarchitectonic subfield Tpt (stippled) are larger in the left than the right hemisphere.

78 per cent of people (a total of 1250 subjects), with an average laterality coefficient, defined as $2(R - L)/(R + L)$, of –0.32; the mean left–right difference in PT area (the paramater most commonly measured) being about 25 per cent (Shapleske *et al.*, 1999). In light of this robustness of evidence, the negative studies likely reflect methodological issues (e.g. imaging protocols, gender, handedness) as well as the problematic and variable definition of the PT (see Barta *et al.*, 1995; Shapleske *et al.*, 1999).

The cytoarchitectural basis of PT asymmetry has been localized to a region called Tpt (Fig. 6.1), an auditory association field which overlaps the posterior part of the STG and PT (Galaburda *et al.*, 1978). Tpt contains more small neurons in layer II on the left than the right (Holinger *et al.*, 1997).

Other temporal lobe asymmetries have been reported. The Sylvian fissure, which forms the boundary between the STG and the frontal and parietal opercula (and which includes the lateral PT border), is longer on the left side (LeMay and Culebras, 1972; LeMay, 1976; Rubens *et al.*, 1976; Steinmetz *et al.*, 1989; Falkai *et al.*, 1992). Not surprisingly, given the left > right size of several of its components, the STG overall may also be larger on the left than the right (Kulynych *et al.*, 1996). Additional cytoarchitectural asymmetries in the STG include a more prominent columnar clustering of neurons (Ong and Garey, 1990) and greater dendritic complexity (Seldon, 1982; Jacobs *et al.*, 1993; Anderson and Rutledge, 1996) in the left hemisphere.

Medial temporal lobe

Hippocampal neuronal number and packing density are symmetrical (Heckers *et al.*, 1991; Zaidel *et al.*, 1997*a*), but the size of neurons is larger in CA2 subfield on the left (Zaidel *et al.*, 1997*b*). A more subtle form of hippocampal asymmetry has also been reported: in the left hippocampus, neuronal density is positively correlated between different pairs of subfields, whereas no such correlations are seen in the right hippocampus (Zaidel *et al.*, 1993, 1995). It is speculated that these asymmetrical correlations are indexing lateralized differences in the organization of the hippocampal circuitry (Zaidel *et al.*, 1995). In the entorhinal cortex, a left-sided excess of pre-α neurons has been reported, albeit with marked individual variation (Heinsen *et al.*, 1994).

Frontal and parietal lobes

Asymmetries have long been demonstrated in the inferior frontal lobe (Eberstaller, 1890), which is larger on the left (Galaburda, 1980; Falzi *et al.*, 1982; Albanese *et al.*, 1989). A population of bigger pyramidal neurons were found in layer III of Brodmann's area 45 in the left hemisphere compared to the right (Hayes and Lewis, 1993, 1995), accompanied by left–right differences in the correlation between the somal size of a neuron and its dendritic arborization (Hayes and Lewis, 1996). These prefrontal asymmetries are, like their counterparts in STG, interpreted with reference to the language functions subserved by these regions. The primary motor cortex shows structural asymmetries which are putative correlates of handedness dominance, being larger on the left than the right (White *et al.*, 1994) and with a greater left-sided neuropil fraction (Amuts *et al.*, 1996, 1997). Moving medially, the anterior cingulate gyrus was reported in a small imaging study to be larger on the right (Albanese *et al.*, 1995), and a recent postmortem study of 40 brains revealed asymmetry of the cingulate sulcus, with a double sulcus commoner on the left than the right side (Ide *et al.*, 1999).

In the parietal lobe, angular gyrus area PG (Brodmann area 39) was found to be larger in the left compared to the right hemisphere (Eidelberg and Galaburda, 1984), an asymmetry which correlated positively with that of the PT. In contrast, area PEG, which is less clearly related to language, tended to be larger on the right, an asymmetry which did not correlate with PT or PG asymmetry. These findings suggest that functionally integrated areas share patterns of asymmetry (Galaburda, 1995). The study of Ide *et al.* (1999) mentioned above also reported asymmetries of parietal fissures.

Thalamus

Eidelberg and Galaburda (1982) reported a left > right size asymmetry for the lateralis posterior and medial geniculate thalamic nuclei, reflecting perhaps their close relationship to temporal lobe language areas. No left–right differences in volume or neuronal density have been found in the mediodorsal (Pakkenberg, 1992) and anterior (Danos *et al.*, 1998) nuclei, which connect primarily with prefrontal cortical areas.

Mechanisms of cerebral asymmetry

Proximate mechanism: cytoarchitectural differences

The proximate explanation for structural asymmetry resides in the cytoarchitecture of the region (Galaburda *et al.*, 1978). *A priori* the larger side of an asymmetrical structure might be due to (a) more neurons (or glia); or (b) the same number of neurons more widely spaced (i.e. a lower packing density). The latter would be accompanied by an increase in the amount of neuropil, in turn reflecting an excess of axons, dendrites, extracellular constituents, or vasculature (Chapter 11). Evidence from animal studies shows that most size asymmetry results from the first possibility, i.e. from changes in total cell number rather than cell packing density (Rosen *et al.*, 1991; Dehay *et al.*, 1993; Cowell *et al.*, 1999). This is perhaps to be expected, since packing density changes large enough to account for significant hemispheric differences would distort cytoarchitectonic appearance, precluding identification of homologous areas (Galaburda *et al.*, 1990).

Though predominant, neuronal number is not the only source of cytoarchitectural asymmetry. The larger side of an asymmetrical region was found to contain parvalbuminergic neurons that were more densely packed as well as being more numerous (Rosen *et al.*, 1993). Differences in cellular composition would suggest that the two sides of an asymmetrical region may differ in their intrinsic and extrinsic connectivity, as well as merely the amount of circuitry putatively dedicated to a particular function. There is also evidence for differences in interhemispheric connectivity between symmetrical and asymmetrical areas (Rosen *et al.*, 1989), consistent with a role for the corpus callosum in generation of asymmetries (Lent and Schmidt, 1993). A further question is whether the asymmetry comes mainly from the smaller or the larger side. The combined volumes of brain regions are greater in symmetrical rather than asymmetrical cases (Galaburda *et al.*, 1990). Moreover, total PT size (right + left) plotted against a directionless asymmetry measure resulted in a significant negative correlation, indicating that total PT area decreased as asymmetry increased (Galaburda *et al.*, 1987). These findings suggest that asymmetry arises from processes whereby the smaller side becomes smaller, though this remains to be shown empirically.

Distal mechanisms: genetic and environmental factors

Fronto-occipital torque is detectable by the 20th week of gestation (Weinberger *et al.*, 1982) and other asymmetries are present at or before term (Witelson and Pallie, 1973; Wada *et al.*, 1975; Chi *et al.*, 1977). Animal data support the interpretation that events early in corticogenesis (during the progenitor cell proliferation stage and/or cell death before birth of the first neuron) are important in formation of asymmetrical areas; that is, cell division and death of progenitor cells change the number of neuroblasts on the two sides (Rosen *et al.*, 1991; Rosen, 1996). Tritiated thymidine labelling studies show that neuroblasts do not divide more on the large side in order to contribute more neurons, nor is there evidence for differential cell death on one side. These findings together suggest that determination of neuronal number asymmetries takes place at the time when the original neuroblasts are assigned to the right and left sides of the midline. This begs the question how such an assignment is made and limited to areas destined to become asymmetrical; because of the early timing of the events, it is likely that the mechanisms are primarily genetic. The recent identification of genes regulating somatic asymmetry (Meno *et al.*, 1996; Isaac *et al.*, 1997) and growth of commissural axons (Kidd *et al.*, 1998) may prove relevant for elucidating genes responsible for cerebral asymmetry. The finding that situs inversus (reversed laterality of visceral position) is associated with reversed fronto-occipital torque gives impetus to this search (Kennedy *et al.*, 1999). Nevertheless, though the genetic contribution may be large, variation in PT asymmetry between monozygotic twins indicates a role for epigenetic and environmental factors (Steinmetz *et al.*, 1995).

Cerebral asymmetry in schizophrenia

Methodological issues

Only a few neuropathological studies of schizophrenia have been designed to address the question of asymmetry. Several methodological issues affect this area in addition to those affecting all neuropathological investigations of schizophrenia (Chapters 13 to 15), and contribute to the inconsistent data to be discussed.

Sampling

Some postmortem studies have only examined one hemisphere from each brain (reflecting the normal procedure in most neuropathology departments and brain banks). Clearly series which have used both hemispheres have considerable advantages, reducing interbrain variation and in some circumstances allowing paired statistical tests.

Statistical issues

The appropriate statistical test of the hypothesis that schizophrenia affects the two hemispheres of the brain differently is an analysis of variance to determine if there is a significant diagnosis-by-side interaction. Some studies have inferred asymmetrical effects from a right–left difference in the magnitude of an alteration, or on the basis of separate comparisons in each hemisphere in which one side reaches significance and the other does not. These are inconclusive demonstrations of lateralized pathology.

In other instances, it has been a matter of interpretation whether a set of data support the presence of a schizophrenia-associated asymmetry or not. This is illustrated by an MRI study of monozygotic twins discordant for schizophrenia. The authors concluded there was no clear difference between them in asymmetry of the temporal lobe (Suddath et al., 1990) or Sylvian fissure (Bartley et al., 1993), whereas the opposite conclusion was drawn by Crow et al. (1991) and Crow (1995; see also response by Weinberger et al., 1991).

Sex differences

Men tend to exhibit greater cerebral asymmetries than women (Bear et al., 1986; Kulynych et al., 1994). Ideally this requires that schizophrenia and control groups are sex-matched and/or that gender is factored into the statistical analysis—especially given data suggesting that males with schizophrenia show more brain abnormalities than females (Flaum et al., 1990). In practice this has rarely been carried out; in any event the size of most studies are inadequately powered to test three-way interactions of diagnosis, hemisphere, and sex (cf. Highley et al., 1998, 1999).

Other variables

Asymmetries can be affected by handedness (Kortesz et al., 1990; Steinmetz et al., 1991; Holinger et al., 1992; Foundas et al., 1995; Shapleske et al., 1999), language dominance (Charles et al., 1994; Foundas et al., 1996), genetic polymorphisms (Soininen et al., 1995), and even musical skills (Schlaug et al., 1995). Such information is rarely if ever available for postmortem studies. Age of onset of schizophrenia may also be a relevant factor (Maher et al., 1998).

With these caveats in mind, Table 6.1 summarizes the key neuropathological studies reporting asymmetrical findings in schizophrenia.

Fronto-occipital torque

Luchins et al. (1979) reported a reversal of the normal fronto-occipital torque in schizophrenia; i.e. patients had frontal lobes which were wider on the left and occipital lobes which were wider on the right. Subsequent imaging and postmortem studies of this index of cerebral asymmetry have had inconsistent results (see Falkai et al., 1995b; De Lisi et al., 1997). However, summation of the data available by 1994, a total of several hundred cases and controls, demonstrates a statistically significant reduction (rather than a reversal) of frontal and occipital asymmetries in schizophrenia (De Lisi et al., 1997). In addition, De Lisi et al. (1997) report a similar finding in a new MRI study, as did

Table 6.1 Key postmortem studies reporting lateralized neuropathological changes in schizophrenia[1]

	Region	Cases/controls	Findings in schizophrenia	Statistical approach to asymmetry
Superior temporal gyrus				
Crow et al., 1992	Sylvian fissure	?/?	Loss of L > R length asymmetry	Not stated
Falkai et al., 1992	Sylvian fissure	35/33	Loss of L > R length asymmetry	Diagnosis × side on ANOVA
Falkai et al., 1995a	PT	24/24	(a) Reduced PT asymmetry coefficient (b) PT shorter and smaller on left	MANOVA, ANOVA
Vogeley et al., 1998	STG	17/20	Decreased volume of middle part of left STG in females	No formal test[2]
Medial temporal lobe				
Brown et al., 1986	Temporal lobe	41/29	Decreased left parahippocampal width	Diagnosis × side on ANOVA
Crow et al., 1989	Lateral ventricle	22/26	Temporal horn enlarged on left	Diagnosis × side on ANOVA
Falkai & Bogerts, 1993	Entorhinal cortex	19/21	Heterotopic pre-α cell clusters (L > R)	Diagnosis × side on ANOVA
Zaidel et al., 1997a	Hippocampus	15/18	(a) Increased neuronal density in right CA3 and CA1 (b) Asymmetrical alteration of neuronal density correlations between subfields	Diagnosis × side on ANOVA Pearson coefficients
Zaidel et al., 1997b	Hippocampus	14/17	(a) Smaller neurons in left CA1 and CA2, right CA3 (b) Altered neuronal shape in left CA1, left subiculum, and right CA3	Diagnosis × side (× subfield) on ANOVA Diagnosis × side (× subfield) on ANOVA
McDonald et al., 2000	PHG and FG	31/27	Reversal of normal L>R asymmetry	ANCOVA, asymmetry coefficient
Other regions				
Albanese et al., 1995	Cingulate gyrus	7/7	Loss of normal R > L asymmetry	Laterality index
Blennow et al., 1996	Thalamus	19/39	Left-sided decrease of rab3a protein	No formal test[2]

[1] Additional references can be found in Falkai and Bogerts (1993).
[2] Inspection of data shows convincing asymmetrical change in schizophrenia.
L, left; R, right; FG, fusiform gyrus; PHG, parahippocampal gyrus; PT, posterior thalamus; STG, superior temporal gyrus.

Falkai *et al.* (1995*b*) using CT; finally, Bilder *et al.* (1994), using volumetric MRI, reported a loss of normal asymmetries in frontal and occipitoparietal regions in first-episode cases. Together the data fairly convincingly demonstrate reduced fronto-occipital torque in schizophrenia.

Planum temporale and superior temporal gyrus

A number of imaging studies have addressed whether PT asymmetry is altered in schizophrenia. The most striking results come from the Johns Hopkins group, who reported a reversal of PT surface area asymmetry in 14 cases compared to 14 controls (Petty *et al.*, 1995). They replicated this in an enlarged series (Barta *et al.*, 1997) but, to complicate matters, they found that the subjects had *bilateral* reductions in PT volume, and no correlation between the areal and volumetric indices; the authors suggest that this combination of findings may arise from changes in the convolution of the PT in schizophrenia. Other MRI studies of the PT in schizophrenia have shown weaker evidence of altered asymmetry, with a mixture of positive (Rossi *et al.*, 1992; Kwon *et al.*, 1999), equivocal (Bartley *et al.*, 1993; Rossi *et al.*, 1994; De Lisi *et al.*, 1997), and negative (Kleinschmidt *et al.*, 1994; Kulynych *et al.*, 1995; Jacobsen *et al.*, 1997) findings. The conflicting data may be attributed to variation in definition of the PT; the mixture of length, area, and volume measurements used (Barta *et al.* 1995); and the uncertain relationship between PT and STG changes (whether lateralized or not) in schizophrenia (Kulynych *et al.*, 1996). Three postmortem studies of PT each found evidence for reduced PT asymmetry in schizophrenia (Table 6.1), either measured in terms of Sylvian fissure length (Crow *et al.*, 1992; Falkai *et al.*, 1992), or by reconstruction of PT volume (Falkai *et al.*, 1995*a*). Having considered all the data, Shapleske *et al.* (1999) conclude that 'patients with schizophrenia show a reliable loss of PT asymmetry', with a mean laterality coefficient of –0.04 (cf. - 0.32 in controls mentioned earlier). The loss is attributed to enlargement of the right PT.

Only one cytoarchitectural study of the PT in schizophrenia has been carried out; it found bilateral decreases in neuronal density in Tpt, with no evidence for a lateralized effect (Holinger *et al.*, 1995, 1997). Given the observations described in the previous paragraph, it will be of interest also to determine the cortical thickness and total neuron number in Tpt in schizophrenia.

It is unclear whether the STG as a whole shows lateralized size changes in schizophrenia. Left-sided decreases (Shenton *et al.*, 1992) and a reversal of the normal STG asymmetry (Pearlson *et al.*, 1997) have been reported, but others have identified bilateral reductions (Barta *et al.*, 1990; Holinger *et al.*, 1999) or no change (Flaum *et al.*, 1995; Kulynych *et al.*, 1996; see Table 13.7 in Chapter 13). The inconsistencies may result from a relationship between the STG and thought disorder (Shenton *et al.*, 1992), auditory hallucinations (Barta *et al.*, 1990), and handedness (Holinger *et al.*, 1999) rather than with schizophrenia itself (Menon *et al.*, 1995). There may also be focal and gender-related decrements in STG volume (Vogeley *et al.*, 1998). There have been no histological investigations of the STG in schizophrenia apart from the PT study mentioned above.

Medial temporal lobe

In contrast to the STG, there have been a large number of postmortem studies of the medial temporal lobe in schizophrenia (Chapter 3), albeit few which have investigated asymmetry meaningfully. Those which have are listed in Table 6.1. The finding of left-sided enlargement of the temporal horn of the lateral ventricle (Crow *et al.*, 1989) has been especially influential (see below). Corresponding findings of decreased size of some or all left medial temporal lobe components have been reported in some MRI studies (Bogerts *et al.*, 1990*a*; Shenton *et al.*, 1992; Kawasaki *et al.*, 1993; Pearlson *et al.*, 1997; Velakulis *et al.*, 1999), but other studies report symmetrical changes (e.g. Altshuler *et al.*, 1990; Bogerts *et al.*, 1990*b*; see also Table 13.6 in Chapter 13).

Evidence for asymmetrical histological changes in medial temporal lobe is sparse. Zaidel and colleagues reported diagnosis-by-side interactions for neuronal density (Zaidel *et al.*, 1997*a*), neuronal size and neuronal shape (Zaidel *et al.*, 1997*b*) in some hippocampal subfields. Since these data reveal lateralized abnormalities affecting both hippocampi, they are not in keeping with a pathological process favoring one side, but instead suggest an alteration in the circuitry of, and perhaps between, medial temporal lobes. Other reports suggesting lateralized histological changes in this region are statistically unconvincing (Jakob and Beckmann, 1986; Jeste and Lohr, 1989).

Other regions

There are few neuropathological data concerning altered asymmetry outside the temporal lobe in schizophrenia (Table 6.1), and a notable absence of studies in lateral prefrontal regions despite their normal asymmetries and putative involvement in the pathophysiology of schizophrenia. The results of Blennow *et al.* (1996) suggest that asymmetrical changes in schizophrenia may extend to the thalamus, affecting left thalamocortical or corticothalamic pathways. However, two stereological studies have found symmetrical reductions of thalamic neurons in schizophrenia, leaving the matter unresolved (Pakkenberg, 1992; Danos *et al.*, 1998).

Other forms of asymmetry in schizophrenia

Studies of asymmetry in schizophrenia have not been limited to structural measures. Table 6.2 lists examples of studies reporting lateralized differences affecting other parameters (reviewed in Cowell *et al.*, 1999; Gur and Chin, 1999; Petty, 1999; Satz and Green, 1999). As with the structural pathology, however, other studies have not found altered asymmetry in these indices in schizophrenia, and the presence of left–right differences in normal subjects must again be taken into account.

Explanation for altered asymmetries in schizophrenia

Altered cerebral asymmetry in schizophrenia has been explained in two ways, which have very different implications for the nature of the disorder.

Table 6.2 Examples of non-structural lateralized changes reported in schizophrenia

Approach	Reference	Finding in schizophrenia
Neurochemistry		
Dopamine content	Reynolds 1983	Left-sided amygdala increase
Kainate receptors	Kerwin et al., 1988	Left-sided hippocampal decrease
Forskolin binding	Kerwin & Beats 1990	Left-sided hippocampal decrease
GABA uptake	Reynolds et al., 1990	Left-sided hippocampal decrease
G protein α subunits	Yang et al., 1998	Left-sided STG decrease
Functional imaging		
^{31}P spectroscopy	Deicken et al., 1995	Left-sided temporal lobe decrease
^{1}H spectroscopy	Deicken et al., 1997	Left-sided frontal lobe decrease of N-accetylaspartate
Electrophysiology		
P300 wave	Faux et al., 1987; Holinger et al., 1992	Left-sided voltage reduction[1]
Neuropsychology		
Tachistoscopic tasks	Gur 1978	Left-sided dysfunction and overactivation
Language	Taylor et al., 1979	Impairment on putative left hemisphere tests
Attention	Carter et al., 1996	Left-sided deficit
Memory	Gruzelier et al., 1988	Impairment on putative left temporohippocampal tasks
Dichotic listening	Løberg et al., 1999	Loss of normal right ear advantage
Miscellaneous		
Handedness	Crow et al., 1996	More ambiguous handedness in pre-schizophrenics
Motor function	Lohr & Cagliuri 1997	R > L hand force instability
Olfactory identification	Good et al., 1998	Left nostril deficit in males

[1] Similar findings reported by several other authors.
STG, superior temporal gyrus.

A manifestation of asymmetrical brain development

One proposal is that altered cerebral asymmetry in schizophrenia is a manifestation of the disorder's neurodevelopmental origin. In this respect the disease process need not be asymmetrical, but merely one which hinders subsequent maturation in a way which alters the pattern of asymmetries in the adult (Bracha, 1991; Roberts, 1991). Since cerebral asymmetries are apparent before birth (see above), this proposal is consonant with the timing at which the pathology of schizophrenia is generally considered to originate (Chapter 8). In passing, the anatomical hypothesis that schizophrenia is a disorder of heteromodal association cortex is in keeping with a developmental explanation of altered asymmetry in schizophrenia, since such cortical regions are the most lateralized (Ross and Pearlson, 1996).

This developmental view of asymmetry has two implications in the current context. Firstly, altered asymmetry has only an epiphenomenal role in the aetiology of schizophrenia, though its consequences may still be critical for its phenomenology and pathophysiology. Secondly, other disorders of early neurodevelopment might be expected also to be associated with aberrant asymmetry. The study of dyslexia has proved valuable, with several studies showing decreased cerebral asymmetry and histological left–right differences (Galaburda, 1993; cf. Rumsey *et al.*, 1997). Moreover, when cortical malformations, such as microgyria, are induced in laboratory rats, changes occur in anatomical asymmetry and inter- and intrahemispheric connectivity (Herman *et al.*, 1997), suggesting that various forms of developmental lesion may compromise formation of cerebral asymmetry.

Whether altered asymmetry is specific to schizophrenia is also raised with regard to other psychotic disorders. The few data suggest asymmetry is not affected in bipolar disorder (Pearlson *et al.*, 1997); for autism the data are unclear (Lotspeich and Ciaranello, 1993).

Schizophrenia as a disorder of the cerebral asymmetry gene

The alternative theory postulates a specific, causal link between altered cerebral asymmetry and schizophrenia (Crow, 1984, 1990, 1995, 1997). It arose from neuropathological, genetic, and epidemiological considerations and has two key premises. Firstly, schizophrenia is a uniquely human disorder and its cause is to be found in the evolutionary change which characterizes the species—language—and its structural correlate, cerebral asymmetry. Altered asymmetry is therefore a cardinal feature of the disorder. Secondly, cerebral asymmetry and schizophrenia are attributable to one and the same gene, putatively located in the X–Y homologous region.

The neuropathological evidence for altered asymmetry is integral to the theory, which had its roots in the finding of left-sided temporal horn changes in schizophrenia (Brown *et al.*, 1986; Crow *et al.*, 1989). The theory predicted in 1989 that 'asymmetry of structural change in schizophrenia will prove to be a general finding' and that 'diagnosis-by-side interactions will be seen; failure to detect such interactions constitutes evidence against the proposal' (Crow *et al.*, 1989). As the current review indicates, the data as a whole provide considerable but incomplete support for these predictions and hence the theory remains neuropathologically speculative. Nevertheless, it has been a major stimulus to research in this field over the past decade, and it continues to be influential—indeed, there are no other comparable hypotheses which integrate the genetic and neuropathological data—and under active investigation.

Conclusions

We have reviewed the evidence for asymmetry in the neuropathology of schizophrenia. There are noteworthy positive studies as well as important equivocal and negative ones. Due to their heterogeneity it is not possible to do a meta-analysis to determine if altered cerebral asymmetry has unequivocally been demonstrated in schizophrenia. Nevertheless, despite the inconsistencies, there is enough evidence to make this a reasonable if tentative conclusion, especially for decreased fronto-occipital torque and decreased PT asymmetry.

The difficulty establishing firmly whether the pathology of schizophrenia is lateralized arises for two main reasons. Firstly, the structural basis of schizophrenia and cerebral asymmetry are both subtle. Demonstrating their interaction is therefore a difficult process with a low signal-to-noise ratio. Secondly, there are limitations to the normative data. Whilst it is clear that asymmetries exist in several areas, their extent and the effects of other factors such as gender and handedness remain poorly understood. Meanwhile, attempts to explain the origins and consequences of aberrant asymmetry in schizophrenia are hampered by the lack of information about the determinants of lateralization and the functional correlates of anatomical asymmetry. Progress in this intriguing aspect of schizophrenia will only come, therefore, from a combination of improved methodologies and greater understanding of the processes involved in cerebral asymmetry itself.

References

Albanese, E., Merlo, A., Albanese, A. and Gomez, E. (1989) Anterior speed region: Asymmetry and weight–surface correlations. *Archives of Neurology*, **47**, 379–380.

Albanese, A. M., Merlo, A. B., Mascitti T. A., Tornese, E., Konopka, V. and Albanese, E. F. (1995) Inversion of the hemispheric laterality of the anterior cingulate gyrus in schizophrenics. *Biological Psychiatry*, **38**, 13–21.

Altshuler, L. L., Casanova, MF., Goldberg, T. E. and Kleinman, J. E. (1990) The hippocampus and parahippocampus in schizophrenic, suicide and control brains. *Archives of General Psychiatry*, **47**, 1029–1034.

Amuts, K., Schlaug, G., Schleicher, A. *et al.* (1996) Asymmetry in the human motor cortex and handedness. *Neuroimage*, **4**, 216–222.

Amuts, K., Schmidt-Passos, F., Schleicher, A. and Zilles, K. (1997) Postnatal development of interhemispheric asymmetry in the cytoarchitecture of human area 4. *Anatomy and Embryology*, **196**, 393–402.

Anderson, B. and Rutledge, V. (1996) Age and hemisphere effects on dendritic structure. *Brain*, **119**, 1983–1990.

Barta, P. E., Pearlson, G. D., Powers, R. E., Richards, S. S. and Tune, L. E. (1990) Auditory hallucinations and smaller superior temporal gyral volume in schizophrenia. *American Journal of Psychiatry*, **147**, 1457–1462

Barta, P. E., Petty, R. G., McGilchrist, I. *et al.* (1995) Asymmetry of the planum temporale: methodological considerations and clinical associations. *Psychiatry Research Neuroimaging*, **61**, 137–150.

Barta, P. E., Pearlson, G. D., Brill II, L. B. *et al.* (1997) Planum temporale asymmetry reversal in schizophrenia: Replication and relationship to gray matter abnormalities. *American Journal of Psychiatry*, **154**, 661–667.

Bartley, A. J., Jones, D. W., Torrey, E. F., Zigun, J. R. and Weinberger, D. R. (1993) Sylvian fissure asymmetries in monozygotic twins: A test of laterality in schizophrenia. *Biological Psychiatry*, **34**, 853–863.

Bear, D., Schiff, D., Saver, J., Greenberg, M. and Freeman, R. (1986) Quantitative analysis of cerebral asymmetries: Fronto-occipital correlation, sexual dimorphism and association with handedness. *Archives of Neurology*, **43**, 598–603.

Bilder, R. M., Wu, H., Bogerts, B. *et al.* (1994) Absence of regional hemispheric volume asymmetries in first-episode schizophrenia. *American Journal of Psychiatry*, **151**, 1437–1447.

Blennow, K., Davidsson, P., Gottfries, C-G., Ekman, R. and Heilig, M. (1996) Synaptic degeneration in thalamus in schizophrenia. *Lancet,* **348**, 692–693.

Bogerts, B., Ashtari, M., Gustav, D. *et al.* (1990*a*) Reduced temporal limbic structure volumes on magnetic resonance images in first episode schizophrenia. *Psychiatry Research*: *Neuroimaging,* **35**, 1–13.

Bogerts, B., Falkaie, P., Haupts, M. *et al.* (1990*b*) Post-mortem volume measurements of limbic system and basal ganglia structures in chronic schizophrenics: Initial results from a new brain collection. *Schizophrenia Research*, **3**, 295–301.

Bracha, H. S. (1991) Etiology of structural asymmetry in schizophrenia: An alternative hypothesis. *Schizophrenia Bulletin,* **17**, 551–553.

Broca, P. (1861) Remarques sur le siege de la faculte du langugage articule, suivies d'une observation d'aphemie. *Bulletin for the Society of Anatomy*, **6**, 137–146.

Brown, R., Colter, N., Corsellis, J. A. *et al.* (1986) Post mortem evidence of structural brain changes in schizophrenia. *Archives of General Psychiatry*, **43**, 36–42.

Carter, C. S., Robertson, L., Nordahi, T., Chaderjian, M. and Oshora-Celaya J. (1996) Perceptual and attentional asymmetries in schizophrenia: further evidence for a left hemisphere deficit. *Psychiatry Research*, **62**, 111–119.

Charles, P. D., Abou-Khalil, R., Abou-Khalil, B. *et al.* (1994) MRI asymmetries and language dominance. *Neurology*, **44**, 2050–2054.

Chi, J. G., Dooling, E. C. and Gilles, F. H. (1977) Left–right asymmetries of the temporal speech areas of the human fetus. *Archives of Neurology*, **34**, 346–348.

Cowell, P. E., Fitch, R. H. and Denenburg, V. H. (1999) Laterality in animals: relevance to schizophrenia. *Schizophrenia Bulletin,* **25**, 41–62.

Crichton Browne, J. (1879) On the weight of the brain and its component parts in the insane. *Brain*, **2**, 42–67.

Crow, T. J. (1984) A re-evaluation of the viral hypothesis: is psychosis the result of retroviral integration at a site close to the cerebral dominance gene? *British Journal of Psychiatry*, **145**, 243–253.

Crow, T. J. (1990) Temporal lobe asymmetries as the key to the etiology of schizophrenia. *Schizophrenia Bulletin*, **16**, 433–443.

Crow, T. J. (1995) The relationship between morphologic and genetic findings in schizophrenia: An evolutionary perspective. In: Fog, R., Gerlach J. and Hemmingsen, R., Eds. *Schizophrenia. Alfred Benzon Symposium 38.* Munksgaard, Copenhagen, pp. 15–25.

Crow, T. J. (1997) Schizophrenia as failure of hemispheric dominance for language. *Trends in Neurosciences,* **20**, 339–343.

Crow, T. J., Ball, J., Bloom, S. *et al.* (1989) Schizophrenia as an anomaly of development of cerebral asymmetry. *Archives of General Psychiatry,* **46**, 1145–1150.

Crow, T. J., Frith, C. D., Johnstone, E. C., Owens, D. G. C., Roberts, G. W. and Colter, N. (1991) Crow's 'lateralization hypothesis' for schizophrenia. *Archives of General Psychiatry,* **48**, 86–87.

Crow, T. J., Brown, R., Bruton, C. J., Frith, C. D. and Gray, V. (1992) Loss of sylvian fissure asymmetry in schizophrenia: findigs in the Runwell 2 series of brains. *Schizophrenia Research,* **6**, 152–153.

Crow, T. J., Done, D. J. and Sacker, A. (1996) Cerebral lateralization is delayed in children who later develop schizophrenia. *Schizophrenia Research,* **22**, 181–185.

Danos, P., Baumann, B., Bernstein, H.-G. *et al.* (1998) Schizophrenia and anteroventral thalamic nucleus: selective decrease of parvalbumin-immunoreactive thalamocortical projection neurons. *Psychiatry Research Neuroimaging,* **82**, 1–10.

Dehay, C., Giroud, P., Berland, M., Smart, L. and Kennedy, H. (1993) Modulation of the cell cycle contributes to the parcellation of the primate visual cortex. *Nature,* **366**, 464–466.

Deicken, R. F., Calabrese, Merrin, E. L., Vinogradov, S., Fein, G. and Weiner, M. W. (1995) Asymmetry of temporal lobe phosphorous metabolism in schizophrenia. A 31phosphorous magnetic resonance spectroscopic imaging study. *Biological Psychiatry,* **38**, 279–286.

Deiken R. F., Zhou, L., Corwin, F., Vinogradov, S. and Weiner, M. W. (1997) Decreased left frontal lobe *N*-acetylaspartate in schizophrenia. *American Journal of Psychiatry,* **154**, 688–690.

DeLisi, L. E., Sakuma, M., Kishner, M., Finer, D. L., Hoff, A. L. and Crow, T. J. (1997) Anomalous cerebral asymmetry and language processing in schizophrenia. *Schizophrenia Bulletin,* **23**, 255–271.

Eberstaller, O. (1890) *Das stirnhirn. Ein beitrag zur anatomie der oberfläche des gehirns.* Urban & Schwarzenberg, Vienna.

Eidelberg, D. and Galaburda, A. M. (1982) Symmetry and asymmetry in the human posterior thalamus. Cytoarchitectonic analysis in normal persons. *Archives of Neurology,* **39**, 325–332.

Eidelberg, D. and Galaburda, A. M. (1984) Inferior parietal lobule. Divergent architectonic asymmetries in the human brain. *Archives of Neurology,* **41**, 843–852.

Falkai, P. and Bogerts, B. (1993) Cytoarchitectonic and developmental studies in schizophrenia. In: Kerwin, R. W., ed. *Neurobiology and psychiatry,* Volume 2. Cambridge University Press, Cambridge, pp. 43–70.

Falkai, P., Bogerts, B., Greve, B. *et al.* (1992) Loss of sylvian fissure asymmetry in schizophrenia. A quantitative post mortem study. *Schizophrenia Research,* **7**, 23–32.

Falkai, P., Bogerts, B., Schneider, T. *et al.* (1995*a*) Disturbed planum temporale asymmetry in schizophrenia. A quantitative post-mortem study. *Schizophrenia Research,* **14**, 161–176.

Falkai, P, Schneider, T., Greve, B., Klieser, E. and Bogerts, B. (1995*b*) Reduced frontal and occipital lobe asymmetry on the CT scans of schizophrenic patients. Its specificity and clinical significance. *Journal of Neural Transmission (General Section),* **99**, 63–77.

Falzi, G., Perrone, P. and Vignolo, L. A. (1982) Right–left asymmetry in anterior speech region. *Archives of Neurology,* **39**, 239–240.

Faux, S. F., Torello, M., McCarley, R. W., Shenton, M. E. and Duffy, F. H. (1987) P300 topographic alterations in schizophrenia: A replication study. *Electroencephalography and Clinical Neurophysiology,* **40**, 688–694.

Flaum, M., Arndt, S. and Andreasen, N. C. (1990) The role of gender in studies of ventricle enlargement in schizophrenia: A predominantly male effect. *American Journal of Psychiatry,* **147**, 1327–1332.

Flaum, M., Swayze, V. W., O'Leary, D. S. *et al.* (1995) Effects of diagnosis, laterality, and gender on brain morphology in schizophrenia. *American Journal of Psychiatry,* **152**, 704–714.

Flor-Henry, P. (1969) Psychosis and temporal lobe epilepsy. A controlled investigation. *Epilepsia,* **10**, 363–395.

Foundas, A. L., Leonard, C. M., Gilmore, R., Fennell, E. and Heilman, K. M. (1994) Planum temporale asymmetry and language dominace. *Neuropsychologia,* **32**, 1225–1231.

Foundas A. L., Leonard, C. M. and Heilman, K. M. (1995) Morphologic cerebral asummetries and handedness: the pars triangularis and planum temporale. *Archives of Neurology,* **52**, 501–508.

Foundas, A. L., Leonard, C. M., Gilmore, R. L., Fennell, E. B. and Heilman, K. M. (1996) Pars triangularis asymmetry and language dominance. *Proceedings of the National Academy of Sciences USA,* **93**, 719–722.

Galaburda, A. M. (1980) La règion de Broca: Observations anatomiques faites un siècle après la mort de son découvreur. *Revue Neurologique,* **136**, 609–616.

Galaburda, A. M. (1993) Neuroanatomic basis of developmental dyslexia. *Neurology Clinics,* **11**, 161–173.

Galaburda, A. M. (1995) Anatomic basis of cerebral dominance. In: Davidson, R. J. and Hugdahl, K., eds. *Brain asymmetry.* MIT Press, Cambridge, MA, pp. 51–73.

Galaburda, A. M., Sanides, F. and Geschwind, N. (1978) Human brain: Cytoarchitectonic left right asymmetries in the temporal speech region. *Archives of Neurology,* **35**, 812–817.

Galaburda, A. M., Corsiglia., J., Rosen, G. D. and Sherman, G. F. (1987) Planum temporale asymmetry: Reappraisal since Geschwind and Levitsky. *Neuropsychologia,* **25**, 853–868.

Galaburda, A. M., Rosen, G. D. and Sherman, G. F. (1990) Individual variability in cortical organization: its relationship to brain laterality and implications to function. *Neuropsychologia,* **28**, 529–546.

Geschwind, N. and Levitsky, W. (1968) Human brain: Left–right asymmetries in temporal speech region. *Science,* **161**, 186–187.

Good, K. P., Martzke, J. S., Honer, W. G. and Kopala, L. C. (1998) Left nostril olfactory identification impairment in a subgroup of male patients with schizophrenia. *Schizophrenia Research*, **33**, 35–43.

Gruzelier, J., Seymour, K., Wilson, L., Jolley, A. and Hirsch, S. (1988) Impairments on neuropsychological tests of temporohippocampal and frontohipppocampal functions and word fluency in remitting schizophrenia and affective disorders. *Archives of General Psychiatry*, **45**, 623–629.

Gur, R. E. (1978) Left hemisphere dysfunction and left hemisphere overactivation in schizophrenia. *Journal of Abnormal Psychology,* **87***, 226–238.*

Gur, R. E. and Chin, S. (1999) Laterality in functional brain imaging studies of schizophrenia. *Schizophrenia Bulletin*, **25**, 141–156.

Harris, L. J. (1999) Early theory and research on hemispheric specialization. *Schizophrenia Bulletin*, **25**, 11–39.

Harrison, P. J. (1995) Cerebral asymmetry. In: Williams, P. L. *et al.*, eds. *Gray's anatomy*, 38th edition. Churchill Livingstone, Edinburgh, pp. 1183–1186.

Hayes, T. L. and Lewis, D. A. (1993) Hemispheric differences in layer III pyramidal neurons of the anterior language area. *Archives of Neurology*, **50**, 501–505.

Hayes, T.L and Lewis, D. A. (1995) Anatomical specialization of the anterior motor speech area: hemispheric differences in magnopyramidal neurons. *Brain and Language*, **49**, 289–308.

Hayes, T. L. and Lewis, D. A. (1996) Magnopyramidal neurons in the anterior motor speech region. Dendritic features and interhemispheric comparisons. *Archives of Neurology,* **53**, 1277–1283.

Heckers, S., Heinsen, H., Geiger, B. and Beckmann, H. (1991) Hippocampal neuron number in schizophrenia. A stereological study. *Archives of General Psychiatry*, **48**, 1002–1008.

Heinsen, H., Henn, R., Eisenmenger, W. *et al.* (1994) Quantitative investigations on the human entorhinal area: Left–right asymmetry and age-related changes. *Anatomy and Embryology,* **190**, 181–194.

Herman, A. E., Galaburda, A. M., Fitch, R. H., Carter, A. R. and Rosen, G. D. (1997) Cerebral microgyria, thalamic cell size and auditory temporal processing in male and female rats. *Cerebral Cortex,* **7**, 453–464.

Highley, J. R., Esiri, M. M., McDonald, B. *et al.* (1998) Anomalies of cerebral asymmetry in schizophrenia interact with gender and age of onset: a post-mortem study. *Schizophrenia Research*, **34**, 13–25.

Highley, J. R., Esiri, M. M., McDonald, B., Cortina-Borja, M., Herron, B. and Crow, T. J. (1999) The size and fibre composition of the corpus callosum with respect to gender and schizophrenia: a post-mortem study. *Brain,* **122**, 99–110.

Holinger, D. P., Faux, S. F., Shenton, M. E. *et al.* (1992) Reversed temporal region asymmetries of P300 topography in left- and right-handed schizophrenic subjects. *Electroencephalography and Clinical Neurophysiology*, **84**, 532–537.

Holinger, D. P., Rosen, G. D. and Galaburda, A. M. (1995) Decreased neuronal density in supragranular layers of area Tpt of the superior temporal gyrus of schizophrenics. *Society for Neuroscience Abstracts,* **21**, 238.

Holinger, D. P., Mori, C. and Galaburda, A. M. (1997) Schizophrenia: Neuronal measures in left and right language and visual cortices. *Society for Neuroscience Abstracts,* **23**, 2198.

Holinger D. P., Shenton, M. E., Wible, C. G. *et al.* (1999) Superior temporal gyrus abnormalities and thought disorder in left-handed schizophrenic males. *American Journal of Psychiatry,* **156**, 1730–1735.

Ide, A., Dolezal, C., Fernandez, M. *et al.* (1999) Hemispheric differences in variability of fissural patterns in parasylvian and cingulate regions of human brains. *Journal of Comparative Neurology,* **410**, 235–242.

Isaac, A., Sargent, M. G. and Cooke, J (1997) Control of vertebrate left-right asymmetry by a snail-related zinc finger gene. *Science,* **275**, 1301–1304.

Jacobs, B., Schall, M. and Scheibel, A. B. (1993) A quantitative dendritic analysis of Wernicke's area in humans. II. Gender, hemispheric, and environmental factors. *Journal of Comparative Neurology,* **327**, 97–111.

Jacobsen, L. K., Giedd, J. N., Tanrikut, C. *et al.* (1997) Three-dimensional cortical morphometry of the planum temporale in childhood-onset schizophrenia. *American Journal of Psychiatry,* **154**, 685–687.

Jakob, H. and Beckmann, H. (1986) Prenatal developmental disturbances in the limbic allocortex in schizophrenics. *Journal of Neural Transmission,* **65**, 303–326.

Jeste, D. V. and Lohr, J. B. (1989) Hippocampal pathologic findings in schizophrenia. A morphometric study. *Archives of General Psychiatry,* **46**, 1019–1024.

Kawasaki, Y., Maeda, Y, Urata, K. *et al.* (1993) A quantitative magnetic resonance imaging study of patients with schizophrenia. *European Archives of Psychiatry and Clinical Neuroscience,* **242**, 268–272.

Kennedy, D. N., O'Craven, K. K., Ticho, B. S., Goldstein A. M., Makris, N. and Henson, J. W. (1999) Structural and functional brain asymmetries in human situs inversus totalis. *Neurology,* **53**, 1260–1265.

Kertesz. A., Polk, M., Black, S. E. and Howell, J. (1990) Sex, handedness, and the morphometry of cerebral asymmetries on magnetic resonance imaging. *Brain Research,* **530**, 40–48.

Kerwin, R. W. and Beats, B. C. (1990) Increased forskolin binding in the left parahippocampal gyrus and CA1 region in post mortem schizophrenic brain determined by quantitative autoradiography. *Neuroscience Letters,* **118**, 164–168.

Kerwin, R. W., Patel, S., Meldrum, B. S., Czudek, C. and Reynolds, G. P. (1988) Asymmetrical loss of glutamate receptor subtype in left hippocampus in schizophrenia. *Lancet,* **i**, 583–584.

Kidd, T., Brose, K., Mitchell, K. J. *et al.* (1998) Roundabout controls axon crossing of the CNS midline and defines a novel subfamily of evolutionarily conserved guidance receptors. *Cell,* **92**, 205–215.

Kleinschmidt, A., Falkai, P., Huang, Y., Schneider, T., Furst, G. and Steinmetz, H. (1994) *In vivo* morphometry of planum temporale asymmetry in first-episode schizophrenia. *Schizophrenia Research,* **12**, 9–18.

Kulynych, J. J., Vladar, K., Jones, D. W. and Weinberger, D. R. (1994) Gender differences in the normal lateralization of the supratemporal cortex: MRI surface-rendering morphometry of Heschl's gyrus and the planum temporale. *Cerebral Cortex,* **4**, 107–118.

Kulynych, J. J., Katalin, V., Bryan, D., Fantie Jones, D. W. Q. and Weinberger, D. R. (1995) Normal asymmetry of the planum temporale in patients with schizophrenia: three-demi-nensional cortical morphometry with MRI. *British Journal of Psychiatry,* **166**, 742–749.

Kulynych, J. J., Vladar, K., Jones, D. and Weinberger, D. R. (1996) Superior temporal gyrus volume in schizophrenia: A study using MRI morphometry assisted by surface rendering. *American Journal of Psychiatry,* **153**, 50–56.

Kwon, J. S., McCarley, R. W., Hirayasu, Y. *et al.* (1999) Left planum temporale volume reduction in schizophrenia. *Archives of General Psychiatry,* **56**, 142–148.

LeMay, M. (1976) Morphological cerebral asymmetries of modern man, fossil man, and nonhuman primate. *Annals of New York Academy of Sciences,* **280**, 349–366.

LeMay, M. and Culebras, A. (1972) Human brain—morphological differences in the hemispheres demonstrable by carotid arteriography. *New England Journal of Medicine,* **287**, 168–170.

LeMay, M. and Kido, D. K. (1978) Asymmetries of cerebral hemispheres on computed tomograms. *Journal of Computer Assisted Tomography,* **2**, 471–476.

Lent, R. and Schmidt, S. L. (1993) The ontogenesis of the forebrain commissures and the determination of brain asymmetries. *Progress in Neurobiology,* **40**, 249–276.

Løberg, E.-M., Hugdahl, H. and Green, M. F. (1999) Hemispheric asymmetry in schizophrenia: A 'dual-deficits' model. *Biological Psychiatry,* **45**, 76–81.

Loftus, W. C., Tramo, M., Thomas, C., Green, R., Nordgern, R. and Gazzaniga, M. S. (1993) Three-dimensional quantitative analysis of hemispheric asymmetry in the human superior temporal region. *Cerebral Cortex,* **3**, 348–355.

Lohr, J. B., Caligiuri, M. P. (1997) Lateralized hemispheric dysfunction in the major psychotic disorders: historical perspectives and findings from a study of motor asymmetry in older patients. *Schizophrenia Research,* **27**, 191–198.

Lotspeich, L. J. and Ciaranello, R. D. (1993) The neurobiology and genetics of infantile autism. *International Review of Neurobiology,* **35**, 87–129.

Luchins, D. J., Weinberger, D. R. and Wyatt, R. J. (1979) Schizophrenia: evidence of a subgroup with reversed cerebral asymmetry. *Archives of General Psychiatry,* **36**, 1309–1311.

McDonald, B., Highley, R., Walker, M. A. *et al.* (2000) Anomalous asymmetry of fusiform and parahippocampal gyrus gray matter in schizophrenia: a postmortem study. *American Journal of Psychiatry,* **157**, 40–47.

Maher, B. A., Manschreck, T. C., Yurgelun-Todd, D. A. and Tsuang, M. T. (1998) Hemispheric asymmetry of frontal and temporal gray matter and age of onset in schizophrenia. *Biological Psychiatry,* **44**, 413–417.

Meno, C., Saijoh, Y., Fujii, H. *et al.* (1996). Left–right asymmetric expression of the TGF family member lefty in mouse embryos. *Nature,* **381**, 151–155.

Menon, R. R., Barta, P. E., Aylward, E. H. *et al.* (1995) Posterior superior temporal gyrus in schizophrenia: Grey matter changes and clinical correlates. *Schizophrenia Research,* **16**, 127–135.

Ong, W. Y. and Garey, L. J. (1990) Neuronal architecture of the human temporal cortex. *Anatomy and Embryology,* **181**, 351–364.

Pakkenberg, B. (1992) The volume of the mediodorsal thalamic nucleus in treated and untreated schizophrenics. *Schizophrenia Research,* **7**, 95–100.

Pearlson, G. D., Barta, P. E., Powers, R. E. *et al.* (1997) Medial and superior temporal gyral volumes and cerebral asymmetry in schizophrenia versus bipolar disorder. *Biological Psychiatry*, **41**, 1–14.

Petty, R. G. (1999) Structural asymmetries of the human brain and their disturbance in schizophrenia. *Schizophrenia Bulletin*, **25**, 121–139.

Petty, R. G., Barta, P. E., Pearlson, G. D. *et al.* (1995) Reversal of asymmetry of the planum temporale in schizophrenia. *American Journal of Psychiatry*, **152**, 715–721.

Pfeiffer, R. A. (1936) Pathologie der Horstrahlung und der corticalen Horsphare. In: Blumke, O. and Foerster, O., eds. *Handbuch der Neurologie*, Springer, Berlin.

Reynolds, G. P. (1983) Increased concentrations and lateral asymmetry of amygdala dopamine in schizophrenia. *Nature*, **305**, 527–529.

Reynolds, G. P., Czudek, C. and Andrews, H. B. (1990) Deficit and hemispheric asymmetry of GABA uptake sites in the hippocampus in schizophrenia. *Biological Psychiatry*, **27**, 1038–1044.

Roberts, G. W. (1991) Schizophrenia. A neuropathological perspective. *British Journal of Psychiatry*, **158**, 8–17.

Rosen, G. D. (1996) Morphometric, ontogenetic and connnectional substrates of anatomical asymmetry. *Neuroscience and Biobehavioral Reviews*, **20**, 607–615.

Rosen, G. D., Sherman, G. F. and Galaburda, A. M. (1989) Interhemispheric connections differ between symmetrical and asymmetrical brain regions. *Neuroscience*, **33**, 525–533.

Rosen, G. D., Sherman, G. F. and Galaburda, A. M. (1991) Ontogenesis of neocortical asymmetry: a [³H] thymidine study. *Neuroscience*, **41**, 779–790.

Rosen, G. D., Sherman, G. F. and Galaburda, A. M. (1993) Neuronal subtypes and anatomic asymmetry: Changes in neuronal number and cell-packing density. *Neuroscience*, **56**, 833–839.

Ross, C. A. and Pearlson, G. D. (1996) Schizophrenia, the heteromodal association neocortex and development: Potential for a neurogenetic approach. *Trends in Neurosciences*, **19**, 171–176.

Rossi, A., Stratta, P., Matteir, P. *et al.* (1992) Planum temporale in schizophrenia: a magnetic resonance study. *Schizophrenia Research*, **7**, 19–22.

Rossi, A., Serio, A., Stratta, P. *et al.* (1994) Planum temporale asymmetry and thought disorder in schizophrenia. *Schizophrenia Research*, **12**, 1–7.

Rubens, A. B., Mahowald, M. W. and Hutton, J. T. (1976) Asymmetry of lateral (Sylvian) fissures in man. *Neurology*, **26**, 620–624.

Rumsey, J. M., Donohue, B. C., Brady, D. R., Nace, K., Giedd, J. N. and Andreason, P. (1997) A magnetic resonance imaging study of planum temporale asymmetry in men with developmental dyslexia. *Archives of Neurology*, **54**, 1481–1489.

Satz, P. and Green, M. F. (1999) Atypical handedness in schizophrenia: some methodological and theoretical issues. *Schizophrenia Bulletin*, **25**, 63–78.

Schlaug, G., Jancke, L., Huang, Y. and Steinmetz, H. (1995) *In vivo* evidence of structural brain asymmetry in musicians. *Science*, **267**, 699–701.

Seldon, H. L. (1982) Structure of human auditory cortex. III. Statistical analysis of dendritic trees. *Brain Research*, **249**, 211–221.

Shapleske, J., Rossell, S. L., Woodruff, P. W. R. and David, A. S. (1999) The planum temporale: a systematic, quantitative review of its structural, functional and clinical significance. *Brain Research Reviews*, **29**, 26–49.

Shenton, M. E., Kikinis, R., Jolesz, F. A. *et al.* (1992) Abnormalities of the left temporal lobe and thought disorder in schizophrenia. A quantitative magnetic resonance imaging study. *New England Journal of Medicine,* **327**, 604–612.

Soininen, H., Partanen, K., Pitkanen, A. *et al.* (1995) Decreased hippocampal volume asymmetry on MRIs in nondemented elderly subjects carrying the apoliproprotein E 4 allele. *Neurology,* **45**, 391–392.

Southard, E. E. (1915) On the topographical distribution of cortex lesions and anomalies in dementia praecox, with some account of their functional significance. *American Journal of Insanity*, **71**, 603–671.

Steinmetz, H., Rademacher, J., Huang, Y. *et al.* (1989) Cerebral asymmetry: MR planimetry of the human planum temporale. *Journal of Computer Assisted Tomography,* **13**, 996–1005.

Steinmetz, H., Rademacher, J., Jancke, L., Huang, Y., Thron, A. and Zilles, K. (1990) Total surface of temporoparietal intrasylvian cortex: Diverging left–right asymmetries. *Brain and Language*, **39**, 357–372.

Steinmetz, H., Volkmann, J., Jancke, L. and Freund, H. J. (1991) Anatomical left–right asymmetry of language-related temporal cortex is different in left- and right-handers. *Annals of Neurology*, **29**, 315–319.

Steinmetz, H., Herzog, A., Schlaug, G., Huang, Y. and Jancke, L. (1995) Brain (a)symmetry in monozygotic twins. *Cerebral Cortex,* **5**, 296–300.

Suddath, R. L., Christison, G. W., Torrey, E. F., Casanova, M. F. and Weinberger, D. R. (1990) Anatomical abnormalities in the brains of monozygotic twins discordant for schizophrenia. *New England Journal of Medicine*, **322**, 789–794.

Taylor, M. A., Greenspan, B. and Abrams, R. (1979) Lateralized neuropsychological dysfunction in affective disorder and schizophrenia. *American Journal of Psychiatry,* **136**, 1031–1034.

Velakulis, D., Pantelis, C., McGorry, P. D. *et al.* (1999) Hippocampal volume in first-episode psychoses and chronic schizophrenia. *Archives of General Psychiatry,* **56**, 133–140.

Vogeley, K., Hobson, T., Schneider-Axmann, T., Honer, W. G., Bogerts, B. and Falkai, P. (1998) Compartmental volumetry of the superior temporal gyrus reveals sex differences in schizophrenia—a post-mortem study. *Schizophrenia Research,* **31**, 83–87.

Von Bonin, G. (1962) Anatomical asymmetries of the cerebral hemispheres. In: Mountcastle, V. B., ed. *Interhemispheric relations and cerebral dominance.* John Hopkins Press, Baltimore.

Wada, J. A., Clarke, R. and Hamm, A. (1975) Cerebral hemispheric asymmetry in humans: Cortical speech zones in 100 adult and 100 infant brains. *Archives of Neurology*, **32**, 239–246.

Weinberger, D. R., Luchins, D. J., Morihisa, J. and Wyatt, R. J. (1982) Asymmetrical volumes of the right and left frontal and occipital regions of the human brain. *Annals of Neurology*, **11**, 97–100.

Weinberger, D. R., Suddath, R. L., Casanova, M. F., Torrey, E. F. and Kleinman, J. E. (1991) Crow's 'lateralisation hypothesis' for schizophrenia. *Archives of General Psychiatry,* **48**, 85.

Weis, S., Haugh, H., Holoubek, B. and Orun, H. (1989) The cerebral dominances: quantitative morphology of the human cerebral cortex. *Journal of Neuroscience,* **47**, 165–168.

White, L. E., Lucas, G., Richards, A. and Purves, D. (1994) Cerebral asymmetry and handedness. *Nature,* **368**, 197–198.

Wigan, A. L. (1844) *A new view of insanity: the duality of mind.* Longman, London.

Witelson, S. F. (1991) Neural sexual mosaicism: Sexual differentiation of the human temporo-parietal region for functional asymmetry. *Psychoneuroendocrinology,* **16**, 131–153.

Witelson, S. F. and Pallie, W. (1973) Left hemisphere specialization for language in the newborn: Anatomical evidence of asymmetry. *Brain,* **96**, 641–646.

Yang, C.-Q., Kitamura, Y., Nishino, N., Shirakawa, O. and Nakai, H. (1998) Isotype-specific G protein abnormalities in the left superior temporal cortex and limbic structures of patients with chronic schizophrenia. *Biological Psychiatry,* **43**, 12–19.

Zaidel, D. W., Esiri, M. M. and Oxbury, J. M. (1993) Regional differentiation of cell densities in the left and right hippocampi of epileptic patients. *Journal of Neurology,* **240**, 322–325.

Zaidel, D. W., Esiri, M. M., Eastwood, S. L. and Harrison, P. J. (1995) Asymmetrical hippocampal circuitry and schizophrenia. *Lancet,* **346**, 656–657.

Zaidel, D. W., Esiri, M. M. and Harrison, P. J. (1997*a*) The hippocampus in schizophrenia: Lateralized increase in neuronal density and altered cytoarchitectural asymmetry. *Psychological Medicine,* **27**, 703–713.

Zaidel D. W., Esiri, M. M. and Harrison, P. J. (1997*b*) Size, shape and orientation of neurons in the left and right hippocampus: Investigation of normal asymmetries and alterations in schizophrenia. *American Journal of Psychiatry,* **154**, 812–818.

7 Functional Imaging and Neural Circuitry in Schizophrenia

Susan K. Schultz and Nancy C. Andreasen

Applied neuroimaging and the neuropathology of schizophrenia
Functional imaging techniques
   Position emission tomography (PET)
   Functional magnetic resonance imaging (fMR)
Functional imaging and neurocircuitry
   PET studies of schizophrenia
   Methodological issues affecting functional imaging
   fMR studies of schizophrenia
   Other functional imaging approaches in schizophrenia
Corticothalamocerebellar circuitry and cognitive dysmetria in schizophrenia
Summary and conclusion

New medical imaging techniques have stimulated exponential advances in the study of brain structure and function. They provide neuroscientists and clinicians with the capacity to see brain structure in a high level of detail and to observe metabolic and neurochemical processes such as cerebral blood flow, glucose utilization, and receptor occupancy. Over recent years these techniques have been applied to schizophrenia, resulting in a veritable revolution in the conceptualization of the illness. In many ways these advances have brought the field back full circle to the emphasis on neurobiology put forth a century ago by such founding fathers as Nissl, Brodmann, Kraepelin, Alzheimer, and Cajal.

Structural MR imaging in schizophrenia is covered comprehensively in Chapter 1. Here we mention selected structural MR results, but the primary focus of the chapter is upon *functional* imaging, and the relationship between findings made using the two modalities. We develop the theme of schizophrenia as a disorder of neural connectivity, particularly affecting the corticocerebellar-thalamocortical circuit.

Applied neuroimaging and the neuropathology of schizophrenia

As detailed in Chapter 1, structural imaging using CT and MR have firmly established that schizophrenia is a brain disease which can be observed at the gross anatomical level when groups of patients are pooled together, averaged, and compared with healthy comparison subjects. As illustrated in Figs 7.1 and 7.2, ventricular enlargement, sulcal enlargement, and decreased cerebral and intracranial size are all confirmed findings in schizophrenia, not explained by factors such as medication or other environmental influences (Ward *et al.*, 1996; Lawrie and Abukmeil, 1998). Examination over a broad age range suggests that ventricular enlargement does not progress over time at a greater rate than would be expected with normal age-related changes, and that structural brain abnormalities are present from the outset of illness (Andreasen *et al.*, 1990; Nopoulos *et al.*, 1995).

Since the advent of volumetric MR, imaging research in schizophrenia has addressed specific brain structures (e.g. cortical regions, grey matter) as opposed to gross brain abnormalities. The earliest MR study of this kind reported a selective decrease in the frontal

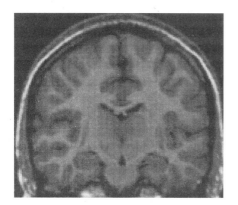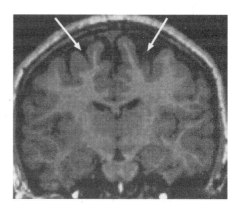

Fig. 7.1 Coronal MRI brain section of healthy control (left) and patient with schizophrenia (right) demonstrating decreased brain tissue volume and increased surface CSF (arrowed). See also Plate 1.

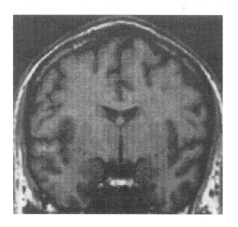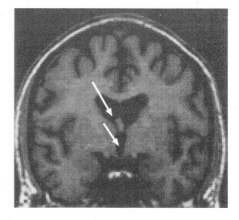

Fig. 7.2 Coronal MRI brain section of healthy control (left) and patient with schizophrenia (right) demonstrating increased ventricular volume (top arrow: lateral ventricles; bottom arrow: third ventricle). See also Plate 2.

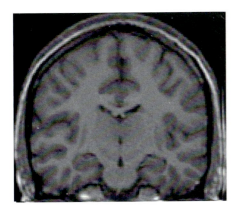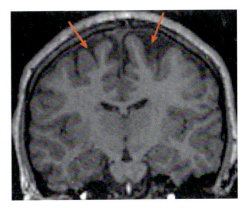

Plate 1 Coronal MRI brain section of healthy control (left) and patient with schizophrenia (right) demonstrating decreased brain tissue volume and increased surface CSF (arrowed).

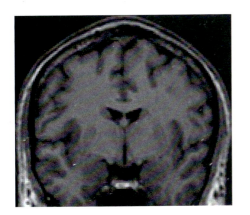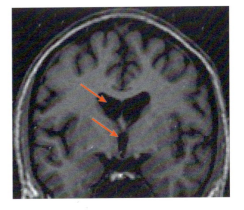

Plate 2 Coronal MRI brain section of healthy control (left) and patient with schizophrenia (right) demonstrating increased ventricular volume (top arrow: lateral ventricle; bottom arrow: third ventricle).

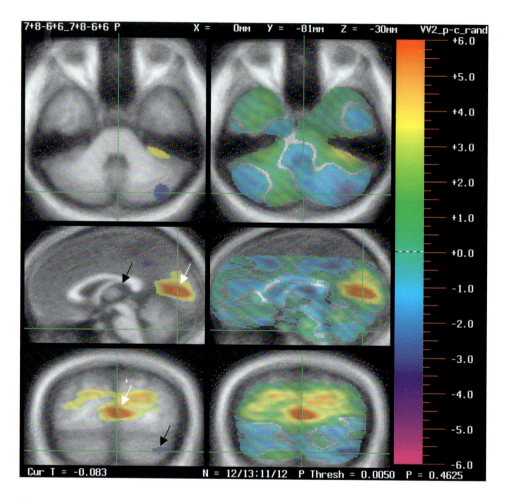

Plate 3 PET images depicting a comparison of 12 patients with schizophrenia with 13 healthy comparison subjects during a visual attention task. A randomization analysis technique was used to generate the comparison images of the visual attention condition, subtracting the resting baseline condition. The regions of significant difference are shown in the left column. The subjects with schizophrenia have greater blood flow than the controls in the occipital cortex, as shown by the white arrows, in the sagittal (middle panel) and coronal (bottom panel) views. The patients have reduced blood flow compared to the controls in the the thalamus (black arrow, middle panel) and in the left cerebellum (black arrow, bottom panel).

cortex, in addition to smaller cerebral and intracranial size, a combination of findings consistent with a neurodevelopmental rather than a neurodegenerative process (Andreasen *et al.*, 1986). The findings suggesting a relatively smaller frontal lobe size in schizophrenia have not been consistently replicated, but hypotheses about frontal dysfunction continue to be widely discussed, particularly in functional imaging studies (see below, also Chapters 10 and 11). The prefrontal cortex performs a large array of higher cortical functions that are disrupted in schizophrenia (e.g. executive functions, abstract thinking, working memory), making it an attractive candidate for study. Yet it is also a large and functionally diverse brain region that was difficult to measure accurately prior to the development of 3D acquisition procedures with MR and volume-rendering techniques that permit visualization of cortical surface anatomy. Four of the five recent studies that used relatively sophisticated measurement techniques have shown decreased frontal size in both chronic and first-episode patients (Breier *et al.*, 1992; Andreasen *et al.*, 1994*b*; Nopoulos *et al.*, 1995; Wible *et al.*, 1995; Gur *et al.*, 1998). If all studies are pooled and those with weaker methods are included, however, negative studies are as frequent as positive ones (see Table 1.5 in Chapter 1). Interestingly there appears to be a gender influence, since the regional cortical tissue decrements are predominantly a male effect (Flaum *et al.*, 1990, 1995).

MR imaging has also been used to explore abnormalities in other brain regions, such as the thalamus, temporal lobes, and basal ganglia (Chapter 1). The thalamus is relatively difficult to measure reliably since it is composed of multiple nuclei, is a mixture of grey and white matter, and has indistinct borders as visualized on nearly all types of MR sequences. Nonetheless, decreased thalamic size has been noted in several studies, and a novel application of image averaging and subtraction methods has indicated that this structure shows the greatest effect size difference when patients are compared to controls (Andreasen *et al.*, 1994*a*). Like the prefrontal cortex, the thalamus is also an interesting candidate region for schizophrenia; although the precise functions of the various thalamic nuclei are still being mapped, it is clearly a major relay station that could serve functions such as gating or filtering or even generating input and output, since it has afferent and efferent projections connecting it with widely distributed cortical and other regions.

Future developments in MR imaging are likely to yield greater insights into the fundamental neuropathology of schizophrenia. For example, more sophisticated analysis techniques, ideally applied in a longitudinal manner in a well-characterized subject sample, are critical to further delineate the anatomy and conceptualization of schizophrenia as a neurodevelopmental process. Such studies will ultimately serve to provide a 'timeline' for both the onset of the aetiological event or process and its trajectory over the lifespan. At the same time, functional imaging will provide another level of understanding, through living representations of how schizophrenia affects interactions between distributed brain regions during specific neuropsychological tasks.

Functional imaging techniques

Functional neuroimaging provides a means to explore inter-relationships between symptomatology and dysfunction in specific brain regions. The pioneering work of Kety *et al.*

(1948) led to the development of models for the measurement of cerebral blood flow and metabolism. The major imaging modalities currently in use include single photon emission CT (SPECT), PET, and functional fMR imaging (Fu and McGuire, 1999). In brief, SPECT permits measurement of cerebral blood flow using tracers (e.g. Tc-HMPAO) externally detected using a rotating gamma camera (Syed et al., 1992); SPECT, like PET may also be used to visualize and measure neuroreceptors. Since PET and fMR are now at the forefront of imaging technology, their principles and applications are considered here in more detail.

Positron emission tomography (PET)

PET permits the evaluation of brain function through the measurement of regional cerebral blood flow (with ^{15}O-H_2O) and glucose utilization (with ^{18}F-2-deoxyglucose (F-DG)). Study of protein synthesis, neurotransmitter synthesis and release, and receptor occupancy, are also possible. The technique is based upon detection by the PET camera of the 'annihilation photons' generated from positrons emitted by the isotope being used (Holcomb et al., 1990). It has a much higher level of resolution than SPECT, and its applications at present are also more flexible. This flexibility that distinguishes PET from SPECT lies in the use of specific, short half-life tracer molecules (e.g. ^{15}O-H_2O), allowing for the assessment of a series of neuropsychological activation tasks that may be quantified and compared relative to one another, as detailed below.

Imaging with PET (and SPECT) also affords the capability to examine receptor function *in vivo* through the use of radioligand binding. The regulation of dopamine activity has been the most extensively studied system, and a recent meta-analysis of 15 studies concluded that the evidence supported an increased dopaminergic activity in schizophrenia both pre- and postsynaptically (Laruelle, 1998). Other systems including 5-hydroxytryptamine (5-HT) and glutamate have also come under recent scrutiny using PET (Soares and Innis, 1999).

Functional magnetic resonance imaging (fMR)

fMR provides another powerful modality for the purpose of exploring brain activity across a variety of conditions. It relies upon MR acquisition techniques based on detection of the paramagnetic effects of deoxyhemoglobin in contrast to the blood oxygen level (Ogawa et al., 1990). This allows for the assessment of relative decrements in deoxyhemoglobin in neuronally active areas, the concept being that an increase in cerebral blood flow due to a neuronal activation results in relatively greater blood oxygen in a given region compared to the deoxyhemoglobin concentration (Latchaw et al., 1995; Raichle, 1998). In this manner investigators may assess the sites of functional activation during neuropsychological activation tasks. fMR affords a continuous measure of brain activity in the context of high resolution MR imaging (though the anatomical measures must be obtained during a separate scanning sequence). There has been a recent surge of interest in fMR, with tremendous potential for new insights into the functional neuropathology of schizophrenia.

Functional imaging and neurocircuitry

PET studies of schizophrenia

Beginning with the work of Ingvar and Franzen (1974), studies of regional cerebral blood flow (rCBF) have been used to investigate functional and metabolic abnormalities in schizophrenia (Fig. 7.3). This early work suggested that subjects with schizophrenia had a relative

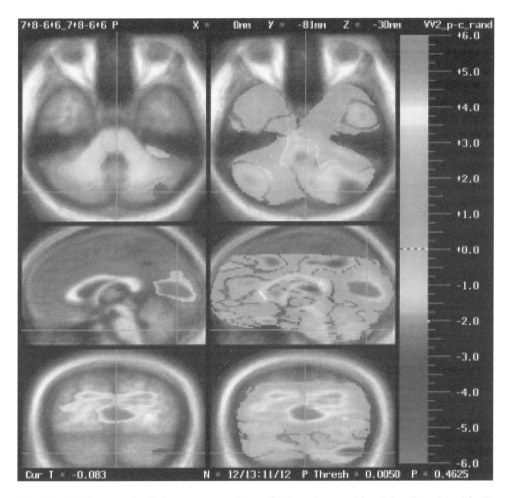

Fig. 7.3 PET images depicting a comparison of 12 patients with schizophrenia with 13 healthy comparison subjects during a visual attention task. A randomization analysis technique was used to generate the comparison images of the visual attention condition, subtracting the resting baseline condition. The regions of significant difference are shown in the left column. The subjects with schizophrenia have greater blood flow than the controls in the occipital cortex, as shown by the white arrows, in the sagittal (middle panel) and coronal (bottom panel) views. The patients have reduced blood flow compared to the controls in the thalamus (black arrow, middle panel) and in the left cerebellum (black arrow, bottom panel). See also Plate 3.

reduction of blood flow to frontal cortex ('hypofrontality'), which was associated with prominent negative symptoms. Functional imaging studies have become steadily more sophisticated, and it is now clear that PET can be used to explore the functional circuitry during performance of a variety of mental tasks. Through comparisons between healthy volunteers and patient populations, investigators may then identify circuits that are dysfunctional in schizophrenia. Much of this work has been facilitated by the maturation of the ^{15}O-H$_2$O technique with PET. ^{15}O-H$_2$O is a tracer with a very short half-life (around 2 minutes), which allows multiple repeated scans (usually 6 to 12) during differing cognitive tasks within a short time period. This permits dissection of the components of cognitive activities (e.g. memory encoding versus retrieval) and visualization of their associated circuitry. ^{18}F-DG is also widely used and has the capability to assess regional metabolic response to cognitive activation tasks, but these tasks must accommodate a 30-minute uptake period.

Current thinking about the mechanisms of schizophrenia, based on functional imaging, postulates a disruption in distributed functional circuits rather than a single abnormality in a single brain region (McGuire and Frith, 1996; Andreasen, 1997). Although no single group of regions has definitively emerged as the 'schizophrenia circuit', a consensus is developing concerning some of the areas most likely to be involved. These areas include a variety of subregions within the frontal cortex (orbital, dorsolateral, medial), anterior cingulate gyrus, thalamus, several temporal lobe subregions, and the cerebellum. The notion of multiple involved areas is consistent with insights gleaned from structural imaging and postmortem studies (see above and elsewhere in this volume), which suggest localized as well as global brain tissue decrements. Identification of the specific circuitry involved has become the charge of functional imaging as discussed below.

The early studies of prefrontal cortex activity in schizophrenia using SPECT tended to examine chronic patients, to evaluate the 'resting state', and to explore small samples. Sometimes patients were studied while neuroleptic free, but not always. As time has evolved, investigators have recognized that study of the resting state has specific limitations—it is difficult to know what the human brain actually does when it is 'resting'—and mental activity may vary between individuals. Consequently, strategies have been employed to produce more consistency. Typically, an experimental task is selected because it is assumed to stimulate the prefrontal cortex. Early examples include the Wisconsin Card Sorting Test, the Continuous Performance Test, the Porteus Mazes, and the Tower of London. A baseline or control task is also selected to control for as many components of the activation task as possible. When the baseline condition is subtracted from the activation condition, selective activation (or failure to activate) certain regions can be identified (Weinberger et al., 1986; Buschbaum, 1995).

One study used a design intended to determine whether hypofrontality is an epiphenomenon caused by long-term treatment with neuroleptic drugs or whether it is a state inherent to schizophrenia (Andreasen et al., 1992). Patients with chronic illness off medication, drug-naive patients, and healthy controls were scanned using the ^{133}xenon method to measure regional cerebral blood flow. Scanning was done under both a baseline condition and an experimental cognitive challenge, the Tower of London task, which is considered to be mediated through the prefrontal cortex (Shallice, 1982). The three groups differed significantly in only two regions: left mesial frontal and right parietal. The normal controls showed an increase in relative left mesial frontal blood flow when given the cognitive challenge, while the two patient groups showed a decrease in flow. The other area showing a significant difference was the right parietal cortex, which had increased flow in the control subjects relative to both of the patient groups. This study suggested that hypoactivity of the frontal cortex may be present in schizophrenia in both drug-naive and chronically treated patients studied while medication free. Similarly, SPECT studies using Tc^{99m}-HMPAO showed decreased frontal activity during the Wisconsin Card Sorting Task among patients receiving neuroleptic medication at the time of imaging, and among never-treated patients (Kawasaki *et al.*, 1993; Catafau *et al.*, 1994).

In addition to examining functional responses to specific cognitive tasks, researchers have used symptom assessments in conjunction with functional imaging in an attempt to understand how imaging measures relate to various symptom clusters (e.g. positive psychotic symptoms, disorganized symptoms, and negative symptoms). Using this approach, Liddle and colleagues (Friston *et al.*, 1992; Liddle *et al.*, 1992) identified increased cerebral blood flow relative to controls in left mesiotemporal structures in patients with positive psychotic symptoms such as hallucinations and delusions as well as increased flow in the right anterior cingulate cortex, left superior temporal gyrus, and dorsomedial thalamus. Additionally, they noted decreased rCBF in the left prefrontal and parietal cortex in patients exhibiting the negative symptom of psychomotor poverty. The total sum of all the symptom measures was most highly associated with parahippocampal blood flow as well as with increased flow in the superior and polar temporal lobe. Separate PET work to assess cerebral blood flow in relation to negative symptom measures by Tamminga and coworkers using ^{18}F-DG, similarly demonstrated decreased cerebral metabolism in frontal and parietal cortex as well as in thalamic areas (Tamminga *et al.*, 1992).

PET imaging is also being used for other, increasingly sophisticated investigations of schizophrenia. For example, to identify symptom correlates of rCBF across several cognitive activation tasks during the same scanning period; to compare patients while symptomatic with the same individuals when non-symptomatic; to simulate symptoms; or to challenge the neural processes thought to be active during symptom production. Using the latter approach, McGuire and colleagues completed a systematic study of hallucinations. They postulated that hallucinations are due to an erroneous attribution of the person's own inner speech to another person, reflecting a defect in self-monitoring. Starting with healthy controls, they developed a task that could potentially mimic this mechanism, whereby subjects were asked to perform a sentence completion task and imagine that the response was spoken in another person's voice. This task led to activation of speech production and perception regions, such as Broca's area, supplementary motor area, and the left superior and middle temporal regions (McGuire *et al.*, 1996*a*). Applying the same task to subjects with schizophrenia and comparing hallucinators to non-hallucinators, they found hallucinators to have decreased flow in the areas used to monitor speech, such as the left middle temporal gyrus and supplementary motor area (McGuire *et al.*, 1996*b*). Moreover, examination of patients while they were actively experiencing auditory hallucinations has revealed increased perfusion, primarily in subcortical regions (thalamus, striatum), limbic and paralimbic regions (anterior cingulate cortex, parahippocampal gyrus), and cerebellum. The authors speculated that activity in subcortical regions may generate or moderate hallucinations, while the content (e.g. auditory, tactile) may be determined by the specific neocortical regions that are engaged (Silbersweig et al., 1995).

Buchsbaum, who conducted the earliest PET studies suggesting hypofrontality, recently utilized an attentional task, the Continuous Performance Test (Schroeder et al., 1994), which has been shown to be impaired in schizophrenia. ^{18}F-DG utilization was measured in 16 regions of interest, and it was observed that patients with schizophrenia were significantly hypoactive in the frontal cortex compared to controls (Buschbaum et al., 1992). These authors also found thalamic abnormalities of glucose metabolism in a sample of 20 never-medicated patients (Buschbaum et al., 1996); interestingly, they additionally reported a diminished cerebellar metabolic rate.

Andreasen and coworkers have provided support for abnormalities in multiple frontal subregions, thalamus, and cerebellum in schizophrenia. In one study comparing patients to healthy volunteers during 'Random Episodic Silent Thought' (REST), they found blood flow abnormalities in medial, orbital, and dorsolateral frontal regions, as well as temporal, cingulate, thalamic, and cerebellar areas (Andreasen et al., 1997). In another study of practiced and novel recall of complex narrative material, abnormalities were present in multiple brain regions, including frontal, thalamic, and cerebellar sites (Andreasen et al., 1996). Similar abnormalities during episodic memory and semantic/working memory tasks have also been observed by others (Gur and Gur, 1995).

Methodological issues affecting functional imaging

PET and SPECT are limited by several factors. Most importantly, radiation exposure restricts the number of studies that can be done per subject. For example, the literature on medication effects is exclusively limited to two studies per patient. Thus medication status is dichotomized as on/off rather than examined in terms of continuous variables such as dose, duration of treatment, or clinical efficacy, which would lend greater insights into the neurobiological manifestations across the course of the illness. Further, these studies have typically compared indices of brain metabolism off medication versus on medication in a resting state or some other specified condition. It would be more informative to examine the degree to which brain activity changes as a function of medication (or clinical) status and the specific brain regions or circuits which appear to be most affected by these variables. To do so requires comparisons of brain function during multiple aspects of cognitive activity, rather than during single conditions. A further issue concerns spatial resolution, which is inherently limited in SPECT and PET. In-plane resolution is ~0.5 to 1 cm for PET and 2 cm for SPECT, whereas the actual effects of interest in schizophrenia may be much more localized.

Despite the tremendous strides made by imaging research to date, the pathoetiology of schizophrenia largely remains a mystery. Perhaps the tools employed remain slightly too crude or they may be guided too empirically at present. The neuropathology of schizophrenia clearly involves complex interactions of brain regions that manifest in a number of symptoms and cognitive deficits. As a result, another important methodological issue concerns structural–functional integration. Structural MR measures have traditionally been used as a template for the localization of regions visualized using PET. This requires special procedures to assimilate the two sets of information, resulting in extremely complex data manipulation techniques which become even more complex when differences between patient and control data are examined. Advances in image analysis and statistical methods are thus at least as important as those affecting the nature of image acquisition.

fMR encompasses a series of techniques that have many potential attractions. The BOLD technique (blood oxygen level dependent contrast; Ogawa *et al.*, 1990) is one prominent and relevant fMR method. The use of deoxygenated hemoglobin as an endogenous tracer represents a key advantage over PET since no radiation exposure is involved, and the technique therefore can be repeated many times on the same subject. Thus subjects can be scanned at baseline (prior to starting medications, or just following a medication discontinuation period), at various intervals, and at various dosages. Additionally, spatial resolution of fMRI is theoretically ~1 mm, and registration with anatomical images is straightforward. As a result of these and other advantages, there has been an explosion of interest in fMR and a number of neuroscience laboratories are in the process of exploring its potential. Like all new techniques, however, there are potential pitfalls and complications that must be systematically worked through, and at least one group has suggested a potential for spurious findings (Callicott *et al.*, 1998). To date, therefore, the capacity of fMR for exploring the neuropathology of schizophrenia has yet to be fully realized. Some of the initial findings are outlined below.

fMR studies of schizophrenia

One of the first reports using fMR in schizophrenia was a case study (Woodruff *et al.*, 1994). This group obtained gradient-echo planar images from a 48-year-old man with paranoid schizophrenia while he was in the state of experiencing auditory hallucinations, and on a separate occasion when he was not. These measures were then compared to a third scan obtained during a non-hallucinating state whilst he was experiencing externally presented speech. It was observed that during the externally presented speech, activation occurred in superior and middle temporal gyrus. Activation in these areas also occurred during auditory hallucinations, with additional activation in the dorsomedial thalamus that had not occurred during the externally presented speech scan (Woodruff *et al.*, 1994). Another group has used fMR to examine activation of sensorimotor cortex and supplemental motor areas during a finger-to-thumb opposition motor task (Wenz *et al.*, 1994; Schroder *et al.*, 1995). The studies suggested a decrease in activation of both areas, as well as a reversed lateralization effect, in patients with schizophrenia compared to controls. However a subsequent study examining a finger motion task using fMR did not find differences between groups in activation of motor cortex (Buckley *et al.*, 1997). Work in this area will almost certainly continue to evolve rapidly, leading to greater validity, consistency, and interpretability of findings.

Other functional imaging approaches in schizophrenia

Other functional imaging techniques include proton magnetic resonance spectroscopy (MRS), which can be used to estimate neuronal markers such as *N*-acetyl aspartate (NAA).

For example, one study examined grey and white matter volumes relative to NAA signal intensity. The group observed a decrement in grey matter volume without a decrement in grey matter NAA; in contrast, white matter volumes were not reduced but white matter NAA signal was (Lim *et al.*, 1998). The authors postulate this may reflect a neurodevelopmental process involving abnormalities of white matter connectivity. Other work using proton MRS has measured regional differences in NAA signal, comparing patients with controls, chronically treated with never-treated patients, and childhood-onset with adult-onset patients (Bertolino *et al.*, 1998a,b). Since NAA measurements are an index of neuronal integrity, neuronal density, and/or neuronal size, they blur the distinction between structural and functional imaging, providing information pertinent to both domains (Harrison, 1999). Similarly, ^{31}P MRS gives information about putative *in vivo* membrane and synaptic pathology (Soares and Innis, 1999). Further evolution of these MR imaging technologies will contribute to a more integrated understanding of the structural and functional neuropathology of schizophrenia.

Corticothalamocerebellar circuitry and cognitive dysmetria in schizophrenia

Whether the modality is fMR, PET, or SPECT, findings from functional imaging are remarkably consistent with the theory that schizophrenia is a disorder of multiple distributed brain regions. Recognition of this has led to strategies to search for abnormalities in specific regions and theories about symptom–region relationships (e.g. negative symptoms in frontal cortex, hallucinations in superior temporal gyrus), which have been examined by a variety of investigators (e.g. Barta *et al.*, 1990; Shenton *et al.*, 1992). As mentioned above, however, this approach may be oversimplified, and it may be more appropriate to develop models that explain clinical symptoms as a consequence of disruptions in anatomically identified circuits that mediate a fundamental cognitive process.

Based on the relatively consistent observations of functional and structural abnormalities in frontal, thalamic, and cerebellar regions described above, Andreasen and colleagues have postulated that the symptoms of schizophrenia arise from impaired connectivity between these regions as a consequence of neurodevelopmental defects (Andreasen *et al.*, 1996, 1997). In this model, the cardinal features of schizophrenia reflect a failure to co-ordinate mental activities, termed 'cognitive dysmetria', a concept closely allied to that of Bleulerian thought disorder (Andreasen, 1999). The word 'metron' literally means 'measure'; i.e. a person with schizophrenia has a core deficit in taking measure of time and space, in making inferences about inter-relationships between himself and others, or between past, present, and future. (S)he cannot accurately time input and output, and therefore cannot co-ordinate the perception, prioritization, retrieval, and expression of experiences and ideas. The cognitive dysmetria is paralleled by motor dysmetria (poor motor co-ordination) which was first described by Kraepelin, and confirmed in contemporary studies (Gupta *et al.*, 1995).

The concept of cognitive dysmetria postulates three key nodes in a feedback loop that involves frontal regions, cerebellum, and thalamus, hence called the corticocerebellar-thalamocortical circuit. Each of these nodes is assumed to have a particular function. The prefrontal node serves the classic 'executive function', which involves prioritizing data, placing data within a broad contextual meaning using information gleaned from other inter-communicating cortical regions, formulating decisions or responses, and initiating their action. The thalamus serves as the filtering site for all these processes, receiving sensory information from multiple sources, simplifying it by excluding redundant or extraneous stimuli, and forwarding on the relevant information. The cerebellum, which remarkably contains half the neurons in the human brain, is composed of cells designed to handle massive amounts of information. The cerebellum may serve as the metron. That is, it co-ordinates the information forwarded to it from cortical and subcortical regions. Its primary role is to match data within the context of time, and perhaps of space, to ensure that the correct pieces of information are connected and co-ordinated with one another. For example, a person carrying on a conversation must hear and understand the words of the other speaker, interpret their implicit and explicit meaning, and generate an appropriate reply. In this simple model, the prefrontal cortex does most of the interpretation, while the thalamus permits the brain to focus on the conversation rather than other stimuli (e.g. ambient back-ground noise). The cerebellum is the site where information from the frontal executive and other sensory regions converge and would perform nearly instantaneous rapid 'on-line' processing. A patient with schizophrenia may manifest impaired verbal and social responses in such situations because of dysfunction in the circuitry that permits prioritizing infor-mation, excluding extraneous information, and performing these functions in an efficient and well co-ordinated manner.

With the same theme that schizophrenia reflects impairment in complex circuitry, Goldman-Rakic and others have proposed a model suggesting that the fundamental deficit in the disorder is an inability to guide behavior by representations, often referred to as a defect in working memory (Goldman-Rakic, 1994). Working memory is the ability to main-tain a meaningful representation of an idea in one's awareness and perform cognitive operations using that awareness. It permits individuals to respond in a flexible manner, to formulate and modify plans, and to base behavior on internally held ideas and thoughts rather than being driven by external stimuli (Goldman-Rakic, 1987). A defect in this ability can explain a variety of symptoms of schizophrenia. For example, the inability to hold a discourse plan in mind and monitor speech output may lead to disorganized speech, or an inability to maintain a plan for behavioral activities could lead to negative symptoms such as avolition or alogia. Overall, the model suports a major role for prefrontal regions and their multiple cortical, thalamic, and striatal connections. These brain regions interact to facilitate a fundamental cognitive function, i.e. representationally guided behavior, that permits individuals to adapt flexibly to a changing environment, and achieve temporal and spatial continuity between past experiences and present and future actions. Future work will continue to better define these models. For example, working memory has been assessed by fMR in an investigation designed to elucidate mechanisms underlying the incongruity of impaired auditory working memory relative to preserved non-auditory memory in schiz-ophrenia (Gur et al., 1998). These authors observed reduced activation in the inferior and medial frontal gyrus, premotor, and anterior temporal areas during verbal memory tasks, which may reflect the subregions mediating this deficit.

Summary and conclusion

Structural brain imaging has provided clear evidence that measurable anatomical differences are present in schizophrenia. Future work will focus increasingly on applying MR techniques to longitudinal studies over the lifespan, allowing researchers to chart the trajectory of regional anatomical brain effects of the illness and their putative neurodevelopmental nature. Meanwhile, functional imaging increasingly permits the structural findings to be placed in the context of circuitry activation and dysfunction: the ability to link mind and brain in the study of schizophrenia is now within the grasp of research (Andreasen, 1997). Once the specific circuitry implicated in schizophrenia is clearly identified, scientists working at the cellular level can begin to tease apart the molecular nature of the interactions and the molecular explanation for the alterations in neuronal and synaptic function. Through this route the neuropathological puzzle of schizophrenia, attacked by many great researchers for over a century, may be ultimately solved.

References

Andreasen NC (1997) Linking mind and brain in the study of mental illnesses: A project for a scientific psychopathology. *Science* **275**, 1586–1593.

Andreasen NC (1999) A unitary model of schizophrenia. Bleuler's 'fragmented phrene' as schizencephaly. *Archives of General Psychiatry* **56**, 782–787.

Andreasen NC, Nasrallah HA, Dunn V, Yuh WTC, Cohen G, Ziebell S (1986) Structural abnormalities in the frontal system in schizophrenia: A magnetic resonance imaging study. *Archives of General Psychiatry* **43**, 136–144.

Andreasen NC, Swayze VW, Flaum M, Yates WR, Arndt S, McChesney C (1990) Ventricular enlargement in schizophrenia evaluated with computed tomographic scanning. *Archives of General Psychiatry* **47**, 1008–1015.

Andreasen NC, Rezai K, Alliger R *et al.* (1992) Hypofrontality in neuroleptic-naive patients and in patients with chronic schizophrenia: Assessment with xenon 133 single-photon emission computed tomography and the Tower of London. *Archives of General Psychiatry* **49**, 943–958.

Andreasen NC, Arndt S, Swayze V *et al.* (1994a) Thalamic abnormalities in schizophrenia visualized through magnetic resonance image averaging. *Science* **266**, 294–298.

Andreasen NC, Flashman L, Flaum M *et al.* (1994b) Regional brain abnormalities in schizophrenia measured with magnetic resonance imaging. *Journal of the American Medical Association* **272**, 1763–1769.

Andreasen NC, O'Leary DS, Cizadlo T *et al.* (1996) Schizophrenia and cognitive dysmetria: A positron-emission tomography study of dysfunctional prefrontal-thalamic-cerebellar circuitry. *Proceedings of the National Academy of Sciences USA* **93**, 9985–9990.

Andreasen NC, O'Leary DS, Flaum M *et al.* (1997) Hypofrontality in schizophrenia: Disturbed dysfunctional circuits in neuroleptic-naive patients. *Lancet* **349**, 1730–1734.

Barta PE, Pearlson GD, Powers RE, Richards SS, Tune LE (1990) Auditory hallucinations and smaller superior temporal gyral volume in schizophrenia. *American Journal of Psychiatry* **147**, 1457–1462.

Bertolino A, Callicott JH, Elman I *et al.* (1998*a*) Regionally specific neuronal pathology in untreated patients with schizophrenia: a proton magnetic resonance spectroscopic imaging study. *Biological Psychiatry* **43**, 641–648.

Bertolino A, Kumra S, Callicott JH *et al.* (1998*b*) Common pattern of cortical pathology in childhood and adult onset schizophrenia as identified by proton magnetic resonance spectroscopic imaging. *American Journal of Psychiatry* **155**, 1376–1383.

Breier A, Buchanan RW., Elkashef A, Munson RC, Kirkpatrick B, Gellad F (1992) Brain morphology and schizophrenia: A magnetic resonance imaging study of limbic, prefrontal cortex, and caudate structures. *Archives of General Psychiatry* **49**, 921–926.

Buckley PF, Friedman L, Wu D *et al.* (1997) Functional magnetic resonance imaging in schizophrenia: initial methodology and evaluation of the motor cortex. *Psychiatry Research: Neuroimaging* **74**, 13–23.

Buschbaum MS (1995) Positron emission tomography studies of abnormal glucose metabolism in schizophrenic illness. *Clinical Neuroscience* **2**, 122–130.

Buchsbaum MS, Haier RJ, Potkin SG *et al.* (1992) Frontostriatal disorder of cerebral metabolism in never-medicated schizophrenics. *Archives of General Psychiatry* **49**, 935–942.

Buchsbaum MS, Someya T, Teng C *et al.* (1996) PET and MRI of the thalamus in never-medicated patients with schizophrenia. *American Journal of Psychiatry* **153**, 191–199.

Callicott JH, Ramsey NF, Tallent K *et al.* (1998) Functional magnetic resonance imaging brain mapping in psychiatry: Methodological issues illustrated in a study of working memory in schizophrenia. *Neuropsychopharmacology* **18**, 186–196.

Catafau AM, Parellada E, Lomena FJ (1994) Prefrontal and temporal blood flow in schziophrenia: resting and activation technetium-99m-HMPAO SPECT patterns in young neuroleptic-naive patients with acute disease. *Journal of Nuclear Medicine* **35**, 935–941.

Flaum M, Arndt S, Andreasen NC (1990) The role of gender in studies of ventricular enlargement in schizophrenia: A predominantly male effect. *American Journal of Psychiatry* **147**, 1327–1332,

Flaum M, Swayze V, O'Leary DS *et al.* (1995) Effects of diagnosis, laterality, and gender on brain morphology in schizophrenia. *American Journal of Psychiatry* **152**, 704–714.

Friston KJ, Liddle PF, Frith CD, Hirsch SR, Frackowiak RSJ (1992) The left medial temporal lobe region and schizophrenia. *Brain* **115**, 367–382.

Fu CHY, McGuire PK (1999) Functional neuroimaging in psychiatry. *Philosophical Transactions of the Royal Society of London[B]* **354**, 1359–1370.

Goldman-Rakic PS (1987) Circuitry of primate prefrontal cortex and regulation of behavior by representational memory. In: Plum F, Mountcastle V, eds. *Handbook of physiology.* Bethesda, MD, American Physiological Society, pp. 373–417.

Goldman-Rakic PS (1994) Working memory dysfunction in schizophrenia. *Journal of Neuropsychiatry and Clinical Neuroscience* **6**, 348–357.

Gupta S, Andreasen NC, Arndt S *et al.* (1995) Neurological soft signs in neuroleptic-naïve and neuroleptic treated schizophrenic patients and in normal comparison subjects. *American Journal of Psychiatry* **152**, 191–196.

Gur RC, Gur RE (1995) Hypofrontality in schizophrenia: RIP. *Lancet* **345**, 1383–1384.

Gur RE, Cowell P, Turetsky BI *et al.* (1998) A follow-up magnetic resonance imaging study of schizophrenia: Relationship of neuroanatomical changes to clinical and neurobehavioral measures. *Archives of General Psychiatry* **55**, 145–152.

Harrison PJ (1999) The neuropathology of schizophrenia. A critical review of the data and their interpretation. *Brain* **122**, 593–624.

Holcomb HH, Links J, Smith C, Wong D (1990) Positron emission tomography: Measuring the metabolic and neurochemical characteristics of the living human nervous system. In: Andreasen NC, ed. *Brain Imaging: applications in psychiatry*. American Psychiatric Press, Washington DC.

Ingvar DH, Franzen G (1974) Abnormalities of cerebral blood flow distribution in patients with chronic schizophrenia. *Acta Psychiatrica Scandinavica* **50**, 425–462.

Kawasaki Y, Maeda Y, Suzuki M *et al.* (1993) SPECT analysis of regional cerebral blood flow changes in patients with schizophrenia during the Wisconsin Card Sorting Test. *Schizophrenia Research* **10**, 109–116.

Kety SS, Woodford RB, Harmel MH, Freyhan FA, Appel KE, Schmidt CF (1948) Cerebral blood flow and metabolism in schizophrenia, The effects of barbiturate semi-narcosis, insulin coma and electroshock. *American Journal of Psychiatry* **104**, 765–770.

Laruelle M (1998) Imaging dopamine transmission in schizophrenia—A review and meta-analysis. *Quarterly Journal of Nuclear Medicine* **42**, 211–221.

Latchaw RE, Ugurbil K, Hu X (1995) Functional MR imaging of perceptual and cognitive functions. *Neuroimaging Clinics of North America* **5**, 193–205.

Lawrie SM, Abukmeil SS (1998) Brain abnormality in schizophrenia. A systematic and quantitative review of volumetric magnetic resonance imaging studies. *British Journal of Psychiatry* **172**, 110–120

Liddle PF, Friston KJ, Frith CD, Hirsch SR, Jones T, Frackowiak RSJ (1992) Patterns of cerebral blood flow in schizophrenia. *British Journal of Psychiatry* **160**, 179–186.

Lim KO, Adalstenisson E, Spielman D, Sullivan EV, Rosenbloom MJ, Pfefferbaum A (1998) Proton magnetic resonance spectroscopy imaging in cortical gray and white matter in schizophrenia. *Archives of General Psychiatry* **55**, 346–352.

McGuire PK, Frith CD (1996) Disordered functional connectivity in schizophrenia. *Psychological Medicine* **26**, 663–667.

McGuire PK, Silbersweig DA , Murray RM (1996*a*) Functional anatomy of inner speech and auditory verbal imagery. *Psychological Medicine* **26**, 29–38.

McGuire PK, Silbersweig DA, Wright I, Murray RM (1996*b*) The neural correlates of inner speech and auditory verbal imagery in schizophrenia: relationship to auditory verbal hallucinations. *British Journal of Psychiatry* **169**, 148–159.

Nopoulos P, Torres I, Flaum M, Andreasen NC, Ehrhardt JC, Yuh WTC (1995) Brain morphology in first-episode schizophrenia. *American Journal of Psychiatry* **152**, 1721–1723.

Ogawa, S. Lee, T-M, Kay AR *et al.* (1990) Brain magnetic resonance imaging with contrast dependent on blood oxygenation. *Proceedings of the National Academy of Sciences USA* **87**, 9898–9872.

Raichle ME (1998) Behind the scenes of functional brain imaging: A historical and physiological perspective. *Proceedings of the National Academy of Sciences USA* **95**, 765–772.

Schroder J, Wenz LR, Schad K, Baudendistel K, Knopp MV (1995) Sensorimotor cortex and supplementary motor area changes in schizophrenia: A study with functional magnetic resonance imaging. *British Journal of Psychiatry* **167**, 197–201.

Schroeder J, Buchsbaum MS, Siegel BV *et al.* (1994) Patterns of cortical activity in schizophrenia. *Psychological Medicine* **24**, 947–955.

Shallice T (1982) Specific impairments of planning. *Philosophical Transactions of the Royal Society of London* **298**, 199–209.

Shenton ME, Kikinis R, Jolesz FA *et al.* (1992) Abnormalities of the left temporal lobe and thought disorder in schizophrenia: A quantitative magnetic resonance imaging study. *New England Journal of Medicine* **327**, 604–612.

Silbersweig DA, Stern E, Frith C *et al.* (1995) A functional neuroanatomy of hallucinations in schizophrenia. *Nature* **378**, 176–179.

Soares JC, Innis RB (1999) Neurochemical brain imaging investigations of schizophrenia. *Biological Psychiatry* **46**, 600–165.

Syed GM, Barrett JJ, Toone BK (1992) What does rCBF-SPECT offer in schizophrenia? *Nuclear Medicine Communications* **13**, 879–884.

Tamminga CA, Thaker GK, Buchanan RW *et al.* (1992) Limbic-system abnormalities identified in schizophrenia using positron emission tomography with fluorodeoxyglucose and neocortical alterations with deficit syndrome. *Archives of General Psychiatry* **49**, 522–530.

Ward KE, Friedman L, Wise A, Schulz SC (1996) Meta-analysis of brain and cranial size in schizophrenia. *Schizophrenia Research* **22**, 197–223.

Weinberger DR, Berman KF, Zec RF (1986) Physiologic dysfunction of dorsolateral prefrontal cortex in schizophrenia I. Regional cerebral blood flow evidence. *Archives of General Psychiatry* **43**, 114–124.

Wenz F, Schad LF, Knopp MV *et al.* (1994) Functional magnetic resonance imaging at 1.5 T: Activation pattern in schizophrenia patients receiving neuroleptic medication. *Magnetic Resonance Imaging* **12**, 975–982.

Wible CG, Shenton ME, Hokama H (1995) Prefrontal cortex and schizophrenia. A quantitative magnetic resonance imaging study. *Archives of General Psychiatry* **52**, 279–288.

Woodruff P, Brammer M, Mellers J, Wright I, Bullmore E, Williams S (1994) Auditory hallucinations and perception of external speech. *Lancet* **346**, 1035–1036.

8 Neuropathology and the Neurodevelopmental Model

Mayada Akil and Daniel R. Weinberger

The neurodevelopmental hypothesis of schizophrenia has been in vogue for over a decade following the emergence of several lines of evidence implicating abnormalities of brain development in this disorder. In this chapter, we summarize the evidence suggesting a neurodevelopmental origin of schizophrenia. We then review the neuropathological findings, asking the question: Are these findings consistent with neurodevelopmental aberrations? Finally, we discuss the limitations of the model and ways it may be refined and tested in the future.

Before proceeding, it is worth noting that several versions of the neurodevelopmental hypothesis have been put forth. For example, some stress a pathological process that affects the brain early in life, probably no later than the second trimester *in utero* (Murray and Lewis, 1987; Weinberger, 1987; Roberts, 1991). Others posit a later abnormality affecting brain maturation during adolescence (Randall, 1980; Feinberg, 1982; Stevens, 1992; DeLisi, 1997) or beyond; such processes may include synaptic pruning and myelination. Since clinical symptoms typically do not manifest until early adulthood, any form of the hypothesis has to account for this delayed onset. The 'late' neurodevelopmental hypothesis posits an aberration occurring in adolescence, around the age of onset of the clinical disorder. While parsimonious, this explanation cannot account for functional deficits and neuroimaging abnormalities detected long before the clinical syndrome is apparent (see below). In contrast, the 'early' form explains these findings, but instead has to account for a longer delay in clinical onset. Pathologically, this delay may be explained in one of two ways: either the early lesion sets the stage for a second neurodevelopmental abnormality which occurs closer to the age of onset, or the early lesion is unmasked by later developmental events or increased functional demands. There are precedents in experimental animal studies for early lesions remaining silent until after puberty whereupon deficits become apparent (Chapter 12). These different speculations regarding the relationship between neurodevelopmental events and the pathophysiology of schizophrenia need not be mutually exclusive. In fact, few *in vivo* or postmortem studies find evidence for a particular alteration in every individual, and heterogeneity in schizophrenia may incorporate different neurodevelopmental models, and other pathogenic processes.

Evidence supporting a neurodevelopmental origin of schizophrenia

Several lines of evidence suggest that there is a neurodevelopmental origin for schizophrenia and its neuropathology (Weinberger, 1995; Harrison, 1997; Table 8.1).

Aetiological evidence

This category includes evidence for insults to the brain that occur during early development and which are hypothesized to be responsible for the later manifestation of symptoms in schizophrenia.

Table 8.1 Categories of evidence for schizophrenia as a neurodevelopmental disorder

Aetiological
Maternal viral infection
Other obstetric and perinatal complications
Phenotypic
Minor physical anomalies
Premorbid childhood intellectual, motor, and behavioural abnormalities
Neuropsychological deficits are non-progressive
Neuropathological
Structural brain changes are present at first episode and are non-progressive[a]
Absence of gliosis excludes degenerative process[b]
Nature of cytoarchitectural findings (e.g. heterotopias)[c]
Increased frequency of focal developmental lesions (e.g. cavum septum pellucidum)[a]

[a] See also Chapter 1.
[b] See also Chapter 5.
[c] See also Chapters 2, 3, 4, 10 and 11.

Obstetric complications

An excess of obstetric complications (OCs) in the histories of schizophrenic patients compared to normal controls, siblings, and non-schizophrenic psychiatric controls has been reported and, on occasion, correlated with poor treatment response, neuropsychiatric abnormalities, and structural brain changes (Pollack *et al.*, 1966; Lewis, 1989; McNeil, 1995). However, the association has not been consistently found (Parnas *et al.*, 1982; Done *et al.*, 1991; McCreadie *et al.*, 1992), and publication bias against negative studies is suspected (Geddes and Lawrie, 1995). With this important caveat in mind, recent meta-analyses show that OCs are associated with a twofold increased risk of schizophrenia (Geddes and Lawrie, 1995), and correlate with early age of onset (Verdoux *et al.*, 1997). A further meta-analysis concluded that the OCs relevant for schizophrenia are: premature rupture of membranes, gestational age less than 37 weeks, and a history of requiring resuscitation or an incubator (Geddes *et al.*, 1999). As such, perinatal hypoxia may be a key mediator, and attention should be paid to its neurodevelopmental and neuropathological sequelae in order to assess the plausibility of the associations between these OCs and schizophrenia (Friede, 1989; Kuchna, 1994; Volpe, 1997; see also Chapter 11). It is also important to consider an alternative explanation for the relationship between OCs and schizophrenia, namely that OCs may result from an already abnormal brain, rather than having a direct causal role (Waddington *et al.*, 1998; McNeill and Cantor-Grae, 1999).

Viral exposure *in utero*

Mednick *et al.* (1988) reported an increased frequency of schizophrenia in the offspring of women who were in their second trimester of pregnancy during the height of an influenza epidemic in Finland in 1957. This finding spurred interest in the possibility that maternal viral infection leads to aberrant neurodevelopment and increases the risk for schizophrenia. A description of 'ectopic nerve cells' in the entorhinal cortex of some schizophrenics that were interpreted as the result of abnormal neuronal migration (Jakob and Beckman 1986) generated a great deal of excitement since neuronal migration occurs during the second trimester. However, this neuropathological evidence has been questioned (see below). Moreover, when other investigators reanalyzed the same epidemiological data from the influenza epidemic of 1957 they found no increased incidence of schizophrenia (Kendell and Kemp, 1989). In addition, the only study that attempted to ascertain that the mothers of the studied individuals had been diagnosed with influenza in their second trimester of pregnancy found no association with schizophrenia (Crow and Done, 1992). Other reports of an association between influenza epidemics and increased risk of schizophrenia appeared (O'Callaghan *et al.*, 1991; Adams *et al.*, 1993), however, reports of no association (Torrey *et al.*, 1988) also emerged. More recently, reports that viral exposure throughout childhood lead to increased risk of psychosis (Rantakallio *et al.*, 1997) put into question the notion that viral infections occurring specifically during early neurodevelopment predispose to schizophrenia. Moreover, prenatal exposure to infectious agents appears to predispose to psychiatric disorders other than schizophrenia (Cannon *et al.*, 1996; Machon *et al.*, 1997). Thus, we can only conclude at this stage that if viral exposure increases the risk for schizophrenia, it does so in a diagnostically non-specific fashion, with no mechanistic explanation, and that little can be said about the importance of the neurodevelopmental stage at which the exposure occurs (see Crow, 1994).

Other prenatal events have been associated with schizophrenia. For example, a twofold increase in risk was reported in male subjects with rhesus antigen incompatibility with their mothers (Hollister *et al.*, 1996). A similar increased risk of schizophrenia was described in the offspring of pregnant women exposed to the Dutch famine in the winter of 1944–45; the authors also provided a putative neurobiological basis for the association of malnutrition with schizophrenia (Brown *et al.*, 1996; Susser *et al.*, 1996). To date, however, these reports have not been independently replicated and the association with rhesus incompatability was not significant in the meta-analysis of Geddes *et al.* (1999).

Phenotypic evidence

This category includes evidence for other physical signs of maldevelopment, and the presence of premorbid neurological and behavioral abnormalities in individuals with schizophrenia.

Minor physical anomalies
It has been suggested that the frequency of minor physical anomalies (MPAs) among schizophrenics is higher than in the general population. MPAs are thought to reflect abnormal brain development since both facial and peripheral structures where these abnormalities are noted share the same origin with the brain, namely the embryonic ectoderm (Buckley, 1998). While theoretically compelling, these findings remain controversial for several reasons. Firstly, MPAs reported to be present in people with schizophrenia range in severity from high palate and low set ears (Kraepelin, 1919) to webbed digits (Green *et al.*, 1989, 1994). It is not clear, therefore, how an 'anomaly' is defined. Secondly, no large studies comparing schizophrenic patients with well-matched controls are available. Finally, the impact of chronic illness and treatment on physical appearance are difficult confounds to take into consideration.

Premorbid neurological and neuropsychological abnormalities
Several studies reported evidence of lower IQ in children who later developed schizophrenia (Albee *et al.*, 1963; Hyde *et al.*, 1994), though others found no difference (Torrey *et al.*, 1994). Abnormalities in motor function were noted in adolescent offspring of schizophrenics (Silverton *et al.*, 1988), and were observed in family home movies of young children who later developed schizophrenia (Walker and Lewine, 1990). In a prospective study of a large, unbiased population sample in the United Kingdom, individuals admitted to hospital for schizophrenia during adult life had evidence of maturational delays in primary motor milestones as early as 6 months of age (Jones *et al.*, 1994). In a separate British cohort, abnormalities in social adjustment were noted during the childhood of adults with schizophrenia compared to both normal controls and those who developed 'neurotic disorders' (Done *et al.*, 1994). In addition, children at risk for schizophrenia exhibit delayed neurological development (Fish *et al.*, 1992). More recently David *et al.* (1997) compared the premorbid IQ of 195 individuals, who were later admitted to hospital for schizophrenia, to those of the remainder of 50 000 males conscripted into the Swedish army. The IQ scores of those who subsequently developed schizophrenia was shifted downward with a

linear relationship between low IQ and risk. Thus the majority of evidence points to the presence of subtle premorbid neurofunctional abnormalities, consistent with a neurodevelopmental predisposition to schizophrenia, at least in some individuals.

Evidence from animal models

Animal models of the neurodevelopmental hypothesis of schizophrenia are described in Chapter 12. Briefly, neonatal lesions of the temporal lobe in both rodents and primates have pharmacological and behavioral consequences that mimic some aspects of schizophrenia, including their delayed emergence until early adulthood (Weinberger and Lipska, 1995).

Evidence against schizophrenia as a neurodegenerative disorder

In terms of fundamental neuropathological processes, the only clear alternative to a neurodevelopmental model is a neurodegenerative one (Chapter 11). Hence whilst evidence against the latter does not directly support the former, it suggests it by default as an explanation for consistent neuropathological findings that are not due to acute agonal events. As such, it is relevant to consider here whether there is evidence for neurodegeneration in schizophrenia. In this regard, two cardinal features of neurodegenerative processes are: the presence of gliosis, and the progression of the pathological changes in parallel with the clinical course of the disease.

Lack of gliosis

If schizophrenia involved an ongoing neuropathological degenerative process one would expect to find evidence of reactive gliosis. In fact, despite some conflicting data and residual controversies, it is widely accepted that there is no gliosis in schizophrenia. The data are reviewed in Chapter 5. The remaining controversies largely concern the certainty with which gliosis has been excluded, and the interpretation of what this negative result means.

In order to appreciate the potential pitfalls of investigating gliosis in schizophrenia, it is important to understand the complexity of the glial response (Kreutzberg *et al.*, 1997). Glial cells in general, and astrocytes in particular, respond to injury and degeneration in a complex fashion. An astrocytic response can manifest in one of several ways: astrocytic swelling is an early response that occurs frequently in hypoxia and other acute conditions. Hypertrophy has also been noted with or without astrocytic proliferation in acute and chronic disease. Once the acute lesion and edema are resolved, extensive formation of astrocytic glial filaments usually follows. Reactive astrocytes show an increase in immunoreactivity for glial fibrillary acidic protein (GFAP), an intermediate filament protein expressed in most if not all reactive astrocytes. In addition, increased GFAP immunoreactivity or mRNA levels are not necessarily disease-related and can occur as a function of development, aging, or other physiological states. For example, GFAP is not expressed in the neonatal rat. Its levels in aged rats are two- to threefold higher than in young adults in the hippocampus, striatum, and cortex. Furthermore, GFAP is regulated at both the transcriptional and translational levels and can be modulated by growth factors, cytokines, thyroid hormones, and adrenal and gonadal steroids in a complex and regionally specific fashion (Laping *et al.*, 1994). In addition to these multiple regulatory factors there are methodological issues affecting the detection and definition of gliosis (Harrison, 1995), which together mean that the possibility of gliosis in schizophrenia, and the circumstances under which it might occur (e.g. Arnold *et al.*, 1996), should remain under review.

The gliotic reaction to brain injury is said to begin in the second trimester *in utero*, and the absence of gliosis in schizophrenia has therefore been used to support the 'early' rather than the 'late' version of the neurodevelopmental model (Roberts, 1991; Weinberger, 1995). However, again this interpretation is subject to limitations. Firstly, there is little firm evidence as to the timing of onset of the glial response in human brain; and secondly, it is theoretically possible that the pathological process of schizophrenia, whenever it occurs, might fail to trigger gliosis.

Non-progressive morphometric abnormalities and intellectual impairment

The *in vivo* brain imaging findings in schizophrenia are summarized in Chapter 1. Relevant to the neurodevelopmental hypothesis, it is clear that enlarged ventricles and decreased cortical volume are present early in the illness, indeed at the onset of symptoms (Weinberger *et al.*, 1982; DeLisi *et al.*, 1991; Lieberman *et al.*, 1993; Hendren *et al.*, 1995). Changes also exist in subjects at high risk of schizophrenia (Keshavan *et al.*, 1997; Lawrie *et al.*, 1999) suggesting that the structural pathology is present premorbidly. Moreover, there is a lack of association between ventricular enlargement and duration of illness in the vast majority of studies (Weinberger *et al.*, 1979), and data from prospective studies following individuals for up to 10 years from the first episode show no progression in ventricular enlargement (Jaskiw *et al.* 1994); there is a similarly static picture for cortical volumes (Chapter 1). In keeping with these imaging findings, there are no correlations reported in postmortem morphometric studies with duration of illness (Chapters 2 to 4). Taken together, these observations suggest that by the time the illness is manifest, the 'lesion' leading to ventricular enlargement, and other pathological features, has already been established.

It should be noted that some neuroimaging studies *have* found evidence for progressive changes in cerebral morphometry over the course of the illness (e.g. Kaplan *et al.*, 1990; Rapoport *et al.*, 1997; Knoll *et al.*, 1998). However, the changes have been remarkably inconsistent from one report to another in terms of the specific structures that appear to lose volume. In addition, the magnitude of the changes is often neuropathologically improbable (e.g. 30 per cent loss of thalamic volume in 2 years; Rapoport *et al.*, 1997). Finally, both volume loss and volume gain have been described in the same samples over time. These findings raise questions about whether the changes are at the level of physiology (e.g. perfusion, blood volume) and not structural neuropathology.

In keeping with the conclusion that the neuropathology of schizophrenia is—at least in most patients—not progressive, adults with schizophrenia have impaired performance on tests of general intellectual functioning which is present at first episode of illness (Hoff *et al.*, 1992; Saykin *et al.*, 1991) and appears largely static thereafter (Offord and Cross, 1971; Goldberg *et al.*, 1993; Aleman *et al.*, 1999). Moreover, the impairment is present premorbidly (Jones *et al.*, 1994; Crow *et al.*, 1995; Russell *et al.*, 1997), leading Russell and colleagues to conclude that deficits of intellectual function are 'lifelong and predate the onset of schizophrenia'. In summary, the lack of progression in both structural pathology and indices of intellectual function provide strong indirect support for the neurodevelopmental hypothesis of schizophrenia.

Neuropathological findings and the neurodevelopmental model

We have considered several lines of evidence which support the neurodevelopmental hypothesis of schizophrenia, notably the presence of premorbid neurological and neuropsychological abnormalities, the non-progressive nature of the pathology in most cases, and the absence of an observable degenerative process. The remaining category of evidence to consider concerns neuropathological findings reported in schizophrenia and how they bear upon the neurodevelopmental hypothesis.

The search for the neuropathology of schizophrenia began over a hundred years ago and was active in the first half of the twentieth century, with a wide range of abnormalities reported. However, by the early 1970s the general view was that no convincing neuropathological features of schizophrenia had been found, and perhaps that there *was* no pathology to be found (Kirch and Weinberger, 1986; see also Chapter 13). However, since the latter view became untenable with the emerging CT and MRI findings in the 1980s (Weinberger, 1995; Chapter 1) there has been an active search for the histological, histochemical, and molecular correlates of these alterations. Findings of postmortem studies have contributed to the formulation of several hypotheses for the pathophysiology of schizophrenia involving neurodevelopment.

A putative failure of the migration of cortical neurons

In a much cited study, Jakob and Beckman (1986) examined the brains from 64 subjects with schizophrenia and compared them to 10 non-schizophrenic controls. They reported abnormal sulcogyral patterns of the temporal lobe in 42 cases and abnormal cytoarchitectonics of the rostral entorhinal cortex in 20 cases. The sulcogyral pattern deviations were not described. As to the cytoarchitectonic differences, the authors noted, the presence of 'heterotopic nerve cells in the third layer pre-β belonging to the second layer pre-α'. They interpreted their findings as evidence of incomplete neuronal migration, presumably occurring during the second trimester of gestation. Some confirmation of this finding was provided by Falkai *et al.* (1988) and by Arnold *et al.* (1991).

These reports, combined with the well-documented decrease in the size of the medial temporal lobe in schizophrenia (Chapter 2) and viewed in the light of the neurodevelopmental model, generated a great deal of excitement because they appeared to offer dramatic neuropathological support for an early developmental aberration. Unfortunately, the reports were fraught with methodological problems (see also Chapters 2 and 13). Jakob and Beckman (1986) selected the sections examined based upon the distance from an external landmark rather than upon cytoarchitectural features. Consequently they are likely to have compared different entorhinal subdivisions in at least some of their schizophrenic and non-schizophrenic groups. This is apparent from the examination of their own illustration where differences in deep cortical layers indicate that more rostral regions were examined in the schizophrenic subjects whereas more caudal areas were examined in the non-schizophrenic subjects. Interestingly, many of the 'abnormal' features they described, such as 'a disordered double row of neurons' are in fact characteristic of the more rostral regions in the normal entorhinal cortex. This mismatching may have resulted from the reduced volume of the medial temporal lobe in schizophrenia, suggesting that the relative location of the entorhinal cortex subdivisions may be altered (Akil and Lewis, 1997). Both studies supporting the Jakob and Beckman report (Falkai et al., 1988; Arnold et al., 1991) provided little detail regarding the exact abnormalities noted and one of them examined six subjects from the Yakovlev collection, each of whom had undergone prefrontal lobotomy (Arnold et al., 1991).

More systematic recent examinations of the rostral entorhinal cortex of schizophrenics have failed to replicate the findings of abnormal sulcogyral patterns or cytoarchitectonic aberrations (Heinsen et al., 1996; Noga et al., 1996; Akil and Lewis, 1997; Krimer et al., 1997). Using cytoarchitectonic criteria, Akil and Lewis (1997) found no qualitative differences in cytoarchitecture of the rostral entorhinal cortex between 10 schizophrenics and 10 matched controls. They also confirmed that there is substantial heterogeneity in the cytoarchitecture of the normal entorhinal cortex. Similarly, Krimer et al. (1997) examined the rostral subdivisions of the entorhinal cortex of 14 pairs of schizophrenic subjects and matched controls, including quantitative analyses of neuronal counts, measures of density, total cortical volume, and laminar depth in a subset of their sample. They noted no consistent cytoarchitectural differences between the two groups, and no statistically significant differences in any of their quantitative measures.

While the recent studies do not support the presence of abnormal migration of neurons in the entorhinal cortex of schizophrenics, it is important to remember that they do not exclude the presence of other alterations in the circuitry of this region (nor of a migrational disturbance elewhere in the cortex). The volume reduction in the medial temporal lobe remains to be explained, and further careful morphometric comparisons may provide important information.

Developmental disturbance of the cortical subplate

In a study of five schizophrenic subjects and five normal controls, Akbarian et al. (1993a) examined white matter neurons in the dorsolateral prefrontal cortex using nicotinamide adenine dinucleotide phosphate-diaphorase (NADPH-D) histochemistry. They reported that the highest density of NADPH-D-containing neurons in normal controls was in the superficial compartment of the subcortical white matter. In the schizophrenic subjects, however, the number of NADPH-D-containing neurons was significantly reduced in the superficial compartments and increased in the deep compartments of the white matter. Since white matter neurons are known survivors of the cortical subplate, these data suggest that a developmental disturbance in the subplate may be present in schizophrenia. The subplate is a transient structure that is critical for the development of normal cortex (Allendoerfer and Shatz, 1994). It contains the first neurons that migrate to the surface of the cerebral hemisphere and, later, neurons migrate through it to form the cerebral cortex. Similarly, afferent and efferent axons grow through the subplate, and patterns of cortical circuitry are thus established. Once these tasks are completed, many subplate neurons undergo programmed cell death and those that survive remain in the white matter. The higher concentration of NADPH-D-containing neurons in the deep portions of the white matter in schizophrenic individuals suggests a developmental abnormality in the subplate involving either abnormal programmed cell death or abnormal migration of subplate neurons. Either way, the abnormality may result in defective connectivity and structure of the overlying cortex.

In a companion study, Akbarian *et al.* (1993*b*) examined the temporal lobe of seven schizophrenic subjects and seven matched controls. The findings differed somewhat from those in the prefrontal cortex. NADPH-D-containing neurons were reduced in the gray matter and increased in the white matter of the middle temporal gyrus. The total number of NADPH-D-containing neurons was reduced by 50 per cent in the hippocampus and unchanged in the entorhinal cortex and the subicular complex. In a later report (Akbarian *et al.*, 1996), the prefrontal cortex was examined in a larger cohort (20 schizophrenics and 20 controls) and using other markers of white matter neurons, namely microtubule associated protein 2 (MAP-2) and non-phosphorylated neurofilament proteins. The schizophrenic group included the five cases in the original report. However, only seven of the 20 schizophrenics included in the second study demonstrated a 'substantial redistribution', suggesting that only two of the added 15 cases showed the same phenomenon. A different group of investigators (Anderson *et al.*, 1996) found that the mean density of MAP-2-labeled neurons was greater in the superficial white matter of schizophrenic subjects compared to controls but did not differ in the deeper white matter. While these findings do not replicate those of Akbarian *et al.* in the prefrontal cortex, they are reminiscent of their findings in the medial temporal lobe and further support the possibility of abnormal development of the cortical subplate. This is an intriguing possibility that requires further investigation.

Loss of neuropil in the cortical mantle

Several lines of evidence point to the possibility that the volume of neuropil may be reduced in the prefrontal cortex, and perhaps in other cortical regions, in schizophrenia (Chapter 3). Firstly, one of the most consistently reported changes in the brains of schizophrenic patients has been the reduction in brain volume and thinning of the cerebral cortex, noted on both neuroimaging and postmortem studies (Chapter 1). For example, the prefrontal and temporal cortices of schizophrenics has been found to be 8 to 10 per cent thinner than that of controls (Brown *et al.*, 1986; Pakkenberg, 1987; Shelton *et al.*, 1988; Breier *et al.*, 1992; Zipursky *et al.*, 1992; Andreasen *et al.*, 1994; Schlaepfer *et al.*, 1994; Selemon *et al.*, 1998; Gur *et al.*, 1999). Secondly, despite some reports of neuronal loss (Benes *et al.*, 1986, 1991), recent careful examinations of the prefrontal cortex found the number of neurons to be unchanged in schizophrenia (Pakkenberg, 1993; Akbarian *et al.*, 1995; Selemon *et al.*, 1995, 1998). Furthermore, preliminary evidence for an increase in the density of pyramidal cells ranging from 10 to 21 per cent in the prefrontal and visual cortices was reported by Selemon *et al.* (1995, 1998). Similarly, a report by Daviss and Lewis (1995) found an increase in calbindin-immunoreactive interneurons in the same areas of the prefrontal cortex.

These data suggest than schizophrenics may have a thinner prefrontal cortex than that of controls with an unaltered number of neurons. What might account for this difference? Reduced neuronal size is one potential contributor that has been examined by Rajkowska *et al.* (1998). They reported a downward shift in neuronal sizes in areas 9 (dorsolateral prefrontal cortex) and 17 (visual cortex) in schizophrenia, particularly in layer III. This reduction in soma size alone could not account, however, for a 20 per cent increase in neuronal density described above. A decrease in the number of other neuronal elements such as dendrites, spines, or axons, which are often collectively referred to as neuropil, has to be considered. Since neuronal soma size has been correlated with volume of dendrites and axons the neuron has to support (Chapter 11), the finding of reduced neuronal soma size—also seen in the hippocampus (Chapter 2)—strengthens the possibility of reduced cortical neuropil in schizophrenia.

The third line of emerging evidence for reduced neuropil comprises a putative reduction in the number of synapses (Chapter 4). Increased phospholipid turnover in the prefrontal cortex of patients with schizophrenia observed with phosphorus magnetic resonance spectroscopy (Pettegrew *et al.*, 1991; Williamson *et al.*, 1991; Deicken *et al.*, 1994; Stanley *et al.*, 1995; Bertolino *et al.*, 1996) may reflect a loss of axons and their terminals. In addition, the number of spines (the major sites of excitatory synapses) on the dendrites of layer III pyramidal neurons in the prefrontal cortex was found to be significantly reduced in schizophrenia (Garey *et al.*, 1998; Glantz and Lewis, 2000). Data from studies of synaptic markers are consistent with the possibility that the prefrontal and temporal cortices have fewer synapses in schizophrenia compared to controls. Synaptophysin is an integral membrane protein which is useful as a marker for synapses because it is present in almost all synaptic terminals (Jahn *et al.*, 1985). Several studies have reported a reduction in the abundance of synaptophysin or its mRNA in schizophrenia (Eastwood and Harrison, 1995; Glantz and Lewis, 1997). Finally, several other synapse-related proteins have been investigated, with the weight of the evidence suggesting reductions in their expression in schizophrenia (Geethabali *et al.*, 1996; Harrison and Eastwood, 1998).

An initial increase and then a decline in synaptic density in layer III of the frontal cortex during late childhood has been reported (Huttenlocher, 1979). In monkey cortex, Rakic *et al.* (1986) also found that synaptic density reaches a peak several months after birth, remains stable until the age of 3, and declines in the following year, corresponding with the time of puberty. By age 4 animals reach the adult level of synaptic density. It appears to be asymmetric synapses, which are generally presumed to be excitatory, which are selectively eliminated during development in monkey cortex (Zecevic *et al.*, 1989; Bourgeois and Rakic, 1993). In contrast to non-human primates, the details of synapse elimination in the human cortex are not well worked out in terms of laminar and regional specificity, types of synapses eliminated, and the time course of this elimination. If

Huttenlocher's evidence for synapse elimination in the human cerebral cortex during puberty is confirmed, then data suggesting a reduction of synapse-related structures or proteins in schizophrenia might be interpreted to reflect an aberration in this event (Keshavan *et al.*, 1994), and support 'late' neurodevelopmental models (see above). However, a cautionary note is necessary concerning speculation that synaptic pruning may be the primary patho-logical substrate of schizophrenia. The molecular evidence indicates that synapses are lost because trophic signals that accompany active connections are diminished. Thus, a loss of synaptic markers presumably reflects a loss or weakening of a functional connection. In this sense, the pruning is not a primary event but the result of the underlying process of maintenance of connectivity. A pathology of the pruning process *per se* would imply some breakdown of the molecular mechanisms of retrograde signaling at synapses. It is unknown if such a pathology exists in any human or experimental condition. It seems more logical to us that observed changes in synaptic markers, both in normal development and possibly in schizophrenia, are secondary to changes in functional connectivity (Chapter 7).

Alterations in glutamatergic and GABAergic neurons

There are two major classes of neurons in the cerebral cortex: (a) output neurons which have pyramidal morphology and are glutamatergic and excitatory; and (b) local circuit neurons (interneurons) of non-pyramidal morphology that use the transmitter GABA and are inhibitory (Chapter 10). Both have been implicated in the pathophysiology of schizo-phrenia (Chapter 3).

Pyramidal neurons and the glutamatergic involvement
Since pyramidal neurons play a central role in cortical function and contain glutamate, several investigators have examined the role of glutamate in schizophrenia. This interest was also sparked by the clinical observation that phencyclidine hydrochloride (PCP) and other NMDA receptor channel antagonists, can produce symptoms reminiscent of this disorder. Furthermore, experimental animal studies have suggested that structural damage due to NMDA antagonists such as PCP is not found until after puberty, consistent with the age of onset in schizophrenia (Henn, 1995). Many findings of altered glutamatergic function in schizophrenia have been reported (see Goff and Wine, 1997; Hirsch *et al.*, 1997), with the weight of the evidence on the side of glutamatergic hypofunction (Halberstadt, 1995; Bachus and Kleinman, 1996). Although altered expression of both NMDA and non-NMDA receptor subtypes has been reported (Chapter 3), particular focus has been on the former, with the hypothesis that NMDA receptor hypofunction is the key mechanism in schizophrenia (Olney and Farber, 1995). Finally, a recent examination in eight brain regions of schizophrenics, controls, and neuroleptic-treated controls revealed reduced glutamate and aspartate concentrations and lower N-acetyl-α-linked acidic dipep-tidase activity in prefrontal cortex and hippocampus of the schizophrenic subjects (Tsai *et al.*, 1995).

These and other reported alterations in glutamatergic neurotransmission in schizophrenia raise several issues, such as the relationship between glutamate and dopamine systems, and whether the glutamatergic changes are primary, or secondary to subtle structural changes affecting pyramidal neurons. For this chapter, the most pertinent question is whether gluta-matergic dysfunction is supportive of a neurodevelopmental model. Unfortunately no clear answer can be given, though it can be argued that the findings are in keeping with a developmental origin (Olney and Farber, 1995; Mohn *et al.*, 1999).

Interneurons and GABAergic involvement

Local circuit neurons constitute 20 to 30 per cent of all neurons in primate cortex and contain the neurotransmitter GABA. Several lines of evidence implicate a disturbance in GABAergic function in schizophrenia. For example, Akbarian and colleagues (1995) reported that the number of neurons expressing glutamic acid decarboxylase (GAD), the synthesizing enzyme for GABA, was reduced in the prefrontal cortex in this disorder. The investigators found no evidence for neuronal loss, however, suggesting that the decrease in GAD mRNA expression was not attributable to a loss of GABAergic neurons.

Morphologically distinct subclasses of local circuit neurons have been identified in both monkey and human cortex. These subpopulations differ in their dendritic and axonal features, their axonal targets, and their neurochemical content (Peters and Jones, 1991). Calcium binding proteins, such as parvalbumin, calbindin, and calretinin, have proven to be useful markers for distinct subpopulations of GABAergic neurons (Chapter 10). Some investigators have reported a decrease in the number of all local circuit neurons (Benes *et al.*, 1991) or of parvalbumin containing neurons (Beasley and Reynolds, 1997). Others, however, did not replicate these findings (Woo *et al.*, 1997). In addition, a study of calbindin containing local circuit neurons in the prefrontal cortex of schizophrenic and control subjects found the density of this subpopulation to be increased (Daviss and Lewis, 1995). Most recently, Woo *et al.* (1998) found that another GABAergic cell population called chandelier cells may be differentially altered in schizophrenia. The role of neurodevelopment in these findings remains unclear but raises interesting questions (Lewis, 1997). For example, the axon terminals of chandelier neurons are arrayed in a morphologically distinct fashion and are referred to as cartridges. The cartridges form inhibitory synapses on the axon initial segment of pyramidal neurons and can be identified by the presence of the calcium binding protein, parvalbumin. The number of parvalbumin-positive cartridges in the monkey prefrontal cortex has been shown to undergo substantial changes during postnatal development (Lewis and Lund, 1990; Akil and Lewis, 1992; Anderson *et al.*, 1995). Perhaps aberrations in these developmental shifts in parvalbumin containing cartridges are related to the observation of reduced numbers of cartridges in the prefrontal cortex in schizophrenia.

The dopaminergic hypothesis

The dopaminergic hypothesis of schizophrenia, in its initial formulation, posited that the disorder was due to a functional excess of dopamine. However, results of more recent studies have led to the suggestion that some symptoms of schizophrenia, particularly those related to cortical dysfunction such as cognitive deficits and negative symptoms, may result from a deficit in cortical dopaminergic neurotransmission. The latter may in fact lead to a functional excess of subcortical dopamine and thus the two alterations are not incompatible in the same system. Evidence for a functional deficit in cortical dopamine includes the following: first, decreased cerebrospinal fluid levels of homovanillic acid, a dopamine metabolite, have been associated with negative symptoms, cortical atrophy, and a subnormal increase in blood flow to the prefrontal cortex during tasks that require its activation (Weinberger *et al.*, 1988). Secondly, depletion of dopamine in the prefrontal cortex of monkeys produces impairments in the performance of delayed response tasks comparable to those seen in schizophrenic patients (Brozoski *et al.*, 1979). Thirdly, binding to the dopamine transporter, a presynaptic marker of dopaminergic axons, was found to be decreased in the anterior cingulate cortex in schizophrenia (Hitri *et al.*, 1995). Finally, the expression of genes encoding the five dopamine receptors is altered in some cortical regions (Schmauss *et al.*, 1993; Meador-Woodruff *et al.*, 1997). More direct evidence for the notion of diminished cortical dopaminergic neurotransmission in schizophrenia comes from postmortem studies indicating a decrease in the density of immunolabeled dopaminergic axons in prefrontal and entorhinal cortices (Akil and Lewis, 1997; Akil *et al.*, 1999, 2000).

From a neurodevelopmental perspective, dopaminergic neurons are thought to migrate and differentiate in the human mesencephalon in the first trimester (Almqvist *et al.*, 1996), with a well-developed dopaminergic innervation of the cerebral cortex by mid-gestation (Verney *et al.*, 1993). However, the dopaminergic innervation of primate cortex undergoes further refinement during adolescence (Rosenberg and Lewis, 1994; Erickson *et al.*, 1998). It is thus possible that dopaminergic innervation of the cerebral cortex might go awry in schizophrenia either in early prenatal life, or around puberty. Unfortunately, this complexity hampers attempts to incriminate a particular neurodevelopmental timepoint in alterations in dopaminergic transmission in schizophrenia.

Alterations in development-related molecules

Postmortem investigations of molecules involved in neurodevelopment (Chapter 9) have emerged as a novel approach for testing the neurodevelopmental hypothesis (Weickert and Weinberger, 1998). For example, cell–cell or cell–matrix interactions are considered essential for the guidance of neuronal migration. A variety of adhesion promoting cell surface receptors have been implicated in cell migration including neural cell adhesion molecule (N-CAM). An N-CAM gene mutation has been shown to inhibit tangential neuronal migration (Ono *et al.*, 1994). The expression of several isoforms of N-CAM, including the embryonic polysialylated isoform PSA-NCAM, were examined in the hippocampus and prefrontal cortex from 10 schizophrenics and 11 matched controls. These investigators found a significant reduction in PSA-NCAM from the dentate gyrus and hilus in the majority of the schizophrenics (Barbeau *et al.*, 1995). In contrast, Vawter *et al.* (1998) found increased N-CAM protein concentrations in the prefrontal cortex and hippocampus in schizophrenia (Chapter 4).

There are preliminary reports of other neurodevelopmentally important molecules in schizophrenia. Limbic associated membrane protein (LAMP), another cell adhesion molecule, has been found to be reduced in the entorhinal cortex compared to controls (Hyde *et al.*, 1997). The expression of brain-derived neurotrophic factor (BDNF), a neurotrophic factor that plays a role in the survival of neurons, is reported to be decreased in the hippocampus (Brouha *et al.*, 1996). Abnormalities of the *Wnt* signalling pathway, implicated in cell proliferation, migration, and fate determination, have also been described in the hippocampus (Cotter *et al.*, 1998). As a final example, there is a decreased expression of reelin in the prefrontal cortex of schizophrenic subjects (Impagnatiello *et al.*, 1998); reelin is the protein disrupted in the *reeler* mouse that shows extensive abnormalities in neuronal migration, consistent with a role for this gene in migration, axonal growth, and synaptogenesis (Borrell *et al.*, 1999).

Despite the preliminary nature of these findings, they represent exciting avenues of direct investigation of the neurodevelopmental hypothesis of schizophrenia at the molecular level. However, the interpretation of findings is not straightforward. The persistence of molecules like N-CAM, LAMP, and BDNF in adult and even elderly brain suggests that these same molecules may subserve different functions at different times of life. Therefore, alterations in the expression of these molecules in schizophrenia may have arisen later in life, rather than necessarily reflecting an early neurodevelopmental origin.

Limitations of the neurodevelopmental model

Limitations of postmortem studies

While postmortem studies provide excellent means for testing hypotheses attempting to explain the neuropathology of schizophrenia, they also suffer from serious limitations. Postmortem evidence for neurodevelopmental abnormalities may be masked by a variety of life events, the consequences of chronic disease and its treatment, the cause of death, not to mention variables that come into play in the aftermath of death (Chapters 14 and 15). Age, chronic illness, and environmental stimulation are known confounders of studies of neuronal morphology and spine numbers. Some, such as age, can be controlled for, while others are more difficult to take into consideration. Obviously, not all postmortem data carry the same weight. Studies that have been designed and executed thoughtfully and have been independently replicated are of greatest value. Even the best postmortem data, however, are greatly enhanced by corroborative *in vivo* results. Such convergence is now becoming feasible with advances in neuroimaging (Chapter 7). For example, proton magnetic resonance spectroscopic imaging has shown that patients with acute schizophrenia have reduced concentrations of *N*-acetyl aspartate (NAA) in the temporal and prefrontal cortical regions bilaterally (Bertolino *et al.*, 1996; see Chapter 7). This finding is strikingly consistent with the postmortem results of Tsai *et al.* (1995) described above.

Conceptual and other limitations

Because much of the evidence supporting the neurodevelopmental hypothesis, both epidemiological and neuropathological, is disputed, inferences should be drawn cautiously from the results. Critical links are missing, such as what neuropathology does a particular OC cause that may account for the development of schizophrenia? Does it reproduce the postmortem data that exist? Another important limitation is that the data which currently support the developmental hypothesis may have alternative, albeit less compelling, explanations. Perhaps the most critical question to ask of the neurodevelopmental hypothesis, in terms of its associated neuropathology, is what neuropathological findings would confirm it or disprove it? Certainly heterotopias or cytoarchitectural disarray that can only be explained by abnormal neuronal migration would provide reasonable confirmation, but such evidence is currently lacking. At the molecular level, if the brains of patients with schizophrenia expressed a developmental molecule not normally found in adulthood, or expressed it in a region where it is not normally found, that would be highly suggestive. Such findings also are lacking. At present, only the absence of gliosis constitutes firm neuropathological evidence for the neurodevelopmental hypothesis—and even here, this is mainly absence of evidence against the neurodegenerative alternative. Clearly, identification of an unambiguously neurodevelopmental genetic or cellular defect abnormality would go a long way towards advancing the neurodevelopmental hypothesis of schizophrenia.

As mentioned at the start of this chapter, the neurodevelopmental hypothesis has variants, with key timeframes ranging from first trimester *in utero* through adolescence to early adulthood. Some recent models advocate progressive, essentially neurodegenerative processes in addition to, or instead of, neurodevelopmental ones (Waddington *et al.*, 1998; Garver *et al.*, 1999; Lieberman, 1999). Whilst such ideas may have heuristic as well as empirical merit, e.g. for explaining heterogeneity and encouraging therapeutic optimism, the broadening of focus in no way diminishes the need to test critically specific aspects of the neurodevelopmental model, along the lines described here. The design and interpretation of these investigations will benefit from the increasing understanding of normal brain developmental processes, as outlined in the next chapter.

References

Adams W, Kendell RE, Hare EH, Munk-Jorgensen P (1993) Epidemiological evidence that maternal influenza contributes to the aetiology of schizophrenia. *British Journal of Psychiatry* **163**, 522–534.

Akbarian S, Bunney WE, Potkin SG *et al.* (1993a) Altered distribution of nicotinamide-adenine dinucleotide phosphate-diaphorase cells in frontal lobe of schizophrenics implies disturbances of cortical development. *Archives of General Psychiatry* **50**, 169–187.

Akbarian S, Viñuela A, Kim JJ, Potkin SG, Bunney WE, Jr, Jones EG (1993b) Distorted distribution of nicotinamide-adenine dinucleotide phosphate-diaphorase neurons in temporal lobe of schizophrenics implies anomalous cortical development. *Archives of General Psychiatry* **50**, 178–187.

Akbarian S, Kim JJ, Potkin SG *et al.* (1995) Gene expression for glutamic acid decarboxylase is reduced without loss of neurons in prefrontal cortex of schizophrenics. *Archives of General Psychiatry* **52**, 258–266.

Akbarian S, Kim JJ, Potkin SG, Hetrick WP, Bunney WE, Jones EG (1996) Maldistribution of interstitial neurons in prefrontal white matter of the brains of schizophrenic patients. *Archives of General Psychiatry* **53**, 425–436.

Akil M, Lewis DA (1992) Differential distribution of parvalbumin-immunoreactive peri-cellular clusters of terminal boutons in developing and adult monkey neocortex. *Experimental Neurology* **115**, 239–249.

Akil M, Lewis DA (1997) Cytoarchitecture of the entorhinal cortex in schizophrenia. *American Journal of Psychiatry* **154**, 1010–1012.

Akil M, Pierri JN, Whitehead RE *et al.* (1999) Lamina-specific alterations in the dopamine innervation of the prefrontal cortex in schizophrenic subjects. *American Journal of Psychiatry* **156**, 1580–1589.

Akil M, Edgar CL, Pierri JN *et al.* (2000) Decreased density of tyrosine hydroxylase-immunoreactive axons in the entorhinal cortex of schizophrenic subjects. *Biological Psychiatry* **47**, 361–370.

Albee G, Corcoran C, Werneke A (1963) Childhood and intercurrent intellectual performance of adult schizophrenics. *Journal of Consultation Psychology* **27**, 364–366.

Aleman A, Hijman R, de Haan EHF, Kahn RS (1999) Memory impairment in schizophrenia: a meta-analysis. *American Journal of Psychiatry* **156**, 1358–1366.

Allendoerfer KL, Shatz CJ. (1994) The subplate, a transient neocortical structure: Its role in the development of connections between thalamus and cortex. *Annual Review of Neuroscience* **17**, 185–218.

Almqvist PM, Akesson E, Wahlberg LU, Pschera H, Seiger A, Sundstrom E (1996) First trimester development of the human nigrostriatal dopamine system. *Experimental Neurology* **139**, 227–237.

Anderson SA, Classey JD, Conde F, Lund JS, Lewis DA (1995) Synchronous development of pyramidal neuron dendritic spines and parvalbumin-immunoreactive chandelier neuron axon terminals in layer III of monkey prefrontal cortex. *Neuroscience* **67**, 7–22.

Anderson S, Volk DW, Lewis DA (1996) Increased density of microtubule associated protein 2-immunoreactive neurons in the prefrontal white matter of schizophrenic subjects. *Schizophrenia Research* **19**, 111–119.

Andreasen NC, Flashman L, Flaum M *et al.* (1994) Regional brain abnormalities in schizophrenia measured with magnetic resonance imaging. *Journal of the American Medical Association* **272**, 1763–1769.

Arnold SE, Hyman BT, Van Hoesen GW, Damasio AR (1991) Some cytoarchitectural abnormalities of the entorhinal cortex in schizophrenia. *Archives of General Psychiatry* **48**, 625–632.

Arnold SE, Franz BR, Trojanowski JQ, Moberg PJ, Gur RE (1996) Glial fibrillary acidic protein-immunoreactive astrocytosis in elderly patients with schizophrenia and dementia. *Acta Neuropathologica* **91**, 269–277.

Bachus SE, Kleinman JE (1996) The neuropathology of schizophrenia. *Journal of Clinical Psychiatry* **57**, 72–83.

Barbeau D, Liang JJ, Robitalille Y, Quirion R, Srivastava L (1995) Decreased expression of the embryonic form of the neural cell adhesion molecule in schizophrenic brains. *Proceedings of the National Academy of Science USA* **92**, 2785–2789.

Beasley CL, Reynolds GP (1997) Parvalbumin-immunoreactive neurons are reduced in the prefrontal cortex of schizophrenics. *Schizophrenia Research* **24**, 349–355.

Benes FM, Davidson J, Bird ED (1986) Quantitative cytoarchitectural studies of the cerebral cortex of schizophrenics. *Archives of General Psychiatry* **43**, 31–35.

Benes FM, McSparren J, Bird ED, San Giovanni JP, Vincent SL (1991) Deficits in small interneurons in prefrontal and cingulate cortices of schizophrenic and schizoaffective patients. *Archives of General Psychiatry* **48**, 996–1001.

Bertolino A, Nawroz S, Mattay VS *et al.* (1996) Regionally specific pattern of neurochemical pathology in schizophrenia as assessed by multislice proton magnetic resonance spectroscopic imaging. *American Journal of Psychiatry* **153**, 1544–1563.

Borrell V, Del Río JA, Alcántara S *et al.* (1999) Reelin regulates the development and synaptogenesis of the layer-specific entorhino-hippocampal connections. *Journal of Neuroscience* **19**, 1345–1358.

Bourgeois JP, Rakic P (1993) Changes of synaptic density in the primary visual cortex of the macaque monkey from fetal to adult stage. *Journal of Neuroscience* **13**, 2801–2820.

Breier A, Buchanan RW, Elkashef A, Munsen RC, Kirkpatrick B, Gellad F (1992) Brain morphology and schizophrenia: a magnetic resonance imaging study of limbic, prefrontal cortex, and caudate structures. *Archives of General Psychiatry* **49**, 921–926.

Brouha AK, Shannon Weickert C, Hyde TM *et al.* (1996) Reductions in brain derived neurotrophic factor mRNA in the hippocampus of patients with schizophrenia. *Society for Neuroscience* **22**, 1680.

Brown R, Colter N, Corsellis J *et al.* (1986) Post-mortem evidence of structural brain changes in schizophrenia. *Archives of General Psychiatry* **43**, 36–42.

Brown AS, Susser E, Butler PD, Andrews RR, Kaufmann CA, Gorman HM (1996) Neurobiological plausibility of prenatal nutritional deprivation as a risk factor for schizophrenia. *Journal of Nervous and Mental Disease* **184**, 71–85.

Brozoski TJ, Brown RM, Rosvoid HE, Goldman PS (1979) Cognitive deficit caused by regional depletion of dopamine in prefrontal cortex of rhesus monkey. *Science* **205**, 929–932.

Buckley PF (1998) The clinical stigmata of aberrant neurodevelopment in schizophrenia. *Journal of Nervous and Mental Disease* **186**, 79–86.

Cannon M, Cotter D, Coffey VP *et al.* (1996) Prenatal exposure to the 1957 influenza epidemic and adult schizophrenia: a follow-up study. *British Journal of Psychiatry* **163**, 368–371.

Cotter D, Kerwin R, Al-Sarraji S *et al.* (1998) Abnormalities of *Wnt* signalling in schizophrenia—evidence for neurodevelopmental abnormality. *Neuroreport* **9**, 1379–1383.

Crow TJ (1994) Prenatal exposure to influenza as a cause of schizophrenia: There are inconsistencies and contradictions in the evidence. *British Journal of Psychiatry* **164**, 588–592.

Crow TJ, Done DJ (1992) Prenatal exposure to influenza does not cause schizophrenia. *British Journal of Psychiatry* **161**, 390–393.

Crow TJ, Done DJ, Sacker A (1995) Childhood precursors of psychosis as clues to its evolutionary origins. *European Archives of Psychiatry and Clinical Neuroscience* **245**, 61–69.

David AS, Malmberg A, Brandt L, Allebeck P, Lewis G (1997) IQ and risk for schizophrenia: a population-based cohort study. *Psychological Medicine* **27**, 1311–1323.

Daviss SR, Lewis DA (1995) Local circuit neurons of the prefrontal cortex in schizophrenia: selective increase in the density of calbindin-immunoreactive neurons. *Psychiatry Research* **59**, 81–96.

Deicken RF, Calbrese G, Merrin EL *et al.* (1994) ^{31}Phosphorus magnetic resonance spectroscopy of the frontal and parietal lobes in chronic schizophrenia. *Biological Psychiatry* **36**, 503–510.

DeLisi LE (1997) Is schizophrenia a lifetime disorder of brain plasticity, growth and aging? *Schizophrenia Research* **23**, 119–129.

DeLisi LE, Hoff AL, Schwartz JE *et al.* (1991) Brain morphology in first-episode schizophrenic-like psychotic patients: a quantitative magnetic resonance imaging study. *Biological Psychiatry* **129**, 159–175.

Done DJ, Johnstone EC, Frith CD, Golding J, Shepherd PM, Crow TJ (1991) Complications of pregnancy and delivery in relation to psychosis in adult life: data from the British perinatal mortality survey sample. *British Medical Journal* **302**, 1576–1580.

Done DJ, Crow TJ, Johnstone EC, Sacker A (1994) Childhood antecedents of schizophrenia and affective illness: social adjustment at ages 7 and 11. *British Medical Journal* **309**, 699–703.

Eastwood SL, Harrison PJ (1995) Decreased synaptophysin in the medial temporal lobe in schizophrenia demonstrated using immunoautoradiography. *Neuroscience* **69**, 339–343.

Erickson SL, Akil M, Levey AI, Lewis DA (1998) Postnatal development of tyrosine hydroxylase and dopamine transporter-immunoreactive axons in monkey rostral entorhinal cortex. *Cerebral Cortex* **8**, 415–427.

Falkai P, Bogerts B, Roberts GW, Crow TJ (1988) Measurement of the alpha-cell-migration in the entorhinal region: a marker for the developmental disturbances in schizophrenia? *Schizophrenia Research* **1**, 157–158.

Feinberg I (1982) Schizophrenia: caused by a fault in programmed synaptic elimination during adolescence? *Journal of Psychiatry Research* **17**, 319–330.

Fish B, Marcus J, Hans SL, Auerbach AG (1992) Infants at risk for schizophrenia: sequelae of a genetic neurointegrative defect: a review and replication analysis of Pandy's maturation in the Jerusalem infant development study. *Archives of General Psychiatry* **49**, 221–235.

Friede RL (1989) *Developmental neuropathology*. Springer Verlag, Berlin.

Garey LJ, Ong WY, Patel TS *et al.* (1998) Reduced dendritic spine density on cerebral cortical pyramidal neurons in schizophrenia. *Journal of Neurology, Neurosurgery and Psychiatry* **65**, 446–453.

Garver DL, Nair TR, Christensen JD, Holcomb J, Ramberg J, Kingsbury S (1999) Atrophic and static (neurodevelopmental) schizophrenic psychoses: premorbid functioning, symptoms and neuroleptic response. *Neuropsychopharmacology* **21**, 82–92.

Geddes JR, Lawrie SM (1995) Obstetric complications and schizophrenia: a meta-analysis. *British Journal of Psychiatry* **167**, 469–472.

Geddes JR, Verdoux H, Takei N *et al.* (1999) Schizophrenia and complications of pregnancy and labor: an individual patient data meta-analysis. *Schizophrenia Bulletin* **25**, 413–423.

Geethabali S, Shannon Weickert C, Hyde TM *et al.* (1996) Decrease in GAP-43 mRNA in the schizophrenic prefrontal cortex. *Society for Neuroscience Abstracts* **22**, 1680.

Glantz LA, Lewis DA (1997) Reduction of synaptophysin immunoreactivity in the prefrontal cortex of subjects with schizophrenia. Regional and diagnostic specificity. *Archives of General Psychiatry* **54** , 943–952.

Glantz LA, Lewis DA (2000) Prefrontal cortical pyramidal neurons exhibit decreased dendritic spine density in subjects with schizophrenia. *Archives of General Psychiatry* **57**, 165–73.

Goff DC, Wine L (1997) Glutamate in schizophrenia: clinical and research implications. *Schizophrenia Research* **27**, 157–168.

Goldberg TE, Hyde TM, Kleinman JE, Weinberger DR (1993) Course of schizophrenia: Neuropsychological evidence for a static encephalopathy. *Schizophrenia Bulletin* **19**, 797–804.

Green MF, Satz P, Gaier DJ, Ganzefl S, Kharabi F (1989) Minor physical anomalies in schizophrenia. *Schizophrenia Bulletin* **15**, 91–99.

Green MF, Bracha HS, Satz P, Christenson CD (1994) Preliminary evidence for an association between minor physical anomalies and second trimester neurodevelopment in schizophrenia. *Psychiatry Research* **53**, 119–127.

Gur RE, Turetsky B, Bilker WB, Gur RC (1999) Reduced gray matter volume in schizophrenia. *Archives of General Psychiatry* **56**, 905–911

Halberstadt AL (1995) The phencyclidine-glutamate model of schizophrenia. *Clinical Neuropharmacology* **18**, 237–249.

Harrison PJ (1995) On the neuropathology of schizophrenia and its dementia: neurodevelopmental, neurodegenerative, or both? *Neurodegeneration* **4**, 1–12.

Harrison PJ (1997) Schizophrenia: a disorder of neurodevelopment? *Current Opinion in Neurobiology* **7**, 285–289.

Harrison PJ, Eastwood SL (1998) Preferential involvement of excitatory neurons in the medial temporal lobe in schizophrenia. *Lancet* **352**, 1669–1673.

Heinsen H, Gossmann E, Rubb U *et al.* (1996) Variability in the human entorhinal region may confound neuropsychiatric diagnoses. *Acta Anatomica* **157**, 226–237.

Hendren RL, Hodde-Vargas J, Yeo RA, Vargas LA, Brooks WM, Ford C (1995) Neuropsychophysiological study of children at risk for schizophrenia: a preliminary report. *Journal of the American Academy of Child and Adolescent Psychiatry* **34**, 1284–1291.

Henn FA (1995) The NMDA receptor as a site for psychopathology. *Archives of General Psychiatry* **52**, 1008–1010.

Hirsch SR, Das I, Garey LJ, de Belleroche J (1997) A pivotal role for glutamate in the pathogenesis of schizophrenia, and its cognitive dysfunction. *Pharmacology Biochemistry and Behavior* **56**, 797–802.

Hitri A, Casanova MF, Kleinman JE, Weinberger DR, Wyatt RJ (1995) Age-related changes in [^{3}H] GBR 12935 binding site density in the prefrontal cortex of controls and schizophrenics. *Biological Psychiatry* **37**, 175–182.

Hoff AL, Riordan H, O'Donnell DW, Morris L, DeLisi LE (1992) Neuropsychological function of first-episode schizophreniform patients. *American Journal of Psychiatry* **149**, 898–903.

Hollister JM, Laing P, Mednick SA (1996) Rhesus incompatibility as a risk factor for schizophrenia in male adults. *Archives of General Psychiatry* **53**, 19–24.

Huttenlocher PR (1979) Synaptic density in human frontal cortex: developmental changes and effects of aging. *Brain Research* **163**, 195–205.

Hyde TM, Nawroz S, Godberg TE *et al.* (1994) Is there cognitive decline in schizophrenia? A cross-sectional study. *British Journal of Psychiatry* **164**, 494–500.

Hyde TE, Bachus SE, Levitt P *et al.* (1997) Reduction in hippocampal limbic system-associated membrane protein (LAMP) mRNA in schizophrenia. *Society for Neuroscience Abstracts* **23**, 2200.

Impagnatiello F, Guidotti AR, Pesold C *et al.* (1998) A decrease of reelin expression as a putative vulnerability factor in schizophrenia. *Proceedings of the National Academy of Sciences USA* **95**, 15718–15723.

Jahn R, Schiebler W, Ouimet C, Greengard P (1985) A 38,000-dalton membrane protein A (p38) present in synaptic vesicles. *Proceedings of the National Academy of Science USA* **82**, 4137–4141.

Jakob H, Beckmann H (1986) Prenatal developmental disturbances in the limbic allocortex in schizophrenics. *Journal of Neural Transmission* **65**, 303–326.

Jaskiw GE, Juliano DM, Goldberg TE *et al.* (1994) Cerebral ventricular enlargement in schizophreniform disorder does not progress. A seven year follow-up study. *Schizophrenia Research* **14**, 23–28.

Jones P, Rodgers B, Murray RM, Marmot M (1994) Child development risk factors for adult schizophrenia in the British 1946 birth cohort. *Lancet* **344**, 1398–1402.

Kaplan MJ, Lazoff M, Kelly K, Lukin R, Garver DL (1990) Enlargment of cerebral third ventricle in psychotic patients with delayed response to neuroleptics. *Biological Psychiatry* **15**, 205–214.

Kendell RE, Kemp IW (1989) Maternal influenza in the etiology of schizophrenia. *Archives of General Psychiatry* **46**, 878–882.

Keshavan MS, Anderson S, Pettegrew JW (1994) Is schizophrenia due to excessive synaptic pruning in the prefrontal cortex? The Feinberg hypothesis revisited. *Journal of Psychiatric Research* **28**, 239–265.

Keshavan MS, Montrose DM, Pierri JN *et al.* (1997) Magnetic resonance imaging spectroscopy in offspring at risk for schizophrenia: preliminary studies. *Progress in Neuropsychopharmacology and Biological Psychiatry* **21**, 1285–1295.

Kirch DG, Weinberger DR (1986) Anatomical neuropathology in schizophrenia: postmortem findings. In Nasrallah HA, Weinberger, DR, Eds. *Handbook of schizophrenia.* Elsevier, Amsterdam, pp. 325–348.

Knoll JL, Garver DL, Ramberg JE, Kingsbury SJ, Croissant D, McDerott B (1998) Heterogeneity of the psychoses: is there a neurodegenerative psychosis? *Schizophrenia Bulletin* **24**, 365–379.

Kraepelin E (1919) *Dementia praecox and paraphrenia.* Livingstone, Edinburgh.

Kreutzberg GW, Blakemore WF, Graeber MB (1997) Cellular pathology of the central nervous system. In Graham DI, Lantos PE, eds. *Greenfield's neuropathology*, 6th edition. Edward Arnold, London, pp. 85–156.

Krimer LS, Herman MM, Saunders RC *et al.* (1997) A qualitative and quantitative analysis of the entorhinal cortex in schizophrenia. *Cerebral Cortex* **7**, 732–739.

Kuchna I (1994) Quantitative studies of human newborns' hippocampal pyramidal cells after perinatal hypoxia. *Folia Neuropathologica* **32**, 9–16.

Laping NJ, Teter B, Nichols NR (1994) Glial fibrillary acidic protein: Regulation by hormones, cytokines, and growth factors. *Brain Pathology* **4**, 259–275.

Lawrie SM, Whalley H, Kestelman JN, Abukmeil SS, Byrne M, Hodges A (1999) Magnetic resonance imaging of the brain in subjects at high risk of developing schizophrenia. Lancet **353**, 30–33.

Lewis DA (1997) Development of the prefrontal cortex during adolescence: insights into vulnerable neural circuits in schizophrenia. *Neuropsychopharmacology* **16**, 385–398.

Lewis DA, Lund JS (1990) Heterogeneity of chandelier neurons in monkey neocortex: Corticotropin-releasing factor and parvalbumin immunoreactive populations. *Journal of Comparative Neurology* **293**, 599–615.

Lewis SW (1989) Congenital risk factors for schizophrenia. *Psychological Medicine* **19**, 5–13.

Lieberman JA (1999) Is schizophrenia a neurodegenerative disorder? A clinical and neuro-biological perspective. *Biological Psychiatry* **46**, 729–739.

Lieberman J, Jody D, Geisler S (1993) Time course and biologic correlates of treatment response in first-episode schizophrenia. *Archives of General Psychiatry* **50**, 369–376.

McCreadie RG, Flail DJ, Berry IJ, Robertson LJ, Ewing JI, Geals MF (1992) The Nithsdale schizophrenia surveys. X. Obstetric complications, family history and abnormal movements. *British Journal of Psychiatry* **161**, 799–805.

Machon RA, Mednick SA, Huttunen MO (1997) Adult major affective disorder after prenatal exposure to an influenza epidemic. *Archives of General Psychiatry* **54**, 322–328.

McNeil TF (1995) Perinatal risk factors and shizophrenia: selective review and methodological concerns. *Epidemiological Review* **17**, 107–112.

McNeil TF, Cantor-Graae E (1999) Does preexisting abnormality cause labor-delivery complications in fetuses who will develop schizophrenia? *Schizophrenia Bulletin* **25**, 425–435.

Meador-Woodruff JH, Haroutunian V, Powchik P, Davidson M, Davis KL, Watson SJ (1997) Dopamine receptor transcript expression in striatum and prefrontal and occipital cortex. Focal abnormalities in orbitofrontal cortex in schizophrenia. *Archives of General Psychiatry* **54**, 1089–1095.

Mednick SA, Machon RA, Huttunen MO, Bonett D (1988) Adult schizophrenia following prenatal exposure to an influenza epidemic. *Archives of General Psychiatry* **45**, 189–192.

Mohn AR, Gainetdinov RR, Caron MG, Koller BH (1999) Mice with reduced NMDA receptor expression display behaviors related to schizophrenia. *Cell* **98**, 427–436.

Murray RM, Lewis SW (1987) Is schizophrenia a neurodevelopmental disorder? *British Medical Journal* **925**, 681–682.

Noga JT, Bartley AJ, Jones DW, Torrey EF, Weinberger DR (1996) Cortical gyral anatomy and gross brain dimensions in monozygotic twins discordant for schizophrenia. *Schizophrenia Research* **22**, 27–40.

O'Callaghan E, Sham P, Takei N, Glover G, Murray RM (1991) Schizophrenia after prenatal exposure to 1957A2 influenza epidemic. *Lancet* **337**, 1248–1250.

Offord DR, Cross LA (1971) Adult schizophrenia with scholastic failure or low IQ in child-hood. A preliminary report. *Archives of General Psychiatry* **24**, 431–436.

Olney JW, Farber NB (1995) Glutamate receptor dysfunction and schizophrenia. *Archives of General Psychiatry* **52**, 998–1007.

Ono K, Tomasiewicz H, Magnuson T, Ruyishauser U (1994) N-CAM mutation inhibits tangential neuronal migration and is phenocopied by enzymatic removal of polysialic acid. *Neuron* **13**, 595–609.

Pakkenberg B (1987) Post-mortem study of chronic schizophrenic brains. *British Journal of Psychiatry* **151**, 744–752.

Pakkenberg B (1993) Total nerve cell number in neocortex in chronic schizophrenics and controls estimated using optical disectors. *Biological Psychiatry* **34**, 768–772.

Parnas J, Shulsinger F, Teasdale TW, Schulsinger H, Feldman PM, Mednick SA (1982) Prenatal complications and clinical outcome within the schizophrenia spectrum. *British Journal of Psychiatry* **140**, 416–420.

Peters A, Jones EG (1991) Classification of cortical neurons. In Jones EG, Peters A. eds. *Cerebral cortex.* New York: Plenum Press, pp. 107–120.

Pettegrew JW, Keshavan MS, Panchalingam K *et al.* (1991) Alterations in brain high-energy phosphate and membrane phospholipid metabolism in first-episode, drug-naive schizophrenics: a pilot study of the dorsal prefrontal cortex by in vivo phosphorus 31 nuclear magnetic resonance imaging. *Archives of General Psychiatry* **48**, 563–568.

Pollack M, Woerner MG, Goodman W, Greenberg IM (1966) Childhood development patterns of hospitalized adult schizophrenic and nonschizophrenic patients and their siblings. *American Journal of Orthopsychiatry* **36**, 510–517.

Rajkowska G, Selemon LD, Goldman-Rakic PS (1998). Neuronal and glial somal size in the prefrontal cortex. A morphometric study of schizophrenia and Huntington disease. *Archives of General Psychiatry* **55**, 215–224.

Rakic P, Bourgeois JP, Eckenoff MF, Zecevic N, Goldman-Rakic P (1986) Concurrent overproduction of synapses in diverse regions of the primate cerbral cortex. *Science* **232**, 232–235.

Randall PL (1980) A neuroanatomical theory on the aetiology of schizophrenia. *Medical Hypotheses* **6**, 645–658.

Rantakallio P, Jones P, Moring J, Von Wendt L (1997) Association between central nervous system infections during childhood and adult onset schizophrenia and other psychoses: a 28-year follow-up. *International Journal of Epidemiology* **26**, 837–843.

Rapoport JL, Giedd J, Kumra S *et al.* (1997) Childhood-onset schizophrenia. Progressive ventricular change during adolescence. *Archives of General Psychiatry* **54**, 897–903.

Roberts GW (1991) Schizophrenia: a neuropathological perspective. *British Journal of Psychiatry* **158**, 8–17.

Rosenberg DR, Lewis DA (1994) Changes in the dopaminergic innervation of monkey prefrontal cortex during late postnatal development: a tyrosine hydroxylase immunohistochemical study. *Biological Psychiatry* **36**, 272–277.

Russell AJ, Munro JC, Jones PB, Hemsley DR, Phil M, Murray RM (1997) Schizophrenia and the myth of intellectual decline. *American Journal of Psychiatry* **154**, 635–639.

Saykin AJ, Gur RC, Gur RE, Mozley PD, Mozley LH, Resnick SM (1991) Neuro-psychological function in schizophrenia. *Archives of General Psychiatry* **48**, 618–24.

Schlaepfer TE, Harris GJ, Tien AY *et al.* (1994) Decreased regional cortical gray matter volume in schizophrenia. *American Journal of Psychiatry* **151**, 842–848.

Schmauss C, Haroutunian V, Davis KL, Davidson M (1993) Selective loss of dopamine D3-type receptor mRNA expression in parietal and motor cortices of patients with chronic schizophrenia. *Proceedings of the National Academy of Sciences USA* **90**, 8942–8946.

Selemon LD, Rajkowska G, Goldman-Rakic PS (1995) Abnormally high neuronal density in the schizophrenic cortex. A morphometric analysis of prefrontal area 9 and occipital area 17. *Archives of General Psychiatry* **52**, 805–18.

Selemon LD, Rajkowska G, Goldman-Rakic PS (1998) Elevated neuronal density in prefrontal area 46 in brains from schizophrenic patients: Application of a three-dimensional, stereologic counting method. *Journal of Comparative Neurology* **392**, 402–412.

Shelton RC, Karson CN, Doran, AR, Pichar D, Bigelow LB, Weinberger DR (1988) Cerebral structural pathology in schizophrenia: evidence for a selective prefrontal cortical defect. *American Journal of Psychiatry* **145**, 154–163.

Silverton L, Harrington ME, Mednick SA (1988) Motor impairment and antisocial behavior in adolescent males at high risk for schizophrenia. *Journal of Abnormal Child Psychology* **16**, 177–186.

Stanley JA, Williamson PC, Drost DJ *et al.* (1995) An in vivo study of the prefrontal cortex of schizophrenic patients at different stages of illness via phosphorus magnetic resonance spectroscopy. *Archives of General Psychiatry* **52**, 399–406.

Stevens JR (1992) Abnormal reinnervation as a basis for schizophrenia: a hypothesis. *Archives of General Psychiatry* **49**, 238–243.

Susser E, Neugebauer R, Hoek H *et al.* (1996) Schizophrenia after prenatal famine. Further evidence. *Archives of General Psychiatry* **53**, 25–31.

Torrey EF, Rawlings R, Waldman IN (1988) Schizophrenic births and viral diseases in two states. *Schizophrenia Research* **1**, 73–77.

Torrey EF, Bowler AE, Taylor EH, Gottesman II (1994) *Schizophrenia and manic depression disorders: the biological roots of mental illness as revealed by a landmark study of identical twins.* New York: Basic Books.

Tsai G, Passani LA, Slusher BS *et al.* (1995) Abnormal excitatory neurotransmitter metabolism in schizophrenic brains. *Archives of General Psychiatry* **52**, 829–836.

Vawter MP, Cannon-Spoor HE, Hemperly JJ, Herman MM, Kleinman JE, Freed WJ (1998) Abnormal expression of cell recognition molecules in schizophrenia. *Experimental Neurology* **149**, 424–432.

Verdoux H, Geddes JR, Takei N *et al.* (1997) Obstetric complications and age at onset in schizophrenia: an international collaborative meta-analysis of individual patient data. *American Journal of Psychiatry* **154**, 1220–1227.

Verney C, Milosevic A, Alvarez C, Berger B (1993) Immunocytochemical evidence of well-developed dopaminergic and noradrenergic innervations in the frontal cerebral cortex of human fetuses at midgestation. *Journal of Comparative Neurology* **336**, 331–344.

Volpe JJ (1997) Brain injury in the premature infant. Neuropathology, clinical aspects, pathogenesis, and prevention. *Clinics in Perinatology* **24**, 567–587

Waddington JL, Lane A, Scully PJ, Larkin C, O'Callaghan E (1998) Neurodevelopmental and neuroprogressive processes in schizophrenia. Antithetical or complementary over a lifetime trajectory of disease? *Psychiatric Clinics of North America*, **21**, 123–149.

Walker E, Lewine RJ (1990) Prediction of adult onset schizophrenia from childhood home movies of the patients. *American Journal of Psychiatry* **147**, 1052–1056.

Weickert CS, Weinberger DR (1998) A candidate molecule approach to defining the developmental pathology in schizophrenia. *Schizophrenia Bulletin* **24**, 303–316.

Weinberger DR (1987) Implications of normal brain development for the pathogenesis of schizophrenia. *Archives of General Psychiatry* **44**, 660–669.

Weinberger DR (1995) Schizophrenia. From neuropathology to neurodevelopment. Lancet **346**, 552–557.

Weinberger DR, Lipska BK (1995) Cortical maldevelopment, anti-psychotic drugs, and schizophrenia: a search for common ground. *Schizophrenia Research* **16**, 87–110.

Weinberger DR, Torrey EF, Neophytides A, Wyatt RJ (1979). Lateral cerebral ventricular enlargement in chronic schizophrenia. *Archives of General Psychiatry* **36**, 735–739.

Weinberger DR, DeLisi LE, Perman G, Targum S, Wyatt RJ (1982) Computed tomography scans in schizophreniform disorder and other acute psychiatric patients. *Archives of General Psychiatry* **39**, 778–783.

Weinberger DR, Berman KF, Illowsky BP (1988) Physiological dysfunction of dorsolateral prefrontal cortex in schizophrenia. III. A new cohort and evidence for a monoaminergic mechanism. *Archives of General Psychiatry* **45**, 609–615.

Williamson P, Drost D, Stanley J, Carr T, Morrison S, Merskey H (1991) Localized phosphorous 31 magnetic resonance spectroscopy in chronic schizophrenic patients and normal controls. *Archives of General Psychiatry* **48**, 578–582.

Woo TU, Miller JL, Lewis DA (1997) Schizophrenia and the parvalbumin-containing class of cortical local circuit neurons. *American Journal of Psychiatry* **154**, 1013–1015.

Woo TU, Whitehead RE, Melchitzky DS, Lewis DA (1998) A subclass of prefrontal gamma-aminobutyric acid axon terminals are selectively altered in schizophrenia. *Proceedings of the National Academy of Sciences USA* **95**, 5341–5346.

Zecevic N, Bourgeois JP, Rakic P (1989) Changes in synaptic density in motor cortex of rhesus monkey during fetal and postnatal life. *Developmental Brain Research* **50**, 11–32.

Zipursky RB, Lim KO, Sullivan EV, Brown BW, Pfefferbaum A (1992) Widespread cerebral gray matter volume deficits in schizophrenia. *Archives of General Psychiatry* **49**, 195–205.

9 Cortical Development and Schizophrenia

Jack Price and Gareth W. Roberts

Molecular basis for the organisation of the forebrain
  Lessons from the hindbrain
  Otx and *Emx* genes
  Boundaries in the telencephalon
  Boundaries in the hippocampal formation
  Differences between rodents and humans
Pattern formation and its functional consequences
  Migration
Fate determination
Concluding remarks

At first sight, the idea that the development of the cerebral cortex might be of more than passing relevance to schizophrenia seems unlikely. Schizophrenia typically emerges during the third decade of life, well after the major events that mould the cerebrum are complete. Moreover, the symptoms and deficits which characterise the disorder persist throughout life for many sufferers. Nonetheless, the 'neurodevelopmental hypothesis', as elaborated in the previous chapter, has become pre-eminent. Partly, this reflects a growing body of data consistent with the hypothesis; partly, it reflects the growing dissatisfaction with older hypotheses and the perceived need for a 'paradigm shift' that might release research into new, profitable areas. Nonetheless, we must not be deceived; the neurodevelopmental hypothesis as currently expounded is scientifically weak. The hypothesis, to quote Waddington (1993), 'takes as the primary event [in the pathogenesis of schizophrenia] changes *in utero* that disrupt the development of fundamental aspects of brain structure and function and that might produce the typical symptoms some two decades later, perhaps only after functional maturation or completion of other, associated, systems or processes'. Some would consider that a brave statement given the inconclusive nature of the evidence concerning the 'primary event'. It also illustrates the weakness of the hypothesis: it accommodates many experimental findings, and it is difficult to conceive of an experiment whose outcome could refute it. This vagueness reflects the fact that we are all feeling our way in a difficult field, and the hypothesis, despite its breadth and shortcomings, at least encourages the gathering of diverse findings in the hope that a credible story might emerge. This chapter is written in the same spirit. Though it is not yet possible to describe the pathogenesis of schizophrenia in terms of specific aberrations in particular processes, we can monitor carefully what modern developmental neuroscience tells us about corticogenesis, and thereby generate more specific, testable hypotheses about the disorder.

The range of findings that support the neurodevelopmental hypothesis were expounded and referenced in Chapter 8. Suffice to note here that they fall into three broad categories as follows.

1. Neuropathological: there are a series of morphological and histological findings whose nature is interpreted as being neurodevelopmental in origin (see below). The absence of glial scarring or of progressive pathology supports a developmental aberration (Chapters 5 and 11).

2. Epidemiological: in keeping with an early, developmental origin, epidemiological studies reveal that maternal exposure to influenza during the second trimester, and obstetric and perinatal complications are risk factors for schizophrenia. Furthermore, longitudinal studies suggest that children who will develop schizophrenia as adults have social, behavioural, and neurological dysfunction.

3. Experimental: lesions in animals indicate that certain types of damage can lead to behavioural consequences that only fully reveal themselves after puberty (Chapter 12).

Several of these findings have suggested discrete deficits that might be the primary cause of schizophrenia. For example, the displacement and disorganisation of pre-α cells in the entorhinal cortex which has been reported (Chapter 2) in schizophrenia, is prima-facia evidence for aberrant neuronal migration. Similarly, the altered distribution of neurons in the subcortical white matter of schizophrenics (Chapter 3) has been taken as evidence for a defect in neuronal migration or apoptotic cell death. The problem, of course, is that these and other pathological features associated with schizophrenia are inconsistent (Chapter 13), and specific hypotheses accommodate this variability with difficulty. A primary deficit in migration, for example, could be extrapolated to cover other findings such as partial agenesis of the corpus callosum, aberrant gyrification, perhaps even the reduced number of thalamic neurons (Pakkenberg, 1990; Danos et al., 1998). But other findings fit much less easily: why, for example, should there be a loss of cerebral asymmetry (Chapter 6)? More to the point, the question is begged: how does one establish which—if any—of these pathologies constitute the primary abnormality of the disorder?

These issues represent some of the problems and conundrums facing the neurodevelopmental hypothesis of schizophrenia. A different perspective may emerge, however, from taking a step backwards. Fortunately, schizophrenia research is not taking place in a vacuum. Developmental neuroscience is currently one of the fastest moving fields in biology, and in the decade or so since the neurodevelopmental hypothesis emerged, our views concerning the development of the cerebral cortex have radically changed. The objective of this chapter is to review some of those advances from the perspective of schizophrenia pathology.

There may be another advantage in looking at schizophrenia from a broader developmental perspective, albeit one that we propose hesitantly. One reason why specific hypotheses regarding the origin of schizophrenia are inadequate may be that they are too mechanistic. Cells might migrate inappropriately because there is a flaw in the migration mechanism, but we already know what such a failure looks like: it produces the radical disturbances which characterise the various heterotopias and dysplasias with which paediatric neurologists are so familiar (Walsh, 1999). It does not produce schizophrenia, as far as one can tell. There are, however, other faults that can give aberrant migration. Cells in the embryonic cerebral cortex migrate radially (for the most part) and form a laminated structure. Neighbouring cells that form the striatum do something quite different. Cortical cells 'know' that they are cortical, and activate the appropriate mechanisms, including that which drives migration. So what would happen if cortical cells 'thought' they were striatal? As discussed below, the answer is unsurprisingly that they do not migrate properly. In fact, several aspects of their behaviour are aberrant. Almost certainly this is not what goes wrong in schizophrenia, but the observation suggests some other thought experiments. What would happen if other cell identities went wrong; e.g. if areas of neocortex were wrongly labelled as limbic, or association cortex as sensory? Surely several aspects of their behaviour would be aberrant—migration, histogenesis, connectivity, cell fate determination, etc. The point is that pattern formation—the process whereby populations of embryonic cells gain a positional identity—underlies all aspects of mechanistic cellular behaviour. A clearer view of schizophrenia pathology might emerge, therefore, from looking at it from this perspective.

Until recently, this suggestion would have been impossible because so little was known about the process of pattern formation in the brain. However, understanding of these fundamental processes has now developed to the stage where testable hypotheses can be entertained about the nature of human forebrain organisation, and about the ways in which it might go wrong. Studies on rodents have led to a number of genes and cellular pathways that appear to direct the primary process whereby regions of the forebrain acquire their identity. Moreover, we are beginning to understand how these primary events interact with the subsequent processes that are of central interest to schizophrenia: cell migration and cell fate determination. In this chapter we follow this logical progression from the molecules that organise the forebrain through to their impact on the identity and behaviour of the cells that go to form the cerebral cortex.

Molecular basis for the organisation of the forebrain

For some time, a detailed morphological description of how the forebrain develops has been available, but little idea of how the development was controlled. While we still have only a partial picture of corticogenesis, we now have a good idea of the identities of some of the genes, and in some cases good models of how they act. We shall consider these candidates in the context of the developmental anatomy of the forebrain.

The cerebral cortex develops from the dorsal telencephalic vesicle, but it develops quite differently from its neighbouring telencephalic structures such as the corpus striatum or the septum. We have become so familiar with the strange and complex cortical form that we tend to overlook the obvious question of how did it grow to become so different from its neighbouring tissue?

The embryonic neuroepithelium from which all central nervous system structures are derived is a continuous layer of undifferentiated cells, but the adult brain is made up of a series of discrete populations of neurons and glia. For this to occur, different areas of the neuroepithelium must somehow gain an identity. How and when these identities arise has been a controversial question, and remains one of the most intensely studied areas of neurodevelopment (Blakemore, 1995). One theory is that at an early stage the neuroepithelium becomes mapped into domains, each of which is specified to transform itself into a particular brain area—the so-called 'protomap' theory. The opposing theory is that specification results from a relatively late interaction between different populations of neurons, which sculpt their own specific role in response to the influences they receive; the so-called 'tabula rasa'. The balance between these alternatives remains contentious. Nonetheless, a substantial body of evidence makes clear that both processes occur to some extent—some properties of cortical cells are determined early, while others do not become determined until the cells begin to interact functionally with their neighbours. From our perspective, two important points need to be made. The first is that an early patterning process most certainly does occur within the telencephalon, and much of this chapter will be concerned with the molecular basis for this early patterning. In fact, this early pattern formation determines much of the patterning of the brain that will become apparent as development unfolds. Second, a number of markers—limbic associated membrane protein (LAMP), latexin, and an enhancer trap transgenic marker—each recognise specific areas within the cortical mantle during embryogenesis (Levitt et al., 1997). There is good experimental evidence that these cortical areas become determined by roughly the middle of corticogenesis in rodents. This is before the major ingrowth of thalamic or corticocortical fibres, so whatever may be subsequently determined by an interaction between cortex and inputs from other brain areas, the cortex appears to have an intrinsic capacity to organise itself into areas.

Lessons from the hindbrain

The first evidence for the type of patterning we want to consider came from the hindbrain. Prior to the generation of neurons and glia, the hindbrain becomes organised into a series of discrete, semi-autonomous units—rhombomeres (Lumsden and Keynes, 1989). This organisation directs all subsequent development of this brain region, including for example, the determination of where brainstem nuclei will develop, where the exit points for each cranial nerve will lie, and the order in which neuronal populations will be generated.

The organisation of the hindbrain depends crucially on a series of genes that encode the *hox* (homeobox) family of transcription factors (Lumsden and Krumlauf, 1996). *Hox* genes do not appear to be important in forebrain development and hence are unlikely to be involved in schizophrenia, but they reveal an organising principle which is of fundamental interest. Each rhombomere carries a distinct identity which is defined by a combinatorial code of *hox* transcription factors (Fig. 9.1). If the code is changed by knocking out a particular component, or by expressing a component ectopically, then rhombomere identity changes appropriately. As transcription factors, *hox* proteins direct the expression of other genes. It seems therefore (although this has proved more difficult to determine experimentally) that the combination of *hox* genes controls the downstream functional genes that direct development along pathways specific for each particular rhombomere. What has been discovered is no less than a fundamental principle of pattern formation in the central nervous system (and, in fact, the rest of the embryo). The *hox* code does not direct a cell to become

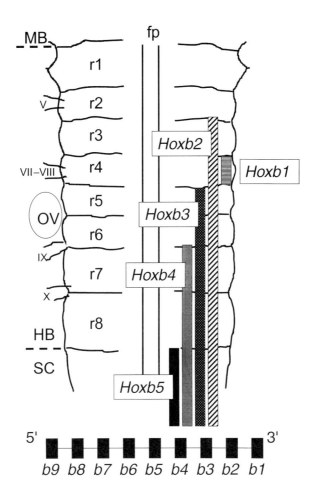

Fig. 9.1 Homeobox genes and hindbrain development. A schematic representation of flattened embryonic hindbrain viewed from the dorsal aspect. The hindbrain develops from a series of rhombomeres (r1 to r8), a series of cellular compartments that arise during the neural plate stage of embryogenesis. The identity of each compartment is determined by the combination of *hox* genes expressed by the cells of which it is composed. This is shown by the shaded bars, each representing the anteroposterior limits of expression of a particular *hox* gene. Hence *hoxb2* is expressed from the spinal cord, through the more caudal rhombomeres to the boundary between r3 and r2, where expression ceases. *Hoxb3* is similar except that its expression stretches only as far as the r5/r4 boundary. The lower part of the figure gives a representation of the linear sequence of the genes in the *hoxb* cluster. Their expression pattern reflects the order of the genes in the cluster. fp, floorplate; HB, hindbrain; MB, midbrain; OV, otic vesicle; SC, spinal cord. (Adapted from Wilkinson *et al.*, 1989.)

a Purkinje cell or a cerebellar astrocyte—that is a result of a different series of control processes—rather it addresses a population of cells and tells them that amongst themselves they must construct a particular piece of brain. Returning to the forebrain, does a similar pattern-forming process occur, and what would the consequences be if it failed?

Otx and *Emx* genes

Naturally, the control of forebrain development is complex, and many genes and cellular mechanisms are involved. Nonetheless, it is clear that *Otx* and *Emx* genes are very close to the key events (Acampora *et al.*, 1996; Ang *et al.*, 1996; Pellegrini *et al.*, 1996; Qiu *et al.*, 1996; Suda *et al.*, 1997; Yoshida *et al.*, 1997). These genes were discovered, like the *hox* genes and most of the other genes to be considered here, from homology with *Drosophila* genes. In *Drosophila*, the *orthodonticle* and *empty-spiracle* genes control head formation. Mammals have two representatives of each family (*Otx-1* and *Otx-2*; *Emx-1* and *Emx-2*, respectively) (Simeone *et al.*, 1992). The functions of these genes are incompletely understood, and are less transparently combinatorial than the *Hox* system in the hindbrain, but some of the same features are beginning to emerge.

Otx-2 is the first to be expressed and is essential for the embryonic patterning by which the rostral brain becomes established. Knock-out mice, homozygous for a null mutation in this gene, have essentially no fore- or midbrain. The expression pattern of each gene as it unfolds is dynamic, but the four genes appear initially to be expressed as a 'nested' set (Fig. 9.2). *Otx-2* has the widest domain of expression, encompassing the domains of the other three genes. The domain of *Otx-1* includes the domains of both *Emx* genes, and the *Emx-2* domain includes the domain of *Emx-1* expression. Gene expression is sequential, with the genes defining the larger domains being expressed before those defining the smaller domains. The simplistic notion emerges therefore that these genes partition the rostral brain into increasingly defined regions.

As might be expected, this partitioning is part of the process that defines the cerebral cortex. The *Emx* genes seem to be particularly important in this regard (Gulisano *et al.*, 1996). *Emx-1* initially demarcates the portion of neuroepithelium that will give rise to the cerebral cortex. Then as development unfolds, *Emx-2* becomes restricted to the precursor cells of the cortical ventricular zone, while *Emx-1* is expressed also in migrating neurons and eventually is expressed in all neurons (but not glia) of the cortical mantle. So we have the first elements of a specification model, in which expression of a set of genes, *Otx* and *Emx* genes being prominent amongst them, defines regions of the brain and gives them a positional identity.

Boundaries in the telencephalon

If the model suggested by *Hox* genes for the hindbrain and by *Emx/Otx* genes for the forebrain is correct, then domains of expression of control genes direct the parcelling up of the neuroepithelium and its derivatives into distinct cell populations. The question then arises: what happens at the borders between neighbouring forebrain regions? Is there a gradual transition from one to another with populations of ambivalent cells falling in the

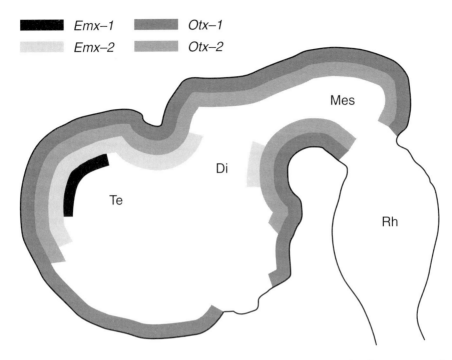

Fig. 9.2 The nested expression pattern of *Otx* and *Emx* genes. The four genes of this set are expressed as a nested set, both temporally and spatially. The earliest to be expressed, *Otx-2*, also has the largest expression domain, and the most profound phenotype when 'knocked-out' in mice. The order in which the other genes are turned on during development—*Otx-1* then *Emx-2* then *Emx-1*—is also reflected in their successively smaller domains of expression, with the latter restricted to the primordium of the cerebral cortex. This temporal and spatial pattern suggests a progressive defining of brain regions as a consequence of some 'combinatorial code' of these genes. Almost certainly, the reality is more complicated, but these data provide an insight into how the brain is organised developmentally. Di, diencephalon; Mes, mesencephalon; Rh, rhombencephalon; Te, telencephalon.

middle, or are there abrupt boundaries? The answer, slightly bizarrely, is that the boundaries are sharp, but cells sometimes appear to ignore them. Certainly, sharp boundaries are clear in the hindbrain, and there are increasingly convincing examples also emerging in the forebrain. The best example is that between the cortex and striatum, for which the principal characters are *Pax-6* and a pair of genes *Dlx-1* and *Dlx-2* (Porteus *et al.*, 1994; Stoykova *et al.*, 1996). During embryogenesis, the cerebral cortex and the corpus striatum are generated from two neighbouring regions of the telencephalic vesicle. The cortex comes from the dorsal wall of the vesicle (the cortical anlage), the striatum from the ventral part (the ganglionic eminence). The boundary between the two appears to be defined by the juxtaposition of the expression domains of the *Pax-6* and the *Dlx* genes (Fig. 9.3). *Pax-6* is expressed in the cortical anlage, with *Dlx-1* and *Dlx-2* having the converse pattern, being expressed in the ganglionic eminence. (Strictly speaking there is a third, intermediate region,

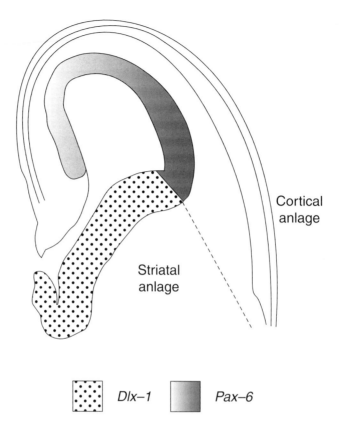

Fig. 9.3 The boundary between *Pax-6* and *Dlx-1* expression. Schematic representation of a frontal section through the forebrain of an embryonic day 14 mouse—approximately equivalent to a 10-week-old human fetus. Dorsal is uppermost and lateral is to the right. The dashed line indicates the approximate position of the boundary between the ganglion eminence (the future corpus striatum) and primordium of the cerebrum. *Dlx-1* labels the cells of the ventricular zone (i.e. the precursor cells) on the striatal side of the boundary, while *Pax-6* is expressed by the equivalent cells on the cerebral side. *Pax-6* is actually expressed as a gradient with its expression highest in the lateralmost cortex, declining medially.

but in mammals it is small, labels with *Pax-6*, and can be considered here to belong to the cerebral anlage; Fernandez *et al.*, 1998.)

How do we know that the expression of these genes defines the boundary rather than itself being the consequence of boundary formation? The best evidence comes from transgenic mice in which the *Pax-6* gene has been knocked out. In wild type mice, the boundary region develops a number of distinctive morphological features, such as a fasciculation of radial glial cells, and expression of the adhesion molecule R-cadherin by cortical but not striatal cells. In the *Pax-6* knock-out mice, these features fail to develop (Stoykova *et al.*, 1997), and cells fail to migrate properly (Caric *et al.*, 1997). Similarly, wild type cortical and striatal cells have distinctive adhesive properties such that if the cells from the two regions are dissociated then encouraged to reaggregate, the two populations tend to segregate into separate aggregates. This tendency is lost in the *Pax-6* knock-out mice. It seems that the cortical cells fail to take on a specific identity distinct from that of the striatal cells, a conclusion supported by the observation that the pattern of *Dlx-1* is also disturbed in the *Pax-6* knock-out mice; it also no longer observes the border and is expressed in cortical cells. Hence it appears that expression of these genes somehow defines the boundary between cortex and striatum.

In keeping with this interpretation, mutations of genes such as *Pax-6* have a profound effect on cortical development. In vertebrates there are eight genes in the *Pax* family (Stuart *et al.*, 1993), and mutations in many of these cause neurological abnormalities. Mutations in *Pax-6* are known as the *small eye* (*sey*) mutation in mice, and cause aniridia in humans (Jordan *et al.*, 1992). Importantly, *Pax-6* influences more than just eye development. Homozygous and heterozygous *Pax-6* mutant mice have severe cortical dysplasia, and at least one family of *Pax-6* aniridia patients have a specific, albeit more subtle, frontal lobe deficit (Heyman *et al.*, 1999). Of note, a *Pax-6* polymorphism has been reported to be associated with paranoid schizophrenia (Stober *et al.*, 1999).

Boundaries in the hippocampal formation

Before considering the significance of these developmental events in terms of their downstream consequences for corticogenesis and schizophrenia pathology, let us look at some other boundaries about which less is known but which might ultimately be of more relevance. How are the borders between neo- and limbic cortex, and between areas within the limbic cortex, prescribed? Knowledge is still thin, but there are a number of studies that may point the way. Several boundaries of gene expression have been described that appear to define limbic cortex and its constituent fields. Some are the genes we have already met. Later in fetal development *Otx-1* marks cortex and *Otx-2* marks hippocampus (Frantz *et al.*, 1994). Within hippocampus, CA1 is marked by members of a different family of transcription factors, the *Pou III* genes, of which three are relevant here: *Brn-1*, *Brn-2*, and *Oct-6* (also known as *SCIP* and *Tst-1*; Alvarez-Bolado *et al.*, 1995). *Brn-1* and *Brn-2* label precursor cells at early stages, but eventually all three of these genes specifically label CA1 cells. The analysis is not yet sufficiently fine grained to see what happens at the boundary between CA1 and CA3, or what occurs in the entorhinal cortex or subiculum which interface between neocortex and hippocampus (see Fig. 2.1, Chapter 2). Given the evidence implicating these regions in schizophrenia, it is to be hoped that clarification of the genes determining their formation will soon emerge.

Differences between rodents and humans

All the data cited so far is from experiments done on rodents. Should that concern us? In one sense the answer is no, since the genes we have discussed have been conserved from fruit flies to mice; they have surely been conserved through primate evolution also. Nonetheless, we should be concerned how little we know about the development of the human forebrain, because there must be fundamental differences between the development of humans and mice. We have two reasons for believing this to be true. Firstly, the timing of developmental events is very different between the two species. Secondly, there are clear differences in how disturbances in forebrain patterning translate into human as opposed to mouse pathology. These issues have relevance for animal models of schizophrenia (Chapter 12).

In rodents, neocortical and hippocampal development are largely synchronous, as are the formation of their connections. In both tissues, primary neurogenesis extends roughly from embryonic day 13 (E13) through to birth, while populations of granule cells continue to be generated postnatally. In humans by contrast, development of the hippocampal formation precedes the neocortex. By 15 weeks of gestation, for example, neurogenesis appears complete in the human hippocampal anlage, whereas the ventricular zone still dominates the neocortex, and will continue producing neurons for several more weeks (Yan and Ribak, 1997). By the same stage, area specification is well advanced in the hippocampal formation, particularly the entorhinal cortex, whereas it is not readily recognisable in the neocortex (Kostovic *et al.*, 1993). Similarly, connections between hippocampal areas form well before those between areas of the neocortex, with robust connections between entorhinal cortex, hippocampus, and subiculum by 19 weeks of gestation (Hevner and Kinney, 1996) but connections between visual cortical areas V1 and V2 not apparent until 37 weeks—over 4 months later (Burkhalter, 1993). It is hard to avoid the conclusion that although the fundamentals of forebrain organisation must be similar across all mammals, profound differences must also exist in the relative control of limbic and neocortical regions between rodents and primates.

There are also species differences in the genetic aspects of neurodevelopment. We have already met one such difference—the more severe cortical phenotype in mice than in humans with *Pax-6* mutations. Another example is *Emx-2*, introduced above, which is of importance for the development of neocortex and hippocampus (Gulisano *et al.*, 1996; Pellegrini *et al.*, 1996; Qiu *et al.*, 1996; Yoshida *et al.*, 1997). Mice carrying homozygous knock-out mutations of *Emx-2* have smaller cerebral hemispheres than normal, and a dramatically reduced hippocampal formation in which the dentate gyrus is almost completely absent. Mouse heterozygotes are phenotypically normal. These findings correlate with the expression pattern of this gene in mouse, since *Emx-2* is expressed in the ventricular zone of both the neocortical and hippocampal primordia, and is particularly highly expressed in the precursor cells that generate the dentate gyrus (Pellegrini *et al.*, 1996). Human mutations for this gene also exist, but the phenotype is quite different. Patients heterozygous for predicted loss-of-function mutations have schizencephaly (Brunelli *et al.*, 1996). In this rare condition there is a dramatic full thickness cleft in the cerebrum (Fig. 9.4). Temporal lobe disturbances have not been reported. This dramatic difference between humans and mice lacking a functional *Emx-2* gene suggests that the normal role of the gene also differs markedly between the two species.

Presumably these two examples of species differences, affecting timing and mutant phenotypes, both point to differences in the control of expression of the genes. If the timing of developmental events is different between two similar species, then assuming the same control genes are involved, these genes must be differentially regulated. Similarly, the different mutant phenotypes must reflect differences in expression. Mouse *Emx-2* heterozygotes probably have a mild phenotype because *Emx-1* is coexpressed with *Emx-2* in the

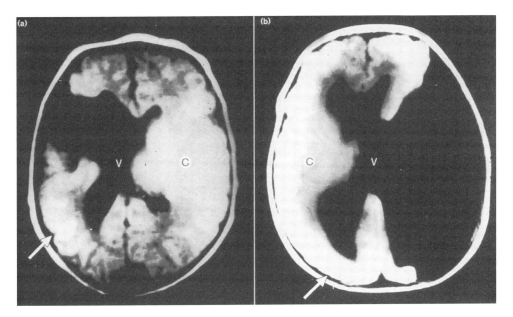

Fig. 9.4 *Emx-2* mutations and schizencephaly. These two MRI images show the consequence of mutation of the *Emx-2* gene in humans. These schizencephalic patients both show large full thickness clefts of the cerebral cortex. (Reproduced with permission from Brunelli *et al.*, 1996.)

ventricular zone cells through most of neurogenesis. Since the proteins are highly homologous, there is likely to be redundancy of function; that is, *Emx-1* covers for the missing *Emx-2*. The clinical phenotype suggests that this does not happen in humans, probably because the two genes are not so broadly coexpressed. These comparisons make clear that it is not sufficient to know that certain classes of genes play a fundamental role in rodent forebrain development. We also need to understand what they do in the human context—how their expression differs, and what the consequences for these differences are. Until we understand how these fundamental genes control *human* cortical development, our grasp of the forebrain pathology in neurodevelopmental disorders will remain primitive.

Pattern formation and its functional consequences

The hypothesis we are driving towards is that the fundamental events underlying forebrain organisation direct downstream processes such as neurogenesis, neuronal migration, and neuronal wiring: if a subtle aberration arose in the process of pattern formation, then this would reveal itself in the disruption of the downstream processes. So far, we have discussed the molecular basis of the primary process. We will now consider the consequences of these discoveries for the downstream processes. We will concentrate on two: migration and fate determination.

Migration

There has been a profound and unexpected change in the conception and understanding of neuronal migration in the past decade. Since the seminal work of Pasko Rakic in the early 1970s, the view had been widely held that neuronal migration in the cortex was purely radial (Rakic, 1972). Neuroblasts were thought to leave the ventricular zone pursuing a radial path through the intermediate zone, following closely the fibres of radial glial cells (Fig. 9.5). Since each cohort of newly generated cells passed through the nascent cortical plate to lie superficial to previously generated cells, the cortical plate grew in an 'inside-

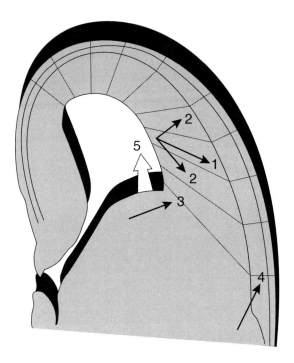

Fig. 9.5 Migration in the cerebral cortex. Neuronal migration in the developing cerebral cortex has long been known to be predominantly radial (path 1) following the radial glial fibres, the trajectories of which are indicated by the radial lines. It is now clear that many migrating neurons disperse tangentially (path 2) during this radial movement. In addition to these pathways followed by the indigenous cortical neurons, there is movement from one telencephalic region to another. Paths 3 and 4 indicate neurons moving from the lateral ganglionic eminence (the presumptive corpus striatum) into the cerebrum. Some of these move in the subventricular zone (path 3), while others are moving in the marginal zone, the future layer I (path 4). Note that these migratory streams occur at an earlier stage of development than that actually drawn here, but for simplicity all these streams are shown in the same diagram. Path 5 is the rostral migratory stream. Cells in the subventricular zone of both ganglionic eminence and cerebrum migrate rostrally (into the plane of the page) to populate the olfactory bulb. This stream originates at a later stage than shown here, and is maintained into adulthood. (See Pearlman et al., 1998 for review of these migratory streams and for the original references.)

out pattern', whereby the oldest cells formed the deepest laminae, and the youngest the most superficial. Not only did this pattern seem to explain the major migrational events, it also appeared to provide a neat explanation of how the cortex came to be organised in a columnar fashion. The 'radial unit hypothesis' proposed that the embryonic cortex embodied a hidden 'protomap' of the adult cortex. The ventricular zone was thought to comprise a series of developmental units, each of which generated a population of neurons, which by virtue of their radial migration, all came to lie in a vertically arranged column. Thus the clone of cells derived from a single neuronal precursor cell belonged to a single functional column (Rakic, 1988).

When the hypothesis was able to be tested in detail, it became apparent that migration is much more complex than originally envisaged by the Rakic model. By the late 1980s, it had become possible to label an individual ventricular zone precursor cell with a retroviral vector and observe the distribution of its daughter cells in the adult cortex (Price and Thurlow, 1988; Walsh and Cepko, 1992; Grove et al., 1993; Mione et al., 1997). The interpretation of these experiments became contentious for a variety of technical reasons, but all researchers were agreed that clones of labelled neurons were certainly not arrayed in a strictly radial fashion. Indeed, the main bone of contention was whether there was any limit at all to the tangential spread of neurons. Some researchers produced evidence for such a wide dispersion of clonally related neurons that they were even found distributed across both hemispheres (Walsh and Cepko, 1992). Confirmation that there is a substantial tangential dispersion of neurons during corticogenesis is provided by cortical slice preparations, which show that many neuroblasts followed in real time migrate tangentially, making only transient, glancing connections with radial glial fibres before continuing tangentially (O'Rourke et al., 1995).

As if these results were not heretical enough, recent studies by a number of laboratories have shown that many cerebral neurons are not even indigenous cortical cells (Gadisseux et al., 1992; Anderson et al., 1997; see Pearlman et al., 1998 for review). In particular, many of the GABAergic neurons of the cortex migrate into the embryonic cortex from the ganglionic eminence—across the boundary between cortex and striatum that was discussed above in relation to Pax-6 function. This population of cells migrate circumferentially around the developing cortex, orthogonal to the conventional radial pathway. The precise number of cells following this route is not clear, but considering tangential migration as a whole—indigenous cells and émigrés—the work of Tan and colleagues is illuminating (Tan and Breen, 1993; Tan et al., 1995). They examined the distribution of cells in the cortices of mosaic mice, generated using an X-inactivated transgenic marker. They estimated that while approximately one-third of the cells appeared to have been dispersed primarily radially, the remaining two-thirds had been dispersed tangentially.

The significance of this series of studies for the neuroscientist is that the pattern of neuronal migration that gives rise to the cerebrum is considerably more complex than might have been thought, and we will return to this point below. From the point of view of the developmental biologist, the more significant point is that the cortex is not a developmental compartment. When we briefly considered the hindbrain earlier, the point was made that the rhombomeres develop as semi-autonomous units. The population of cells that will generate each rhombomeric structure becomes identified, and from each population is generated all the structures to which that particular rhombomere will give rise. Each rhombomere is therefore a 'compartment'; a population of cells with a common developmental identity. (This use of the term 'compartment' is quite distinct from its usage as applied to the histology of the striatum; Nothias *et al.*, 1998.) Whether there is a similar organisation anywhere else in the embryonic central nervous system is a moot point, but the cerebrum clearly is not such a compartment. The precursor cells of the ventricular zone appear to observe the boundary between cortex and striatum and do not cross it (Fishell *et al.*, 1993), but this is not true for a variety of neuronal populations. In fact, we already knew that cells moved between telencephalic regions during development. It has been known for some time (and was recently confirmed) that there is a stream of cells moving rostrally from the subventricular zone of the cerebrum into the olfactory bulb (Goldman and Luskin, 1998). This migration begins in the embryo but continues into adulthood, and is one of the few active areas of neurogenesis in the adult mammalian nervous system. So, just as cells move from the cerebrum to the olfactory bulb, so they move from the striatum into the cerebrum.

Where this leaves the radial unit hypothesis is open to debate. Clearly, a column of cortical cells is not the progeny of a protocortical unit in any meaningful sense. Nonetheless, the data suggest that while many cortical neurons disperse tangentially, many migrate radially, the old-fashioned way. So long as a population of cells retain the same relative distribution in the cortical plate that they held in the ventricular zone, then it remains possible that the positional information held in a 'protomap' underlies the construction of the cortex. Whether this is in fact how the cortex is built, is still unclear, but there is good evidence that the different populations of ventricular zone cells that will give rise to different cortical areas can have distinct cell cycle properties (Polleux *et al.*, 1997). This would argue that such pre-patterning does exist. Pre-patterning in the form of neat cortical columns probably appears less likely now than it once did, if only because cortical anatomists and physiologists now seem less certain than they once were that the column is a fundamental cortical unit anyway (Swindale, 1998).

The importance of this work for human pathology is broader than just a consideration of schizophrenia. Taking the radial unit hypothesis as their starting point, neurologists have tended to classify disorders of neuronal proliferation as the result of either a 'diminished number of proliferative cortical units', or as a 'diminished size of proliferative units'—the so-called microencephaly vera (e.g. Volpe, 1995). A basic distinction probably still holds between the two types of pathology, even if proliferative units do not really exist as such. Nonetheless, it is probably time the logic behind this classification were rethought.

The significance for schizophrenia lies mainly in appreciating that there are multiple populations of migrating cells that could be affected by the disease process, and the paths they take are considerably more complex than simply radial. Equally, there are many genes involved in migration which could be affected (Hatten, 1999). It also carries a more arcane message. The considerable 'to-ing' and 'fro-ing' of cortical cells during development probably means that patterning information is carried by specific subsets of cells. If the patterning of connectivity goes awry in schizophrenia, then specific subsets of cells are more likely to be involved than the population of cortical neurons as a whole. Which those populations might be is currently guesswork, but the evidence implicating cells of the primordial plexiform layer origin is tantalising. These studies have recently been reviewed by Jones (Jones, 1997; see also Chapters 3, 8, and 13), from whose laboratory much of the interesting work has emerged (Akbarian *et al.*, 1993*a,b*). It will not therefore be reiterated here, except to say that cells of the primordial plexiform layer are the earliest cerebral cells to emerge. They are now being discovered to have complex origins and migration patterns, and though many of them are transient cells that disappear during later development, others remain in the adult layer I and subcortical white matter. Most importantly, a subset of the cells—those that form the subplate—have a proven role in cortical patterning, specifically in guiding thalamocortical projections (Ghosh *et al.*, 1990). Further understanding of the processes of migration, and the regulatory genes involved, will be necessary if their putative involvement in schizophrenia is to be clarified.

Fate determination

The final process to consider is that of fate determination, and its link to area specification within the telencephalon. Given that the adult cerebrum is composed of various cell types (Chapter 10), two questions arise. Firstly, what is the process by which these cell types are generated? This is the cell lineage question: for instance, are neurons and glia both generated by the same population of multipotential precursor cells, or are each generated by separate populations of committed cells? Secondly, how is this process integrated into the process of positional specification that we have just considered?

In the rodent cerebral cortex, fate determination appears to be a biphasic process. The early stage is dominated by multipotential precursor cells, which apparently have the potential to generate all cortical cell types (Davis and Temple, 1994; Williams and Price, 1995). These are the cells that are sometimes called 'neural stem cells', even though they are a transient, quickly-dividing population quite unlike the adult cells that usually carry that name. They can be recognised by their potential to generate the entire range of cerebral cell types—neurons, astrocytes, and oligodendrocytes. This early phase is remarkably short lived. By the time the cortical plate is six to 10 cells thick (E16 in the rat), the multipotential cells may represent as little as 5 per cent of the precursor cell population (Williams and Price, 1995). Most of the remainder appear to be committed to the generation of just a single cell type, with less than 10 per cent having some intermediate capacity (Williams *et al.*, 1991; Grove *et al.*, 1993). It appears that by this stage the ventricular zone has become a mosaic of precursor cell types, each with a different determined fate. The majority are committed neuronal precursor cells, with subpopulations of glial precursors that are relatively small but grow over the subsequent period of corticogenesis. If this finding extrapolates to humans, it would mean that after roughly 10 weeks of embryonic development, the primary determination of cell fate was well advanced. Needless to say, this extrapolation is a big one given that cortical neurogenesis is delayed in primates compared to rodents, and part of the mechanism for this delay might be the timing of this phase switch (Finlay and Darlington, 1995).

Once a population of precursor cells is committed to the generation of neurons, the next, more fine-grained question, is whether within this population there are different subpopulations each committed to the production of subsets of neurons. For example, do there exist committed 'pyramidal neuron precursors' and 'non-pyramidal neuron precursors'? The data on this point are ambiguous. A number of studies have implied that there are clones composed of either pyramidal or non-pyramidal neurons (Lavdas et al., 1996; Mione et al., 1997), but other data indicate that some clones are composed of both neuronal types (Gotz et al., 1995). The conclusion from the latter study was that indigenous cortical neurons are probably generated by a single population of neuronal precursor cells, and that the fate of each neuron (pyramidal versus non-pyramidal) was determined postmitotically by influences on each individual cell.

A similar conclusion has been drawn concerning laminar fate. The cortical lamina to which a cortical neuron migrates correlates strongly with its 'birthday'. Cells that become postmitotic early during corticogenesis are fated to migrate to the deeper layers; those generated later take up successively more superficial locations. In principle, this could be explained in a number of different ways. There could be different subpopulations of precursor cells for each of the laminae, with the sequential birthdays reflecting their sequential activation. At the opposite extreme, all neurons could be equal when they left the ventricular zone, programmed to migrate as far as they could (i.e. to the marginal zone) then stop. That would ensure the 'inside-out' pattern of development that we observe. In fact, neither of these alternatives is correct. In a very elegant study, McConnell and Kaznowski (1991) showed that a neuron acquires its laminar identity shortly after it goes through its final S phase of the cell cycle. If cortical cells were labelled with tritiated thymidine (TdR) at a time when they were generating lamina VI cells, and immediately transplanted into a later stage animal whose precursor cells were generating lamina II/III cells, then most labelled cells turned into lamina II/III neurons. Thus, although they were fated to give rise to lamina VI neurons, they were not committed to do so and would generate lamina II/III cells if placed in the appropriate environment. If, however, the labelled cells were left undisturbed for 4 hours before transplantation, they retained their lamina VI fate, and migrated to lamina VI even though the host cells around them migrated to lamina II/III. This means that during that 4 hours, they had become determined to adopt the lamina VI fate. As TdR incorporation takes place during S phase, fate determination must have occurred some time during the 4 hours following the cell's final S phase.

Other studies show that many aspects of neuronal fate are determined at the time a cell passes through its final mitosis. Much of its subsequent behaviour, including appropriate migration, will follow from this set of decisions, which therefore have many downstream implications.

In the context of this chapter, it is interesting that there is evidence that the process of fate determination differs between telencephalic areas. The cell cycle differences between different cortical areas have already been mentioned (Polleux et al., 1997). Comparing cells across the cortical–striatal boundary discussed above, other differences arise. Cortical cells respond to different growth factors from striatal cells (Birling and Price, 1995), express different helix–loop–helix genes (a class of transcription factor known to be important in fate determination; Gradwohl et al., 1996), express different cell surface receptors (Hecht et al., 1996), and may even be composed of different subpopulations of neural precursor cells. This latter point relates to the observations that cortical oligodendrocytes may not be derived from indigenous precursors (Birling and Price, 1998). Rather, like the neuronal émigrés discussed above, they are derived from precursor cells that migrate into the cortex from ventral telencephalon.

Concluding remarks

In this chapter, we have considered what is known about the developmental organisation of the forebrain with a view to suggesting new avenues for research into the developmental deficit that putatively underlies schizophrenia (Chapter 8). Primarily, it has been driven by the conviction that the pathology of schizophrenia might make more sense if viewed in this light, a conviction accompanied by a suspicion that schizophrenia may actually be a failure of telencephalic pattern formation; we pointed out that a number of aspects of the pathology fit this hypothesis somewhat better than they fit more mechanistic failures of migration, cell death, or synapse formation. We recognise this is a weak argument, since most of the current evidence fits a wide range of theories. Currently, we know very little about the expression in humans of the genes discussed in this chapter, either in normal or pathological situations. The little that we do know—the work on *Emx-2* and *Pax-6* particularly—has proved of considerable interest, and is surely an area worthy of further investigation.

References

Acampora, D., Mazan, S., Avantaggiato, V. *et al.* (1996) Epilepsy and brain abnormalities in mice lacking the Otx1 gene. *Nature Genetics* **14**, 218–222.

Akbarian, S., Bunney, W. E. Jr, Potkin, S. G. *et al.* (1993*a*) Altered distribution of nicotinamide-adenine dinucleotide phosphate-diaphorase cells in frontal lobe of schizophrenics implies disturbances of cortical development. *Archives of General Psychiatry* **50**, 169–177.

Akbarian, S., Vinuela, A., Kim, J. J., Potkin, S. G., Bunney, W. E., Jr, Jones, E. G. (1993*b*) Distorted distribution of nicotinamide-adenine dinucleotide phosphate-diaphorase neurons in temporal lobe of schizophrenics implies anomalous cortical development. *Archives of General Psychiatry* **50**, 178–187.

Alvarez-Bolado, G., Rosenfeld, M. G., Swanson, L. W. (1995) Model of forebrain regionalization based on spatiotemporal patterns of POU-III homeobox gene expression, birthdates, and morphological features. *Journal of Comparative Neurology* **355**, 237–295.

Anderson, S. A., Eisenstat, D. D., Shi, L., Rubenstein, J. L. (1997) Interneuron migration from basal forebrain to neocortex: dependence on Dlx genes. *Science* **278**, 474–476.

Ang, S. L., Jin, O., Rhinn, M., Daigle, N., Stevenson, L., Rossant, J. (1996) A targeted mouse Otx2 mutation leads to severe defects in gastrulation and formation of axial mesoderm and to deletion of rostral brain. *Development* **122**, 243–252.

Birling, M. C., Price, J. (1995) Influence of growth factors on neuronal differentiation. *Current Opinion in Cell Biology* **7**, 878–884.

Birling, M. C., Price, J. (1998) A study of the potential of the embryonic rat telencephalon to generate oligodendrocytes. *Developmental Biology* **193**, 100–113.

Blakemore, C. (1995) Introduction: mysteries in the making of the cerebral cortex. In: Bock, G. R. and Cardue, G., Eds. *Development of the cerebral cortex*, pp. 1–20. Chichester, UK: John Wiley.

Brunelli, S., Faiella, A., Capra, V. *et al.* (1996) Germline mutations in the homeobox gene EMX2 in patients with severe schizencephaly. *Nature Genetics* **12**, 94–96.

Burkhalter, A. (1993) Development of forward and feedback connections between areas V1 and V2 of human visual cortex. *Cerebral Cortex* **3**, 476–487.

Caric, D., Gooday, D., Hill, R. E., McConnell, S. K., Price, D. J. (1997) Determination of the migratory capacity of embryonic contical cells lacking the transcription factor Pax-6. *Development* **124**, 5087–5096.

Danos, P., Baumann, B., Bernstein, H.-G. *et al.* (1998) Schizophrenia and anteroventral thalamic nucleus: selective decrease of parvalbumin-immunoreactive thalamocortical projection neurons. *Psychiatry Research: Neuroimaging* **82**, 1–10

Davis, A. A., Temple, S. (1994) A self-renewing multipotential stem cell in embryonic rat cerebral cortex. *Nature* **372**, 263–266.

Fernandez, A. S., Pieau, C., Reperant, J., Boncinelli, E., Wassef, M. (1998) Expression of the Emx-1 and Dlx-1 homeobox genes define three molecularly distinct domains in the telencephalon of mouse, chick, turtle and frog embryos: implications for the evolution of telencephalic subdivisions in amniotes. *Development* **125**, 2099–2111.

Finlay, B. L., Darlington, R. B. (1995) Linked regularities in the development and evolution of mammalian brains. *Science* **268**, 1578–1584.

Fishell, G., Mason, C. A., Hatten, M. E. (1993) Dispersion of neural progenitors within the germinal zones of the forebrain. *Nature* **362**, 636–638.

Frantz, G. D., Weimann, J. M., Levin, M. E., McConnell, S. K. (1994) Otx1 and Otx2 define layers and regions in developing cerebral cortex and cerebellum. *Journal of Neuroscience* **14**, 5725–5740.

Gadisseux, J. F., Goffinet, A. M., Lyon, G., Evrard, P. (1992) The human transient subpial granular layer: an optical, immunohistochemical, and ultrastructural analysis. *Journal of Comparative Neurology* **324**, 94–114.

Ghosh, A., Antonini, A., McConnell, S. K. (1990) Requirement for subplate neurons in the formation of thalamocortical connections. *Nature* **347**, 179–181.

Goldman, S. A., Luskin, M. B. (1998) Strategies utilized by migrating neurons of the postnatal vertebrate forebrain. *Trends in Neurosciences* **21**, 107–114.

Gotz, M., Williams, B. P., Bolz, J., Price, J. (1995) The specification of neuronal fate: a common precursor for neurotransmitter subtypes in the rat cerebral cortex in vitro. *Euopean Journal of Neuroscience* **7**, 889–898.

Gradwohl, G., Fode, C., Guillemot, F. (1996) Restricted expression of a novel murine atonal-related bHLH protein in undifferentiated neural precursors. *Developmental Biology* **180**, 227–241.

Grove, E. A., Williams, B. P., Li, D. Q., Hajihosseini, M., Friedrich, A., Price, J. (1993) Multiple restricted lineages in the embryonic rat cerebral cortex. *Development* **117**, 553–561.

Gulisano, M., Broccoli, V., Pardini, C., Boncinelli, E. (1996) Emx1 and Emx2 show different patterns of expression during proliferation and differentiation of the developing cerebral cortex in the mouse. *European Journal of Neuroscience* **8**, 1037–1050.

Hatten, M. E. (1999) Central nervous system migration. *Annual Review of Neuroscience* **22**, 511–539.

Hecht, J. H., Weiner, J. A., Post, S. R., Chun, J. (1996) Ventricular zone gene-1 (vzg-1) encodes a lysophosphatidic acid receptor expressed in neurogenic regions of the developing cerebral cortex. *Journal of Cell Biology* **135**, 1071–1083.

Hevner, R. F., Kinney, H. C. (1996) Reciprocal entorhinal-hippocampal connections established by human fetal midgestation. *Journal of Comparative Neurology* **372**, 384–394.

Heyman, I., Frampton, I., van Heyningen, V., Hanson, I., Taylor, I., Simonoff, E. (1999) Psychiatric disorder and cognitive function in a family with an inherited novel mutation of the developmental control gene PAX6. *Psychiatric Genetics* **9**, 85–90

Jones, E. G. (1997) Cortical development and thalamic pathology in schizophrenia. *Schizophrenia Bulletin* **23**, 483–501.

Jordan, T., Hanson, I., Zaletayev, D. *et al.* (1992) The human PAX6 gene is mutated in two patients with aniridia. *Nature Genetics* **1**, 328–332.

Kostovic, I., Petanjek, Z., Judas, M. (1993) Early areal differentiation of the human cerebral cortex: entorhinal area. *Hippocampus* **3**, 447–458.

Lavdas, A. A., Mione, M. C., Parnavelas, J. G. (1996) Neuronal clones in the cerebral cortex show morphological and neurotransmitter heterogeneity during development. *Cerebral Cortex* **6**, 490–497.

Levitt, P., Barbe, M. F., Eagleson, K. L. (1997) Patterning and specification of the cerebral cortex. *Annual Review of Neuroscience* **20**, 1–24.

Lumsden, A., Keynes, R. (1989) Segmental patterns of neuronal development in the chick hindbrain. *Nature* **337**, 424–428.

Lumsden, A., Krumlauf, R. (1996) Patterning the vertebrate neuraxis. *Science* **274**, 1109–1115.

McConnell, S. K., Kaznowski, C. E. (1991) Cell cycle dependence of laminar determination in developing neocortex. *Science* **254**, 282–285.

Mione, M. C., Cavanagh, J. F. R., Harris, B., Parnavelas, J. G. (1997) Cell fate specification and symmetrical/asymmetrical divisions in the developing cerebral cortex. *Journal of Neuroscience* **17**, 2018–2029.

Nothias, F., Fishell, G., Ruiz (1998) Cooperation of intrinsic and extrinsic signals in the elaboration of regional identity in the posterior cerebral cortex. *Current Biology* **8**, 459–462.

O'Rourke, N. A., Sullivan, D. P., Kaznowski, C. E., Jacobs, A. A., McConnell, S. K. (1995) Tangential migration of neurons in the developing cerebral cortex. *Development* **121**, 2165–2176.

Pakkenberg, B. (1990) Pronounced reduction of total neuron number in mediodorsal thalamic nucleus and nucleus accumbens in schizophrenics. *Archives of General Psychiatry* **47**, 1023–1028.

Pearlman, A. L., Faust, P. L., Hatten, M. E., Brunstrom, J. E. (1998) New directions for neuronal migration. *Current Opinion in Neurobiology* **8**, 45–54.

Pellegrini, M., Mansouri, A., Simeone, A., Boncinelli, E., Gruss, P. (1996) Dentate gyrus formation requires Emx2. *Development* **122**, 3893–3898.

Polleux, F., DeHay, C., Moraillon, B., Kennedy, H. (1997) Regulation of neuroblast cell-cycle kinetics plays a crucial role in the generation of unique features of neocortical areas. *Journal of Neuroscience* **17**, 7763–7783.

Porteus, M. H., Bulffone, A., Liu, J.-K., Puelles, L., Lo, L.-C., Rubenstein, J. L. (1994) DLX-2, MASH-1, and MAP-2 expression and bromodeoxyuridine incorporation define molecularly distinct cell populations in the embryonic mouse forebrain. *Journal of Neuroscience* **14**, 6370–6383.

Price, J., Thurlow, L. (1988) Cell lineage in the rat cerebral cortex: a study using retro-viral-mediated gene transfer. *Development* **104**, 473–482.

Qiu, M., Anderson, S., Chen, S. *et al.* (1996) Mutation of the Emx-1 homeobox gene disrupts the corpus callosum. *Developmental Biology* **178**, 174–178.

Rakic, P. (1972) Mode of cell migration to the superficial layers of fetal monkey neocortex. *Journal of Comparative Neurology* **145**, 61–84.

Rakic, P. (1988) Specification of cerebral cortical areas. *Science* **241**, 170–176.

Simeone, A., Acampora, D., Gulisano, M., Stornaiuolo, A., Boncinelli, E. (1992) Nested expression domains of four homeobox genes in developing rostral brain. *Nature* **358**, 687–690.

Stober, G., Syagailo, Y. V., Okladnova, O. *et al.* (1999) Functional Pax-6 gene-linked poly-morphic region: potential association with paranoid schizophrenia. *Biological Psychiatry* **45**, 1585–1591.

Stoykova, A., Fritsch, R., Walther, C., Gruss, P. (1996) Forebrain patterning defects in small eye mutant mice. *Development* **122**, 3453–3465.

Stoykova, A., Gotz, M., Gruss, P., Price, J. (1997) Pax6-dependent regulation of adhesive patterning, R-cadherin expression and boundary formation in developing forebrain. *Development* **124**, 3765–3777.

Stuart, E. T., Kiossi, C., Gruss, P. (1993) Mammalian Pax genes. *Annual Review of Genetics* **27**, 219–236.

Suda, Y., Matsuo, I., Aizawa, S. (1997) Cooperation between Otx1 and Otx2 genes in developmental patterning of rostral brain. *Mechanisms of Development* **69**, 125–141.

Swindale, N. V. (1998) Cortical organization: modules, polymaps and mosaics. *Current Biology* **8**, R270–R273.

Tan, S. S., Breen, S. (1993) Radial mosaicism and tangential cell dispersion both contribute to mouse neocortical development. *Nature* **362**, 638–640.

Tan, S. S., Faulkner, J. B., Breen, S. J., Walsh, M., Bertram, J. F., Reese, B. E. (1995) Cell dispersion patterns in different cortical regions studied with an X-inactivated trans-genic marker. *Development* **121**, 1029–1039.

Volpe, J. J. (1995) *Neurology of the newborn,* 3rd edition. Philadelphia: W. B. Saunders.

Waddington, J. L. (1993) Schizophrenia: developmental neuroscience and pathobiology. *Lancet* **341**, 531–536.

Walsh, C. A. (1999) Genetic malformations of the human cerebral cortex. *Neuron* **23**, 19–29.

Walsh, C. A., Cepko, C. L. (1992) Widespread dispersion of neuronal clones across func-tional regions of the cerebral cortex. *Science* **255**, 434–440.

Wilkinson, D. G., Bhatt, S., Cook, M., Boncinelli, E., Krumlauf, R. (1989) Segmental expression of Hox-2 homeobox-containing genes in the developing mouse hindbrain. *Nature* **341**, 405–409.

Williams, B. P., Price, J. (1995) Evidence for multiple precursor cell types in the embryonic rat cerebral cortex. *Neuron* **14**, 1181–1188.

Williams, B. P., Read, J., Price, J. (1991) The generation of neurons and oligodendrocytes from a common precursor cell. *Neuron* **7**, 685–693.

Yan, X. X., Ribak, C. E. (1997) Prenatal development of nicotinamide adenine dinucleotide phosphate-diaphorase activity in the human hippocampal formation. *Hippocampus* **7**, 215–231.

Yoshida, M., Suda, Y., Matsuo, I. *et al.* (1997) Emx1 and Emx2 functions in development of dorsal telencephalon. *Development* **124**, 101–111.

10 The Organization of Cortical Circuitry

David A. Lewis

Among the various signs and symptoms of schizophrenia, some appear to be attributable to dysfunction of a specific brain region, and to be associated with evidence of altered synaptic neurotransmission therein. For example, convergent lines of evidence from *in vivo* neuroimaging and postmortem studies support the view that the impairments in working memory seen in schizophrenia (Chapter 7) may reflect alterations in the synaptic connectivity (Chapter 4) of the dorsolateral prefrontal cortex (PFC). The gray matter volume of the PFC has been found to be decreased in schizophrenia in many MRI studies (Chapter 1), and MR spectroscopic investigations have found evidence for a decrease in synaptic building blocks in the PFC (Pettegrew *et al.*, 1991; Stanley *et al.*, 1995). Reduced levels of *N*-acetyl aspartate, a putative marker of neuronal and/or axonal integrity, in the PFC of schizophrenic subjects (Bertolino *et al.*, 1996; Deicken *et al.*, 1997) may also reflect disturbances in axon terminals or dendrites.

In postmortem studies of the PFC in schizophrenia (Chapter 3), cell packing density has been reported to be increased and cortical thickness decreased (Pakkenberg, 1987; Daviss and Lewis, 1995; Selemon *et al.*, 1995). The total number of PFC neurons does not appear to be altered (Pakkenberg, 1993), although decreased numbers of certain populations of prefrontal neurons have been observed (Benes *et al.*, 1991). Increased cell packing density without a change in neuron number suggests that PFC neuropil, which includes the axon terminals, small dendrites, and dendritic spines that are the components of most cortical synapses, is diminished in schizophrenia. Consistent with this interpretation, levels of the synapse-associated protein synaptophysin have been reported to be decreased in the PFC in subjects with schizophrenia (Chapter 4). However, understanding the potential aetiological and pathophysiological significance of alterations in synaptic connectivity requires an understanding of which elements of PFC circuitry are preferentially affected.

Similarly, because the function of all neurotransmitter systems is determined by the morphological constraints that govern the location of the synthesis, release, and sites of action of the neurotransmitter, understanding the significance of alterations in neurotransmitters and their receptors is dependent on an appreciation of their roles in specific neural circuits. For example, much evidence points to abnormalities in γ-aminobutyric acid (GABA) transmission in the PFC in schizophrenia (Chapter 3). However, since there are at least a dozen different classes of PFC GABA neurons (Condé *et al.*, 1994), many of which are highly specialized in terms of their synaptic targets, knowledge of which GABA cell class(es) is/are affected is critical to understanding the functional consequences of an alteration in GABA neurotransmission.

Finally, a circuitry analysis approach to the study of schizophrenia is of particular importance because it seems clear that brain dysfunction in this disorder is not restricted to a single region or neurotransmitter system. Consequently, the pathophysiological significance of any specific abnormality can only be understood within the context of the neural circuitry that is affected. Furthermore, knowledge of the functional relationships between components of a neural circuit is required in order to determine whether a given abnormality is more likely to represent a cause, consequence, or compensation for other abnormalities in the same circuit. Thus, the goal of this chapter is to provide an overview of some principles of neural circuitry organization that can be used to guide the conduct and interpretation of postmortem studies of schizophrenia. The discussion will focus on the dorsolateral PFC (DLPFC) as a prototypical brain region implicated in schizophrenia.

A model system for circuitry analysis: the primate dorsolateral prefrontal cortex

A distinguishing feature of the primate brain is the marked expansion of the PFC. The PFC has been estimated to occupy less than 4 per cent of the total cerebral cortex in cats; in macaque monkeys, it comprises 12 per cent of an expanded cortical mantle, and in the much larger human brain, the PFC constitutes approximately 30 per cent of cortical volume (Fuster, 1997). This increase in both relative and absolute size is associated with an increased complexity and differentiation of structure and organization of the primate PFC. For example, the PFC in rodents is agranular (lacks an internal granular layer 4), whereas monkey and human PFC are granular and can, in part, be parcellated into different regions by the degree of differentiation of this layer (Barbas and Pandya, 1989). In addition to other cytoarchitectural differences (Walker, 1940; Barbas and Pandya, 1989), rodent and primate PFC vary in the organization and sources of intrinsic and extrinsic connections. Such species differences may reflect their ontogenic differences discussed in Chapter 9.

In contrast to these differences between rodents and primates, the characteristics of monkey PFC appear, on current data, to reflect accurately the organization of human PFC. For example, the density and laminar distribution of somatostatin-containing neurons and fibres is regionally heterogeneous but comparable in both species (Lewis *et al.*, 1986; Hayes *et al.*, 1991), whereas this intrinsic neuropeptide system is uniform across the rodent cerebral cortex (Campbell *et al.*, 1987). Similarly, the dopaminergic projection to the rat cerebral cortex is very restricted, whereas every region of the primate neocortex receives a projection (Lewis *et al.*, 1987; Berger *et al.*, 1991). In addition, the regional density, laminar distribution, and synaptic targets of dopamine axons appear to be common to monkey and human neocortex (Lewis and Sesack, 1997).

These distinctive features of the primate PFC, in concert with the fact that information about many aspects of cortical circuitry cannot currently be obtained in humans (Crick and Jones, 1993), indicates that knowledge of monkey PFC circuitry is both valuable and necessary for interpreting the functional significance of abnormalities observed in the PFC in schizophrenia; consequently, most of the information in the following sections is derived from studies in monkeys. In addition, it is worth pointing out that, although focusing on the DLPFC, the issues have a broader relevance because the cell types and patterns of circuitry organization to be described for the DLPFC apply generally to other cortical association areas implicated in schizophrenia (Pearlson *et al.*, 1996).

Cortical neuron types

Pyramidal neurons

Pyramidal neurons constitute about 70 per cent of all cortical neurons (Powell, 1981). As a group, pyramidal neurons have several distinguishing morphological features (Fig.10.1). The majority have a characteristically shaped cell body that gives rise to a single apical dendrite, which ascends vertically toward the cortical surface and frequently ends in a terminal tuft. Pyramidal neurons also have an array of shorter basilar dendrites that spread laterally from the base of the cell. The dendrites of pyramidal neurons are coated with short protrusions, called spines, that are the sites of most of the excitatory synaptic inputs to these neurons. Consequently, the density of dendritic spines provides a good estimate of the number of excitatory inputs that a pyramidal neuron receives (Mates and Lund, 1983). Typically, it possesses 6000 to 10 000 dendritic spines (DeFelipe and Farinas, 1992). In addition to receiving one excitatory input, a fraction of dendritic spines also receive a synapse with the features suggestive of an inhibitory input. Inhibitory terminals also synapse on the dendritic shafts, cell body, and axon initial segment of pyramidal neurons. As a rule of thumb, each neuron receives about 2000 inhibitory (Gray's type II; see below) synapses on dendritic shafts, 200 on the cell soma, and 20 on the axon initial segment (DeFelipe and Farinas, 1992). Most pyramidal neurons are projection neurons, meaning that their principal axon enters the white matter and travels to another brain region. However, before reaching the white matter, these axons give rise to intrinsic collaterals which travel either horizontally or vertically within the gray matter. The connections furnished by these collaterals are discussed in detail below. Pyramidal neurons are the principal class of cortical

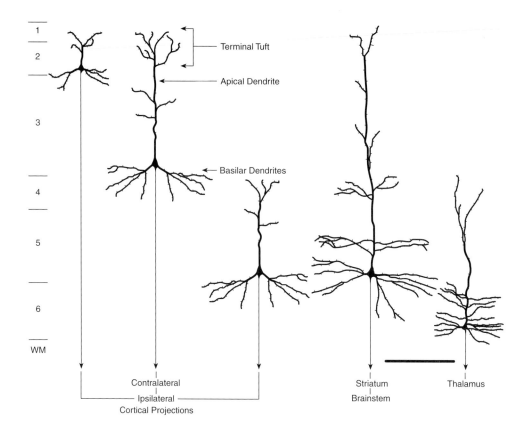

Fig. 10.1 Schematic drawing illustrating the characteristic morphological features of pyramidal neurons in different cortical layers. Note that the laminar location of the cell soma tends to be associated with the major projection target of the principal axon. Arabic numbers indicate the cortical layers and WM indicates white matter. (Adapted from Jones, 1984).

excitatory neurons and utilize excitatory amino acids, such as glutamate, as their transmitter. In addition, the synapses formed by the boutons of pyramidal neuron axons have the characteristic morphology associated with excitatory neurotransmission (Gray's type I; see Chapter 4 for discussion of synaptic morphology).

Non-pyramidal neurons

These cells are generally small, and also known as local circuit neurons or interneurons, meaning that their axonal arbor remains within the cortical gray matter. Over 90 per cent of non-pyramidal neurons utilize the inhibitory neurotransmitter GABA. Their axons form Gray's type II synapses (characterized by pleomorphic vesicles in the axon terminal and symmetric pre- and postsynaptic densities; Chapter 4). As a group, GABA neurons constitute approximately 25 per cent of neurons in the primate neocortex (Hendry *et al.*, 1987), and are comprised of a variety of distinct subtypes (Fairen *et al.*, 1984). Although the differences among subtypes can be described on the basis of the morphological features of the cell body and proximal dendrites (e.g. bipolar, multipolar, bitufted), the most discriminating and functionally meaningful classification system is based on the organization of the axonal arbor and the synaptic targets of the axon terminals. For example, at least 12 different morphological subclasses of local circuit neurons have been identified in the primate neocortex (Lund, 1973; Jones, 1975; Fairen *et al.*, 1984), with most of these subtypes found in both monkey and human PFC (Mrzljak *et al.*, 1988; Lund and Lewis, 1993). GABA neurons are also chemically heterogeneous, and separate subpopulations can be identified by the presence of specific neuropeptides or calcium-binding proteins (Condé *et al.*, 1994; Gabbott and Bacon, 1996).

Together, these features define subpopulations of GABA neurons that appear to have different biophysical properties and different roles in PFC circuitry (Fig. 10.2). For example, GABA neurons of the chandelier class, which may also express either the neuropeptide corticotropin-releasing factor (Lewis *et al.*, 1989) or the calcium-binding protein parvalbumin (DeFelipe *et al.*, 1989; Lewis and Lund, 1990), are found primarily in cortical layers 2 to 5 (Lund and Lewis, 1993). The axon terminals of these neurons, which are arrayed as distinct vertical structures (termed 'cartridges'), form inhibitory synapses exclusively with the axon initial segment of pyramidal neurons (Szentagothai and Arbib, 1974; Jones, 1975; Somogyi, 1977; Fairen and Valverde, 1980; Peters *et al.*, 1982; DeFelipe *et al.*, 1985), the site of action potential generation in pyramidal neurons. Each chandelier cell may contact up to 300 pyramidal neurons within a radius of 100 to 150 μm from its cell body (Peters, 1984), hence exerting critical inhibitory control over the activity of a localized group of pyramidal neurons. In contrast, the axons of wide arbor (basket) neurons, which form inhibitory synapses with the cell bodies, dendritic shafts, and dendritic spines of pyramidal neurons (Jones and Hendry, 1984), spread horizontally for considerable distances (up to 1.0 mm) within the PFC (Lund and Lewis, 1993). These neurons may be specialized to provide inhibitory constraints over the activity of spatially segregated populations of PFC pyramidal neurons (Levitt *et al.*, 1993; Lund *et al.*, 1993). A third example of a GABA neuron, double bouquet cells, which contain the calcium-binding proteins calbindin or calretinin (Condé *et al.*, 1994), have radially restricted axonal arbors that synapse with the dendritic shafts of both pyramidal and local circuit neurons (Somogyi and Cowey, 1984).

Laminar arrangement of neurons

Most neocortical association areas are composed of six layers which can be identified based on the size and packing density of their constituent neurons (Fig. 10.3). Layer 1, located just below the pial surface, is cell sparse but 90 per cent of the neurons in this layer contain GABA. Layers 2 and 4 are thin and densely packed with small 'granular' cells. The majority of these neurons are small pyramidal cells, with GABA neurons constituting approximately 30 and 15 per cent of all neurons in layers 2 and 4, respectively (Hendry *et al.*, 1987).

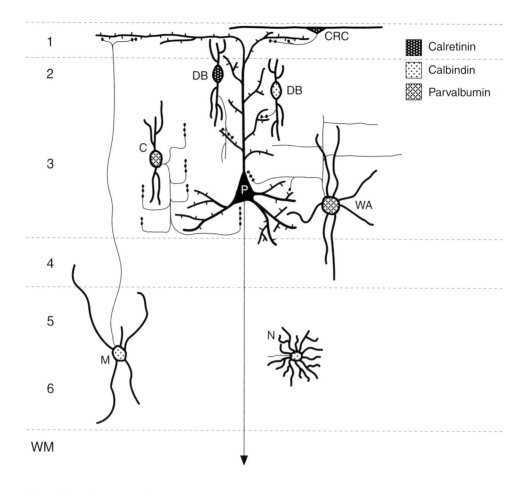

Fig. 10.2 Schematic drawing of the synaptic interactions between different classes of local circuit neurons and a layer 3 pyramidal neuron (P) in monkey prefrontal cortex. C indicates a parvalbumin (PV)-labeled chandelier neuron; CRC: calretinin (CR)- and/or calbindin (CB)-labeled Cajal–Retzius neuron; DB: CR- or CB-labeled double-bouquet neuron; M: CB-labeled Martinotti cell; N: CB-labeled neurogliaform neuron; WA: PV-labeled wide arbor (basket) neuron. (Modified from Condé *et al.*, 1994.)

Layers 3 and 5 are the thickest cortical layers and contain prominent pyramidal neurons with a classical morphology (described above). In both of these layers, the size and packing density of the pyramidal neurons is greater near their borders with layer 4. These patterns make it possible to subdivide layers 3 and 5 into two or three subdivisions, usually designated by the suffixes a, b, and c. In layer 6, many of the pyramidal cells have a modified or atypical appearance leading to the designation of this layer as the pleomorphic layer. In most neocortical regions, GABA cells comprise 20 to 30 per cent of the neurons in layer 3, and about 15 per cent of the neurons in layers 5 and 6 (Hendry *et al.*, 1987).

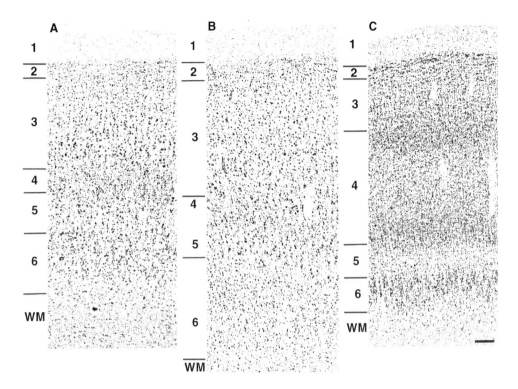

Fig. 10.3 Nissl-stained sections showing laminar and regional differences in cell size in packing density in areas 46 (A) and 9 (B) of the human prefrontal cortex and area 17, primary visual cortex (C). WM, white matter. Calibration bar = 200 μm.

As indicated below, afferents to the PFC innervate neural elements in certain cortical layers, and projections from the PFC to other brain regions generally originate from pyramidal neurons in specific laminae. Thus, the laminar specificity of any neural abnormalities in schizophrenia may reveal significant information about alterations in particular types of inputs or outputs. However, due to the vertical spread of the dendrites of many neurons (Figs 10.1 and 10.2) , alterations in afferents to one layer can affect the function of neurons whose cell body is located in a different layer.

Organization of efferent projections

Pyramidal neurons in each cortical layer tend to furnish characteristic types of projections (Fig. 10.1; Jones, 1984). For example, many pyramidal neurons located in layers 2 and the superficial part of layer 3 (3a) project to nearby ipsilateral cortical regions, whilst those in deep layer 3 (3b) project to more distant ipsilateral areas, or across the corpus callosum to contralateral cortical regions. Projections within the same hemisphere are termed associational whereas those to the contralateral hemisphere are termed callosal. In layer 5, pyramidal neurons project to the striatum, superior colliculus, and other subcortical structures, whereas cells located in layer 6 preferentially project to the thalamus. The efferent axons of pyramidal neurons tend to terminate in just one brain region, although a small percentage of these neurons do give rise to collateral projections (Schwartz and Goldman-Rakic, 1984; Barbas, 1995). In contrast to these extrinsic projections, the small pyramidal cells in layer 4 tend to project just within the gray matter and relatively few send axons into the underlying white matter.

Although these patterns describe the general organization of cortical efferents, they are a first approximation and there are many exceptions. For example, 25 to 30 per cent of the pyramidal neurons furnishing associational projections are located in the infragranular layers (layers 5 and 6; Schwartz and Goldman-Rakic, 1984), and 15 to 20 per cent of neurons projecting to the striatum are located in layer 3 (Arikuni and Kubota, 1986). In addition, the nature of the cortical output to a given region may vary with the location of the cell body of origin. For example, neurons in layer 6 have been proposed to provide 'modulatory' inputs to cells in higher order thalamic nuclei (such as the mediodorsal nucleus, the principal source of thalamic afferents to the PFC) as well as inputs to the reticular nucleus, which regulates thalamocortical interactions. In contrast, thalamic projections originating in layer 5 do not innervate the reticular nucleus and appear to provide 'driving' afferent inputs to higher order nuclei (Guillery et al., 1998).

As well as their primary extrinsic projections, pyramidal neurons give rise to local axon collaterals that provide different patterns of intrinsic connectivity (Levitt et al., 1993). For example, as illustrated in Fig. 10.4, pyramidal neurons in layers 2 and 3 furnish horizontal axons that spread for considerable distances and then give rise to discrete clusters of axon terminals in the supragranular layers. Although pyramidal neurons in layers 5 and 6 also send horizontal intrinsic collaterals, these have a more limited spread and do not terminate in spatially segregated clusters. In contrast, pyramidal cells in layer 4 furnish predominantly vertically oriented axons which appear to be specialized for interlaminar connections.

Organization and termination of afferent projections

Cortical afferents

Inputs from other cortical regions terminate across all cortical layers, though different layers tend to be preferentially innervated depending upon the source of the inputs. For example, inputs from cortical regions that have a well-developed layer 4 terminate more prominently

Fig. 10.4 (See opposite page.) Schematic diagram illustrating the typical projection patterns of intrinsic axon collaterals of pyramidal neurons in different layers (A–E) of monkey prefrontal cortex as revealed by small injections of anterograde tracers (filled circles). Note that the pyramidal neurons in layers 2 and 3 (A, B) give rise to horizontally oriented axon collaterals which spread for considerable distances before forming discrete clusters of terminals that span the supragranular layers. In contrast, pyramidal neurons in layers 5 and 6 (D, E) give rise to intrinsic axon collaterals with a more restricted horizontal spread, whereas the pyramidal neurons in layer 4 (C) tend to be oriented vertically. (Adapted from Levitt et al., 1993.)

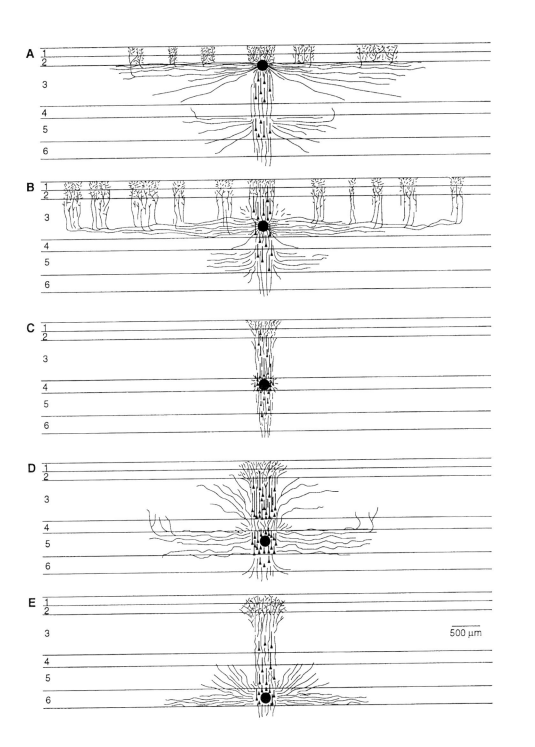

in layers 4 to 6, whereas those that originate in regions with a poorly developed layer 4 tend to terminate in layers 1 to 3 (Barbas and Rempel-Clower, 1997). In some cases, afferents from different regions (e.g. callosal inputs from the contralateral PFC and associational inputs from the posterior parietal cortex) are distributed into interdigitated columns (Goldman-Rakic and Schwartz, 1982).

Thalamic and amygdalar afferents

In contrast to these cortical inputs, afferents from thalamic relay nuclei such as the mediodorsal nucleus project dominantly to layers 3b and 4, with a minor projection to layer 6 (Giguere and Goldman-Rakic, 1988). Afferents from the amygdala project more densely to orbital than dorsal PFC, but in both regions tend to terminate in layers 1 and 6 (Amaral and Price, 1984).

Monoaminergic and cholinergic afferents

Subcortical nuclei containing monoamines or acetylcholine also exhibit distinct laminar patterns of termination in the PFC, along with substantial regional differences in relative density. In most regions, dopamine-containing projections from the ventral mesencephalon have a bilaminar distribution (Lewis and Sesack 1997), with dopaminergic axons forming a dense band in layers 1, 2, and superficially in 3a, with a band of lower density in deep layer 5 and 6 (Fig. 10.5A). In more densely innervated regions, such as motor cortices and dorsomedial PFC (area 9), labelled dopamine axons are also present in high density in the middle cortical layers, forming a third distinctive band in deep layer 3. These innervation patterns contrast with sensory regions, such as primary visual cortex, where dopaminergic axons are restricted to layer 1.

The dopamine innervation differs from the other catecholamine-containing afferent system, the noradrenergic projection from the locus coeruleus. Across the monkey PFC, though the regional distribution of noradrenergic axons is quite similar to that exhibited by dopaminergic axons (Lewis and Morrison, 1989), noradrenergic fibres have a substantially lower overall density and exhibit less regional variation. Dopaminergic and noradrenergic afferents also exhibit different, and in some ways complementary, laminar innervation patterns. For example, the density of noradrenergic axons is greater in the deep cortical layers, especially layer 5 (Fig. 10.5B) whereas particularly few are present in layer 1 which receives a dense dopaminergic innervation. Similar differences in innervation between these two catecholamine systems occur in human neocortex (Gaspar et al., 1989).

The specificity of the patterns of cortical innervation are further illustrated by comparisons with other extrathalamic cortical afferent systems, such as the acetylcholine-containing projection from the nucleus basalis of Meynert and the serotonin-containing projections from the raphe nuclei. Within the PFC, there is a relatively uniform regional distribution of cholinergic (Lewis, 1991) and serotonergic (Lewis, 1990) axons, unlike the dopamine and noradrenergic inputs mentioned above. In addition, although dopaminergic, cholinergic, and serotonergic axons are heavily represented in layers 1 and 2, the latter two afferent systems also innervate the middle cortical layers in regions where DA axons are relatively sparse in these layers (Fig. 10.5C and D).

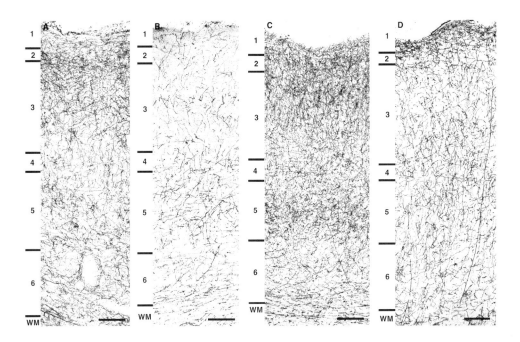

Fig. 10.5 Distribution of dopamine (A), noradrenaline (B), acetylcholine (C), and serotonin (D) axons in macaque monkey prefrontal cortex. Note the differences in relative density and the distinctive laminar distribution of each afferent system. Scale bars = 200 μm. (Modified from Lewis *et al.*, 1992.)

Vulnerable prefrontal cortex circuitry in schizophrenia

As mentioned at the start of this chapter, an understanding of PFC organization is essential both for making predictions about the elements of PFC circuitry that are dysfunctional in schizophrenia and for interpreting the functional significance of abnormalities observed in the PFC of subjects with the disorder. To illustrate the point, this section provides one example of such an analysis. As introduced in Chapter 7, the DLPFC is a critical component of the neural network that mediates working memory (Goldman-Rakic, 1987; Fuster, 1997), a basic cognitive function that is disturbed in subjects with schizophrenia (Park and Holzman, 1992). In macaque monkeys, a substantial proportion of DLPFC neurons exhibit sustained firing during the delay period of delayed-response tasks, and this delay period activity appears to be critical for the active maintenance of information needed to perform the task correctly (Kubota and Niki, 1971; Fuster *et al.*, 1982; Funahashi *et al.*, 1989). Thus, the sustained firing of DLPFC neurons in the absence of continued sensory input has been proposed to constitute the cellular basis of working memory (Goldman-Rakic, 1995; Fuster, 1997).

The maintenance of neuronal activity during the delay period has been suggested to be subserved, at least in part, by reverberating excitatory circuits (Funahashi and Kubota,

1994). Although the available data are limited, several findings suggest that this circuitry is likely to involve DLPFC layer 3 pyramidal neurons, since sustained neuronal firing during the delay period of working memory tasks is most commonly observed in this layer (Fuster *et al.*, 1985; Friedman and Goldman-Rakic, 1994). As subjects with schizophrenia are frequently impaired on working memory tasks, identifying the neural circuitry of the DLPFC that subserves working memory may reveal the interconnected neural elements particularly vulnerable to the pathophysiology of the disorder. Based on our work and that of

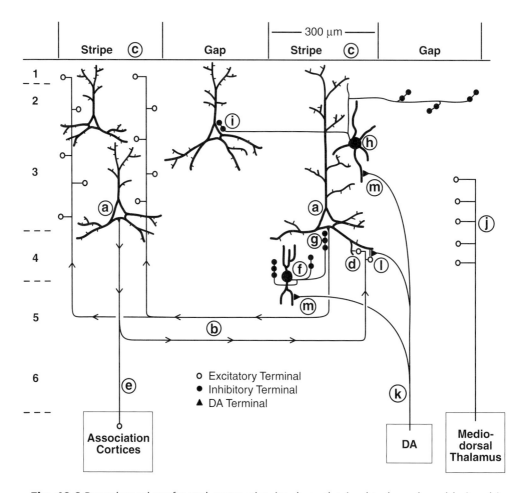

Fig. 10.6 Dorsolateral prefrontal cortex circuitry hypothesized to be vulnerable in schizophrenia. a: layer 3 pyramidal neuron; b: horizontal axon collateral from a layer 3 pyramidal neuron; c: stripe-like clusters of intrinsic projections between segregated pyramidal neurons; d: input to a dendritic spine; e: association axon projection; f: chandelier cell; g: input to a pyramidal neuron initial axon segment; h: wide arbor neuron; i: input to a pyramidal neuron soma; j: input from mediodorsal thalamus; k: dopamine (DA) projection from ventral mesencephalon; l: DA input to a dendritic spine; m: DA input to GABA cell dendrites.

other investigators, we have suggested that the following elements (Fig. 10.6) are essential components.

Layer 3 pyramidal neurons

These neurons (label a in Fig. 10.6) furnish horizontal intrinsic axon collaterals (label b in Fig. 10.6) that form stripe-like clusters (label c in Fig. 10.6) of axon terminals in layers 1 to 3 (Fig. 10.4). Over 95 per cent of these terminals form excitatory synapses on the dendritic spines of other pyramidal neurons (label d in Fig. 10.6; Melchitzky *et al.*, 1998). The presence of reciprocal connections between spatially segregated clusters of layer 3 pyramidal neurons may provide an anatomical substrate for a reverberating excitatory circuit that subserves the maintenance of sustained activity in specific modules (groups of interconnected stripe-like clusters) of DLPFC neurons during the delay period of working memory tasks (Lewis and Anderson, 1995; Pucak *et al.*, 1996). This interpretation is supported by findings from electrophysiological studies indicating that the vast majority of layer 3 pyramidal neurons receive excitatory input from the intrinsic, horizontal axons furnished by other layer 3 pyramidal neurons, and that this input constitutes a large proportion of their excitatory drive (Gonzalez-Burgos *et al.*, 2000).

The principal axons (label e in Fig. 10.6) of layer 3 pyramidal neurons project through the white matter to connect with other cortical regions. These projections innervate in a reciprocal fashion clusters of neurons in other regions of the PFC (Fig. 10.7) and presumably in other association regions of the neocortex. These findings indicate that a given DLPFC module of interconnected stripe-like clusters participates in a larger neural network of cortical connections that may play different roles in the sensory, memory, and motor

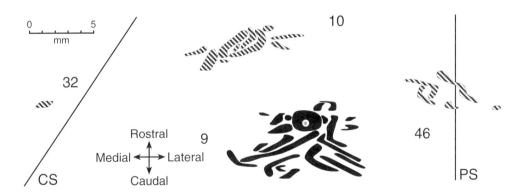

Fig. 10.7 View, on an unfolded map of the surface of the dorsolateral prefrontal cortex, of the stripe-like clusters of layer 3 pyramidal cells that are interconnected via horizontal intrinsic axon collaterals (solid stripes) or associational projections through the white matter (cross-hatched stripes). Asterisk indicates the location of the injection site. This figure illustrates that the intrinsic and associational projections furnished by layer 3 pyramidal cells link spatially segregated groups of neurons both locally and in other cortical regions. Numerals indicate the locations of PFC areas 9, 10, 32, and 46. CS: cingulate sulcus; PS: principal sulcus. (Adapted from Pucak *et al.*, 1996.)

components of working memory tasks. These patterns of corticocortical connectivity raise questions regarding the relative role in working memory of sustained neuronal firing in the DLPFC versus that in other brain regions. In particular, since delay period neuronal activity is also common in parietal and temporal association cortices, it is possible that the long-range excitatory connections between the DLPFC and posterior cortical regions subserve sustained neuronal activity. Although this may be the case, it is interesting that the stripe-like clustering of intrinsic horizontal connections in DLPFC contrasts with the smaller, patch-like clusters in visual association cortices such as V4 and TE (Yoshioka *et al.*, 1992; Lund *et al.*, 1993; Tanigawa *et al.*, 1998). The larger size of the interconnected stripes in the DLPFC could mean that more cells are involved in recurrent excitation in these regions than in more posterior regions. If a greater number of neurons contributing to such inter-actions produces more robust sustained firing, then these regional differences in intrinsic excitatory connections could explain why delay-related activity of neurons is less likely to be interrupted by intervening stimuli in the DLPFC than in temporal or parietal cortices (Miller *et al.*, 1996). Thus, although sustained neuronal activity in the DLPFC during working memory tasks may be the consequence of more than one type of reciprocal circuit, the data suggest an important and unique role for the intrinsic excitatory connections between spatially segregated clusters of DLPFC layer 3 pyramidal neurons.

Chandelier class of GABA interneurons

The axon terminals of chandelier cells (label f in Fig. 10.6) form distinctive vertical arrays (termed 'cartridges') that provide inhibitory input exclusively to the axon initial segment of pyramidal neurons (label g in Fig. 10.6). Interestingly, the spread of the axon arbor (approximately 200 to 300 μm diameter) of chandelier neurons in monkey DLPFC (Lund and Lewis, 1993) is similar to the width of the stripes formed by layer 3 pyramidal cells, suggesting that chandelier cells may be specialized to inhibit the output of pyramidal neurons within a given stripe, and thus to regulate activity within a given module of interconnected stripes.

Wide arbor class of GABA interneurons

A substantial portion of the axon terminals of wide arbor cells—the large GABA interneu-rons (label h in Fig. 10.6) found most commonly in layers 3 and 5 (Lund and Lewis, 1993), synapse on the soma of pyramidal neurons (label i in Fig. 10.6). Although the dendritic field width of wide arbor neurons (approximately 300 μm; Lund and Lewis, 1993) indi-cates that their afferent drive is limited to axon terminals within a stripe, the size (approximately 800 to 1000 μm) and spatial arrangement (thought to be elongated in one plane) of their axon arbor (Lund and Lewis, 1993), suggests that they may be specialized to inhibit the activity of pyramidal neurons located in the gaps between the interconnected stripes that form a particular module of layer 3 pyramidal neurons (Pucak *et al.*, 1996; Melchitzky *et al.*, 1998). Consequently, while activation of a given stripe-like cluster(s) of supragranular pyramidal neurons is predicted to lead to sustained firing in pyramidal neurons distributed across a module of interconnected stripes, activation of the wide arbor neurons within these stripes would result in the suppression of firing in the pyramidal neurons located in the intervening areas. This inhibition would thus help to maintain the fidelity of the information coded by the activity in the interconnected stripes.

Afferents from the mediodorsal thalamic nucleus

Afferents from the mediodorsal thalamic nucleus (MDTN) (label j in Fig. 10.6) also play a key role in working memory (Shulman, 1964; Isseroff *et al.*, 1982). We saw earlier that the excitatory projections from MDTN terminate in layers 3b and 4 (Giguere and Goldman-Rakic, 1988) of DLPFC, primarily upon the dendritic spines of pyramidal neurons (Melchitzky *et al.*, 1999). In addition, the dendrites of interneurons, at least some of which have the biochemical features of chandelier and wide arbor neurons, also receive synapses from MDTN axons. These findings suggest that the basilar dendrites of deep layer 3 pyramidal neurons (label a in Fig. 10.6) and the dendrites of chandelier and/or wide arbor local circuit neurons (labels f and h in Fig. 10.6) are among the targets of the inputs from MDTN, providing additional support for the role of these components of the DLPFC in the circuitry that mediates working memory.

Two other lines of evidence suggest that the circuitry illustrated in Fig. 10.6 plays a critical role in working memory tasks. Firstly, working memory depends upon an intact dopminergic innervation of the DLPFC (Brozoski *et al.*, 1979; Roberts *et al.*, 1994), and a certain degree of stimulation of D1 dopamine receptors is required for optimal functioning of the DLPFC (Sawaguchi *et al.*, 1986; Sawaguchi and Goldman-Rakic, 1991; Cohen and Servan-Schreiber, 1992; Arnsten *et al.*, 1994; Williams and Goldman-Rakic, 1995; Murphy *et al.*, 1996). Interestingly, dopaminergic afferents from the mesencephalon (label k in Fig. 10.6; see also Fig. 10.5A) provide synaptic input to both pyramidal neurons (label l in Fig. 10.6) and the dendrites (label m in Fig. 10.6) of parvalbumin-containing interneurons (which include the chandelier and wide arbor neurons) in the middle cortical layers (Sesack *et al.*, 1998). In contrast, parvalbumin-labeled neurons in the superficial layers and the calretinin-containing class of GABA neurons do not appear to be synaptic targets of dopaminergic terminals (Sesack *et al.*, 1995). Given the critical role of dopamine in working memory, these observations are consistent with the notion that layer 3 pyramidal neurons, and the associated chandelier and wide arbor neurons, contribute to working memory processes.

The second line of evidence is that the time course of postnatal maturation of the circuitry regulating the function of DLPFC layer 3 pyramidal neurons parallels the improvement in performance on working memory tasks (see Lewis, 1997 for review). For example, dendritic spines, markers of excitatory inputs to layer 3 pyramidal neurons, increase substantially in number during late prenatal development and the first few months of postnatal life, and then undergo a substantial regression during adolescence (Anderson *et al.*, 1995). These changes in excitatory inputs to layer 3 pyramidal neurons during puberty preferentially involve the intrinsic projections between stripes as opposed to associational inputs from other cortical regions (Woo *et al.*, 1997). A virtually identical developmental profile occurs in the number of parvalbumin-positive chandelier neuron axon cartridges, markers of inhibitory inputs to the axon initial segment of pyramidal neurons in deep layer 3 of the DLPFC (Anderson *et al.*, 1995; Condé *et al.*, 1996). In addition, the density of dopaminergic axons in layer 3 in monkey increases during the first few postnatal months (Rosenberg and Lewis, 1995), paralleling the increase in densities of pyramidal neuron dendritic spines and chandelier neuron axon cartridges. After a plateau period, dopaminergic axons in layer 3 undergo a second marked increase in density to reach peak values during adolescence before declining to relatively stable adult levels. These refinements in the dopaminergic innervation of the primate DLPFC are highly specific in that densities of dopaminergic axons in the superficial and deep cortical layers do not change during adolescence (Rosenberg and Lewis, 1995).

Together, these findings support the hypothesis that the circuitry illustrated in Fig. 10.6 may be vulnerable to pathophysiological alterations in schizophrenia. To test this hypothesis, we have evaluated the integrity of the axon terminals of chandelier cells in the DLPFC of subjects with schizophrenia (Woo *et al.*, 1998) using an antibody against the GABA membrane transporter (GAT-1). The density of GAT-1-labeled axon cartridges was decreased on average by 40 per cent in subjects with schizophrenia compared to both normal controls and subjects with non-schizophrenic psychiatric disorders. In over 70 per cent of the cases, cartridge density was decreased in the schizophrenic subject relative to both of the matched comparison subjects. In addition, the density of labeled cartridges did not differ between normal controls and subjects who had been treated with antipsychotic medications for other psychotic disorders. These changes also appeared to be selective for the axon terminals of the chandelier class of GABA neurons since the density of axon terminals immunoreactive for calretinin, a calcium binding protein found in other GABA neurons, was not altered in schizophrenia. A follow-up study has indicated that the alterations in chandelier neuron axon cartridges may be greatest in magnitude and frequency in the middle cortical layers (Pierri *et al.*, 1999). Additional studies will be required to determine whether these changes in chandelier neuron axon cartridges in schizophrenia represent a primary pathological disturbance, a downstream consequence of some more primary abnormality, or a compensatory response. Regardless, knowledge of the relationship of chandelier neurons to other aspects of DLPFC circuitry, as illustrated here, will make it possible to design experiments capable of addressing these questions.

Acknowledgements

Work by the author cited in this chapter was supported by USPHS grants MH00519, MH45156, MH51234, and MH43784.

References

Amaral, D. G., Price, J. L. (1984) Amygdalo-cortical projections in the monkey (*Macaca fascicularis*). *Journal of Comparative Neurology*, **230**, 465–496.

Anderson, S. A., Classey, J. D., Condé, F., Lund, J. S., Lewis, D. A. (1995) Synchronous development of pyramidal neuron dendritic spines and parvalbumin-immunoreactive chandelier neuron axon terminals in layer III of monkey prefrontal cortex. *Neuroscience*, **67**, 7–22.

Arikuni, T., Kubota, K. (1986) The organization of prefrontal caudate projections and their laminar origin in the Macaque monkey: a retrograde study using HRP-gel. *Journal of Comparative Neurology*, **244**, 492–510.

Arnsten, A. F. T., Cai, J. X., Murphy, B. L., Goldman-Rakic, P. S. (1994) Dopamine D1 receptor mechanisms in the cognitive performance of young adult and aged monkeys. *Psychopharmacology*, **116**, 143–151.

Barbas, H. (1995) Pattern in the cortical distribution of prefrontally directed neurons with divergent axons in the rhesus monkey. *Cerebral Cortex*, **2**, 158–165.

Barbas, H., Pandya, D. N. (1989) Architecture and intrinsic connections of the prefrontal cortex in the rhesus monkey. *Journal of Comparative Neurology*, **286**, 353–375.

Barbas, H., Rempel-Clower, N. (1997) Cortical structure predicts the pattern of cortico-cortical connections. *Cerebral Cortex*, **7**, 635–646.

Benes, F. M., McSparren, J., Bird, E. D., SanGiovanni, J. P., Vincent, S. L. (1991) Deficits in small interneurons in prefrontal and cingulate cortices of schizophrenic and schizoaffective patients. *Archives of General Psychiatry*, **48**, 996–1001.

Berger, B., Gaspar, P., Verney, C. (1991) Dopaminergic innervation of the cerebral cortex: Unexpected differences between rodents and primates. *Trends in Neuroscience*, **14**, 21–27.

Bertolino, A., Nawroz, S., Mattay, V. S. *et al.* (1996) Regionally specific pattern of neuro-chemical pathology in schizophrenia as assessed by multislice proton magnetic resonance spectroscopic imaging. *American Journal of Psychiatry*, **153**, 1554–1563.

Brozoski, T. J., Brown, R. M., Rosvold, H. E., Goldman, P. S. (1979) Cognitive deficit caused by regional depletion of dopamine in prefrontal cortex of rhesus monkeys. *Science*, **205**, 929–932.

Campbell, M. J., Lewis, D. A., Benoit, R., Morrison, J. H. (1987) Regional heterogeneity in the distribution of somatostatin-28- and somatostatin-28(1–12)-immunoreactive profiles in monkey neocortex. *Journal of Neuroscience*, **7**, 1133–1144.

Cohen, J. D., Servan-Schreiber, D. (1992) Context, cortex, and dopamine: A connectionist approach to behavior and biology in schizophrenia. *Psychological Review*, **99**, 45–77.

Condé, F., Lund, J. S., Jacobowitz, D. M., Baimbridge, K. G., Lewis, D. A. (1994) Local circuit neurons immunoreactive for calretinin, calbindin D-28k, or parvalbumin in monkey prefrontal cortex: Distribution and morphology. *Journal of Comparative Neurology*, **341**, 95–116.

Condé, F., Lund, J. S., Lewis, D. A. (1996) The hierarchical development of monkey visual cortical regions as revealed by the maturation of parvalbumin-immunoreactive neurons. *Developmental Brain Research*, **96**, 261–276.

Crick, F., Jones, E. (1993) Backwardness of human neuroanatomy. *Nature*, **361**, 109–110.

Daviss, S. R., Lewis, D. A. (1995) Local circuit neurons of the prefrontal cortex in schiz-ophrenia: Selective increase in the density of calbindin-immunoreactive neurons. *Psychiatry Research*, **59**, 81–96.

DeFelipe, J., Farinas, I. (1992) The pyramidal neuron of the cerebral cortex: Morphological and chemical characteristics of the synaptic inputs. *Progress in Neurobiology*, **39**, 563–607.

DeFelipe, J., Hendry, S. H. C., Jones, E. G., Schmechel, D. (1985) Variability in the termi-nations of GABAergic chandelier cell axons on initial segments of pyramidal cell axons in the monkey sensory-motor cortex. *Journal of Comparative Neurology*, **231**, 364–384.

DeFelipe, J., Hendry, S. H. C., Jones, E. G. (1989) Visualization of chandelier cell axons by parvalbumin immunoreactivity in monkey cerebral cortex. *Proceedings of the National Academy of Sciences USA*, **86**, 2093–2097.

Deicken, R. F., Zhou, L., Corwin, F., Vinogradov, S., Weiner, M. W. (1997) Decreased left frontal lobe *N*-acetylaspartate in schizophrenia. *American Journal of Psychiatry*, **154**, 688–690.

Fairen, A., Valverde, F. (1980) A specialized type of neuron in the visual cortex of cat: A Golgi and electron microscope study of chandelier cells. *Journal of Comparative Neurology*, **194**, 761–779.

Fairen, A., DeFelipe, J., Regidon, J. (1984) Nonpyramidal neurons, general account. In: A. Peters and E. G. Jones, eds. *Cerebral cortex*, Volume 1, pp. 201–245. Plenum Press, New York.

Friedman, H. R., Goldman-Rakic, P. S. (1994) Coactivation of prefrontal cortex and inferior parietal cortex in working memory tasks revealed by 2DG functional mapping in the rhesus monkey. *Journal of Neuroscience*, **14**, 2775–2788.

Funahashi, S., Kubota, K. (1994) Working memory and prefrontal cortex. *Neuroscience Research*, **21**, 1–11.

Funahashi, S., Bruce, C. J., Goldman-Rakic, P. S. (1989) Mnemonic coding of visual space in the monkey's dorsolateral prefrontal cortex. *Journal of Neurophysiology*, **61**, 331–349.

Fuster, J. M. (1997) *The prefrontal cortex: anatomy, physiology, and neuropsychology of the frontal lobe*. Lippincott-Raven, Philadelphia.

Fuster, J. M., Bauer, R. H., Jervey, J. P. (1982) Cellular discharge in the dorsolateral prefrontal cortex of the monkey in cognitive tasks. *Experimental Neurology*, **77**, 679–694.

Fuster, J. M., Bauer, R. H., Jervey, J. P. (1985) Functional interactions between inferotemporal and prefrontal cortex in a cognitive task. *Brain Research*, **330**, 200–307.

Gabbott, P. L. A., Bacon, S. J. (1996) Local circuit neurons in the medial prefrontal cortex (areas 24a, b, c, 25 and 32) in the monkey: I. Cell morphology and morphometrics. *Journal of Comparative Neurology*, **364**, 567–608.

Gaspar, P., Berger, B., Fabvret, A., Vigny, A., Henry, J. P. (1989) Catecholamine innervation of the human cerebral cortex as revealed by comparative immunohistochemistry of tyrosine hydroxylase and dopamine-beta-hydroxylase. *Journal of Comparative Neurology*, **279**, 249–271.

Giguere, M., Goldman-Rakic, P. S. (1988) Mediodorsal nucleus: Areal, laminar, and tangential distribution of afferents and efferents in the frontal lobe of rhesus monkeys. *Journal of Comparative Neurology*, **277**, 195–213.

Goldman-Rakic, P. S. (1987) Circuitry of primate prefrontal cortex and regulation of behavior by representational memory. In: F. Plum and V. Mountcastle, eds. *Handbook of physiology*, pp. 373–417. American Physiological Society, Bethesda, MD.

Goldman-Rakic, P. S. (1995) Cellular basis of working memory. *Neuron*, **14**, 477–485.

Goldman-Rakic, P. S., Schwartz, M. L. (1982) Interdigitation of contralateral and ipsilateral columnar projections to frontal association cortex in primates. *Science*, **216**, 755–757.

Gonzalez-Burgos, G., Barrionuevo, G., Lewis, D. A. (2000) Horizontal synaptic connections in monkey prefrontal cortex: An in vitro electrophysiological study. *Cerebral Cortex*, **10**, 82–92.

Guillery, R. W., Feig, S. L., Lozsádi, D. A. (1998) Paying attention to the thalamic reticular nucleus. *Trends in Neuroscience*, **21**, 28–32.

Hayes, T. L., Cameron, J. L., Fernstrom, J. D., Lewis, D. A. (1991) A comparative analysis of the distribution of prosomatostatin-derived peptides in human and monkey neocortex. *Journal of Comparative Neurology*, **303**, 584–599.

Hendry, S. H. C., Schwark, H. D., Jones, E. G., Yan, J. (1987) Numbers and proportions of GABA-immunoreactive neurons in different areas of monkey cerebral cortex. *Journal of Neuroscience*, **7**, 1503–1519.

Isseroff, A., Rosvold, H. E., Galkin, T. W., Goldman-Rakic, P. S. (1982) Spatial memory impairments following damage to the mediodorsal nucleus of the thalamus in rhesus monkeys. *Brain Research*, **232**, 97–113.

Jones, E. G. (1975) Varieties and distribution of nonpyramidal cells in the somatic sensory cortex of the squirrel monkey. *Journal of Comparative Neurology*, **160**, 205–268.

Jones, E. G. (1984) Laminar distribution of cortical efferent cells. In: A. Peters and E. G. Jones, eds. *Cerebral cortex,* Volume 1, pp. 521–553. Plenum Press, New York.

Jones, E. G., Hendry, S. H. C. (1984) Basket cells. In: A. Peters and E. G. Jones, eds. *Cerebral cortex,* Volume 1, pp. 309–336. Plenum Press, New York.

Kubota, K., Niki, H. (1971) Prefrontal cortical unit activity and delayed alternation performance in monkeys. *Journal of Neurophysiology*, **34**, 337–341.

Levitt, J. B., Lewis, D. A., Yoshioka, T., Lund, J. S. (1993) Topography of pyramidal neuron intrinsic connections in macaque monkey prefrontal cortex (areas 9 and 46). *Journal of Comparative Neurology*, **338**, 360–376.

Lewis, D. A. (1990) The organization of chemically-identified neural systems in primate prefrontal cortex: Afferent systems. *Progress in Neuro-Psychopharmacology and Biological Psychiatry*, **14**, 371–377.

Lewis, D. A. (1991) Distribution of choline acetyltransferase immunoreactive axons in monkey frontal cortex. *Neuroscience*, **40**, 363–374.

Lewis, D. A. (1997) Development of the prefrontal cortex during adolescence: Insights into vulnerable neural circuits in schizophrenia. *Neuropsychopharmacology*, **16**, 385–398.

Lewis, D. A., Anderson, S. A. (1995) The functional architecture of the prefrontal cortex and schizophrenia. *Psychological Medicine*, **25**, 887–894.

Lewis, D. A., Lund, J. S. (1990) Heterogeneity of chandelier neurons in monkey neocortex: Corticotropin-releasing factor and parvalbumin immunoreactive populations. *Journal of Comparative Neurology*, **293**, 599–615.

Lewis, D. A., Morrison, J. H. (1989) The noradrenergic innervation of monkey prefrontal cortex: A dopamine-beta-hydroxylase immunohistochemical study. *Journal of Comparative Neurology*, **282**, 317–330.

Lewis, D. A., Sesack, S. R. (1997) Dopamine systems in the primate brain. In: F. E. Bloom, A. Björklund, and T. Hökfelt, eds. *Handbook of chemical neuroanatomy*, pp. 261–373. Elsevier Science, Amsterdam.

Lewis, D. A., Campbell, M. J., Morrison, J. H. (1986) An immunohistochemical characterization of somatostatin-28 and somatostatin-28 (1–12) in monkey prefrontal cortex. *Journal of Comparative Neurology*, **248**, 1–18.

Lewis, D. A., Campbell, M. J., Foote, S. L., Goldstein, M., Morrison, J. H. (1987) The distribution of tyrosine hydroxylase-immunoreactive fibers in primate neocortex is widespread but regionally specific. *Journal of Neuroscience*, **7**, 279–290.

Lewis, D. A., Foote, S. L., Cha, C. I. (1989) Corticotropin releasing factor immunoreactivity in monkey neocortex: An immunohistochemical analysis. *Journal of Comparative Neurology*, **290**, 599–613.

Lewis, D. A., Hayes, T. L., Lund, J. S., Oeth, K. M. (1992) Dopamine and the neural circuitry of primate prefrontal cortex: Implications for schizophrenia research. *Neuropsychopharmacology*, **6**, 127–134.

Lund, J. S. (1973) Organization of neurons in the visual cortex, area 17, of the monkey (*Macaca mulatta*) *Journal of Comparative Neurology*, **147**, 455–496.

Lund, J. S., Lewis, D. A. (1993) Local circuit neurons of developing and mature macaque prefrontal cortex: Golgi and immunocytochemical characteristics. *Journal of Comparative Neurology*, **328**, 282–312.

Lund, J. S., Yoshioka, T., Levitt, J. B. (1993) Comparison of intrinsic connectivity in different areas of macaque monkey cerebral cortex. *Cerebral Cortex*, **3**, 148–162.

Mates, S. L., Lund, J. S. (1983) Spine formation and maturation of type 1 synapses on spiny stellate neurons in primate visual cortex. *Journal of Comparative Neurology*, **221**, 91–97.

Melchitzky, D. S., Sesack, S. R., Pucak, M. L., Lewis, D. A. (1998) Synaptic targets of pyramidal neurons providing intrinsic horizontal connections in monkey prefrontal cortex. *Journal of Comparative Neurology*, **390**, 211–224.

Melchitzky, D. S., Sesack, S. R., Lewis, D. A. (1999) Parvalbumin-immunoreactive axon terminals in monkey and human prefrontal cortex: Laminar, regional and target specificity of Type I and Type II synapses. *Journal of Comparative Neurology*, **408**, 11–22.

Miller, E. K., Erickson, C. A., Desimone, R. (1996) Neural mechanisms of visual working memory in prefrontal cortex of the macaque. *Journal of Neuroscience*, **16**, 5154–5167.

Mrzljak, L., Uylings, H. B. M., Kostovic, I., Van Eden, C. G. (1988) Prenatal development of neurons in the human prefrontal cortex: I. A qualitative Golgi study. *Journal of Comparative Neurology*, **271**, 355–386.

Murphy, B. L., Arnsten, A. F. T., Goldman-Rakic, P. S., Roth, R. H. (1996) Increased dopamine turnover in the prefrontal cortex impairs spatial working memory performance in rats and monkeys. *Proceedings of the National Academy of Sciences USA*, **93**, 1325–1329.

Pakkenberg, B. (1987) Post-mortem study of chronic schizophrenic brains. *British Journal of Psychiatry*, **151**, 744–752.

Pakkenberg, B. (1993) Total nerve cell number in neocortex in chronic schizophrenics and controls estimated using optical disectors. *Biological Psychiatry*, **34**, 768–772.

Park, S., Holzman, P. S. (1992) Schizophrenics show spatial working memory deficits. *Archives of General Psychiatry*, **49**, 975–982.

Pearlson, G. D., Petty, R. G., Ross, C. A., Tien, A. Y. (1996) Schizophrenia: A disease of heteromodal association cortex? *Neuropsychopharmacology*, **14**, 1–17.

Peters, A. (1984) Chandelier cells. In: A. Peters and E. G. Jones, eds. *Cerebral cortex*, Volume 1, pp. 361–380. Plenum Press, New York.

Peters, A., Proskauer, C. C., Ribak, C. E. (1982) Chandelier neurons in rat visual cortex. *Journal of Comparative Neurology*, **206**, 397–416.

Peters, A., Palay, S. L., Webster, D. F. (1991) *The fine structure of the nervous system*. Oxford University Press.

Pettegrew, J. W., Keshavan, M. S., Panchalingam, K. *et al.* (1991) Alterations in brain high-energy phosphate and membrane phospholipid metabolism in first-episode, drug-naive schizophrenics. *Archives of General Psychiatry*, **48**, 563–568.

Pierri, J. N., Chaudry, A. S., Woo, T. U., Lewis, D. A. (1999) Alterations in chandelier neuron axon terminals in the prefrontal cortex of schizophrenic subjects. *American Journal of Psychiatry*, **156**, 1709–1719.

Powell, T. P. S. (1981) Certain aspects of the intrinsic organisation of the cerebral cortex. In: O. Pompeiano and C. A. Marsan, eds. *Brain mechanisms and perceptual awareness*, pp. 1–19. Raven Press, New York.

Pucak, M. L., Levitt, J. B., Lund, J. S., Lewis, D. A. (1996) Patterns of intrinsic and associational circuitry in monkey prefrontal cortex. *Journal of Comparative Neurology*, **376**, 614–630.

Roberts, A. C., DeSalvia, M. A., Wilkinson, L. S. *et al.* (1994) 6-Hydroxydopamine lesions of the prefrontal cortex in monkeys enhance performance on an analog of the Wisconsin Card Sort Test: Possible interactions with subcortical dopamine. *Journal of Neuroscience*, **14**, 2531–2544.

Rosenberg, D. R., Lewis, D. A. (1995) Postnatal maturation of the dopaminergic innervation of monkey prefrontal and motor cortices: A tyrosine hydroxylase immuno-histochemical analysis. *Journal of Comparative Neurology*, **358**, 383–400.

Sawaguchi, T., Goldman-Rakic, P. S. (1991) D1 dopamine receptors in prefrontal cortex: Involvement in working memory. *Science*, **251**, 947–950.

Sawaguchi, T., Matsumura, M., Kubota, K. (1986) Dopamine modulates neuronal activities related to motor performance in the monkey prefrontal cortex. *Brain Research*, **371**, 404–408.

Schwartz, M. L., Goldman-Rakic, P. S. (1984) Callosal and intrahemispheric connectivity of the prefrontal association cortex in rhesus monkey: Relation between intraparietal and principal sulcal cortex. *Journal of Comparative Neurology*, **226**, 403–420.

Selemon, L. D., Rajkowska, G., Goldman-Rakic, P. S. (1995) Abnormally high neuronal density in the schizophrenic cortex: A morphometric analysis of prefrontal area 9 and occipital area 17. *Archives of General Psychiatry*, **52**, 805–818.

Sesack, S. R., Bressler, C. N., Lewis, D. A. (1995) Ultrastructural associations between dopamine terminals and local circuit neurons in the monkey prefrontal cortex: A study of calretinin-immunoreactive cells. *Neuroscience Letters*, **200**, 9–12.

Sesack, S. R., Hawrylak, V. A., Melchitzky, D. S., Lewis, D. A. (1998) Dopamine innervation of a subclass of local circuit neurons in monkey prefrontal cortex: Ultrastructural analysis of tyrosine hydroxylase and parvalbumin immunoreactive structures. *Cerebral Cortex*, **8**, 614–622.

Shulman, S. (1964) Impaired delayed response from thalamic lesions. *Archives of Neurology*, **11**, 477–499.

Somogyi, P. (1977) A specific axo-axonal interneuron in the visual cortex of the rat. *Brain Research*, **136**, 345–350.

Somogyi, P., Cowey, A. (1984) Double bouquet cells. In: A. Peters and E. G. Jones, eds. *Cerebral cortex*, pp. 337–360. Plenum Press, New York.

Stanley, J. A., Williamson, P. C., Drost, D. J. *et al.* (1995) An *in vivo* study of the prefrontal cortex of schizophrenic patients at different stages of illness via phosphorus magnetic resonance spectroscopy. *Archives of General Psychiatry*, **52**, 399–406.

Szentagothai, J., Arbib, M. (1974) Conceptual models of neural organization. *Neuroscience Research Program Bulletin*, **12**, 307–510.

Tanigawa, H., Fujita, I., Kato, M., Ojima, H. (1998) Distribution, morphology, and γ-aminobutyric acid immunoreactivity of horizontally projecting neurons in the macaque inferior temporal cortex. *Journal of Comparative Neurology*, **401**, 129–143.

Walker, A. E. (1940) A cytoarchitectural study of the prefrontal area of the macaque monkey. *Journal of Comparative Neurology*, **73**, 59–86.

Williams, G. V., Goldman-Rakic, P. S. (1995) Modulation of memory fields by dopamine D1 receptors in prefrontal cortex. *Nature*, **376**, 572–575.

Woo, T.-U., Pucak, M. L., Kye, C. H., Matus, C. V., Lewis, D. A. (1997) Peripubertal refinement of the intrinsic and associational circuitry in monkey prefrontal cortex. *Neuroscience*, **80**, 1149–1158.

Woo, T.-U., Whitehead, R. E., Melchitzky, D. S., Lewis, D. A. (1998) A subclass of prefrontal GABA axon terminals are selectively altered in schizophrenia. *Proceedings of the National Academy of Sciences USA*, **95**, 5341–5346.

Yoshioka, T., Levitt, J. B., Lund, J. S. (1992) Intrinsic lattice connections of macaque monkey visual cortical area V4. *Journal of Neuroscience*, **12**, 2785–2802.

11 Perspectives from other Diseases and Lesions

Margaret M. Esiri and R. Carl A. Pearson

Neuropathology and diagnostic issues
Diseases sharing non-specific pathological features with schizophrenia
   Neurodegenerative disorders
   Neurodevelopmental disorders
Disorders in which schizophrenia-like symptoms may occur
   Metabolic diseases
   Epilepsy
   Psychosis in neurodegenerative disorders
Normal determinants of neuronal parameters and the effects of experimental lesions
Suggestions for future studies

The aims of this chapter are twofold. Firstly, to set the neuropathological findings reported in schizophrenia in the context of other neurological and neuropsychiatric disorders; and secondly, to consider what light experimental studies of the nervous system can shed on the interpretation of the schizophrenia findings, especially those concerning alterations in neuronal structure.

Neuropathology and diagnostic issues

Despite the body of work reviewed in this volume it is not yet possible to point to neuropathological changes that are specific for schizophrenia. This limitation is separate from that of the uncertain reliability of the reported findings (Chapter 13). Specific neuropathological changes are those distinctively associated with a disease. They may exist at the macroscopic, microscopic, or ultrastructural levels, and may be non-specific at one level but distinctive at another. They may depend essentially on quantitative, not qualitative, differences from the normal state. And they should go some way to explaining the clinical manifestations of the disease.

These points can be illustrated if we look at a range of neuropathological conditions. A large acoustic neuroma is visible to the naked eye, has a distinctive microscopic appearance, and interrupts function of the VIIIth cranial nerve, providing a clear explanation for why the patient is deaf. This is a qualitatively distinct lesion that may lack macroscopic specificity if its connection with the VIIIth nerve cannot be discerned, since there are other tumours that may grow in a similar location. However, it possesses microscopic specificity in its cellular architecture and it explains disturbed function. A colloid cyst of the third ventricle is macroscopically distinctive though not microscopically so, and again its presence and location explain disturbed function, if present (e.g. headache, unconsciousness). Adrenoleucodystrophy is an inherited defect of peroxisome metabolism which causes diffuse cerebral demyelination indistinguishable from other causes of sudanophilic myelin degeneration at macroscopic and microscopic levels, but with distinctive trilaminar inclusions in cells detectable with the electron microscope. Again, this is a qualitatively distinct disease which produces white matter damage to which the clinical features of progressive motor and mental deficits are plausibly attributable. Alzheimer's disease produces non-specific macroscopic (cerebral atrophy, ventricular dilatation) and microscopic (neuronal loss, gliosis) changes, together with more specific microscopic features (amyloid plaques, neurofibrillary tangles) which are more numerous than similar changes seen in normal ageing, and are localised in parts of the cerebral cortex and interconnected subcortical nuclei (Pearson and Powell, 1989). Their location convincingly explains the cognitive and behavioural features of the disease (Esiri, 1996; Grabowski and Damasio, 1997). In addition there are some diseases, traditionally considered under the rubric of organic psychiatric disorders (Lishman, 1998) which have a well-defined biochemical or genetic aetiology but no specific neuropathology despite characteristic clinical signs of central nervous system dysfunction. Porphyria is a good example. However, even a disorder of this kind differs from schizophrenia, for while both show brain dysfunction without demonstrable neuropathology, porphyria at least has a distinctive biochemical pathology whereas schizophrenia does not.

These examples illustrate the types of neuropathology that may be encountered in different disorders, and the variable manner in which they can be related to aetiology and to altered functioning. With this preamble we can now examine in more detail the similarities and differences between the described changes in schizophrenia and those in other pathological conditions.

Diseases sharing non-specific pathological features with schizophrenia

Neurodegenerative disorders

Some of the changes discussed in schizophrenia, notably ventricular enlargement and reduction in brain weight or volume (Chapter 1), are reproducible but lack specificity. Perhaps the most obvious of the diseases that share this non-specific pathology with schizophrenia are neurodegenerative conditions such as Alzheimer's disease and Pick's disease. (It is also worth pointing out, *vis-à-vis* the neurodevelopmental theory of schizophrenia (Chapter 8), that the same features are seen with normal ageing). As noted above, the crucial difference from schizophrenia is that the neurodegenerative disorders also show specific microscopic features. Furthermore, these occur in the parts of the brain that are functionally impaired, and the severity of pathology is strongly correlated with the severity of dementia (Wilcock and Esiri, 1982; Arriagada *et al.*, 1992; Nagy *et al.*, 1995, 1996). This imparts confidence in the assumption that the structural changes are responsible for the functional deficits.

In schizophrenia, attempts at equivalent correlations are hampered both because the functional impairments are less precisely localisable, and because of the lack of specific microscopic pathology. However, some progress has been made in localising functional impairments in schizophrenia, both from lesioning experiments in animals which roughly parallel the neuropsychological deficits of the disorder, and from functional neuroimaging studies. Thus, lesions in monkey dorsolateral prefrontal cortex mimic deficits in working memory observed in schizophrenia (Goldman-Rakic *et al.*, 1994; see Chapters 7 and 10), whilst reduced cerebral blood flow and metabolism are seen in the same regions in schizophrenia (Chapter 7). Complementing these findings are the histological data suggesting cytoarchitectural differences in dorsolateral prefrontal cortex in schizophrenia (Chapter 3), such as increased neuronal packing density and decreased neuronal size, which may reflect a loss of cortical neuropil, including synapses (Selemon *et al.*, 1995; Rajkowska *et al.*, 1998). These frontal studies represent a start on the task of correlating symptoms with pathology in schizophrenia, but there is a long way to go. The symptoms of schizophrenia are attributable to a very extensive range of functional systems that are widely distributed in the brain. However, the same may also be said of the dementias, and here the explanation is that the cardinal pathological changes are also widely, albeit somewhat selectively, distributed. It remains to be seen whether reduced numbers of synapses and increased packing cell density—the prevailing histological explanation put forward for frontal lobe deficits in schizophrenia—can also explain disturbed function in other parts of the brain. It is already clear that alterations in synaptic markers are not confined to the frontal lobes (Chapter 4), and that the increased neuronal density, but not the decreased neuronal size, mentioned above are seen in primary visual cortex (Selemon *et al.*, 1995; Rajkowska *et al.*, 1998).

In neurodegenerative disorders, as well as the relatively specific pathology noted above, there are non-specific reactive changes in astrocytes and microglial cells. The extent to which these changes are secondary or primary is debated, but there is no real argument about their occurrence. In contrast, the lack of reproducible glial cell reaction (Chapter 5) has been seized upon as an important clue to the likely neurodevelopmental, as opposed to neurodegenerative, origin of schizophrenia (Chapters 5 and 8). This view is supported by the lack of good evidence for progression in the pathology of schizophrenia during the course of the disease.

In summary, the presence of relatively specific microscopic abnormalities and the accompanying gliosis mark neurodegenerative conditions out as different from schizophrenia with respect to their neuropathological nature. It is therefore appropriate now to consider whether more convincing neuropathological similarities exist between schizophrenia and known neurodevelopmental diseases, which can also show the same non-specific features of ventricular enlargement and decreased brain size.

Neurodevelopmental disorders

Neurodevelopmental disorders vary enormously in their neuropathological severity. At one extreme are the gross cerebral malformations of holoprosencephaly and lissencephaly; in the middle are readily demonstrable but clinically much less apparent states such as agenesis of the corpus callosum, and, at the other extreme, mild abnormalities such as cortical dysplasia, neuronal heterotopias, and Rett's syndrome. Clearly the more severe abnormalities bear little resemblance to schizophrenia and are generally associated with severe mental and motor retardation. However, the milder forms of developmental malformation are worth examining and comparing with schizophrenia.

Cortical dysplasia and cerebrocortical microdysgenesis

Cortical dysplasia and cortical microdysgenesis are increasingly recognised to be a cause of primary epilepsy. Cortical microdysgenesis may also be found in neurologically normal subjects (Kaufman and Galaburda, 1989) and in some people with developmental dyslexia (Galaburda *et al.*, 1985; see Chapter 6). In cortical dysplasia the only macroscopic abnormality is a focal blurring of the margin between cortical grey and white matter. Microscopically the cortex shows disordered lamination with some large, abnormally shaped neurons scattered within it. Abnormal neurons are also found in subcortical white matter wherein there may be enlarged astrocytes with pleomorphic nuclei. Some cells express both neuronal and glial cell markers (Vinters *et al.*, 1992; Vital *et al.*, 1994), and there appears to be a reduction in the number of GABAergic interneurons immunoreactive for parvalbumin and calbindin (Ferrer *et al.*, 1992; Chapter 10). Cortical microdysgenesis is a similar but milder condition without macroscopic abnormalities in which the significant features are disordered lamination with blurring of the demarcation between layers 1 and 2 and more neurons in layer 1, but preserved normal appearances of individual neurons and glia. Some authors include small grey matter heterotopias, increased neuronal satellitosis, and small aggregates of glial cells as features (Armstrong, 1993). Increased numbers of white matter neurons have also been described (Meencke and Janz, 1984).

Cortical dysplasia and microdysgenesis are considered to result from genetically influenced neocortical maldevelopment occurring during fetal life (Walsh, 1999). Similarities to the changes found in schizophrenia include the presence of increased numbers of neurons in white matter, parallelling the excess number of white matter neurons reported in schizophrenia (Akbarian *et al.*, 1993, 1996). Likewise, a reduction in presumed cortical GABAergic interneurons has been described in schizophrenia (Benes *et al.*, 1991; Chapter 3) as well as in cortical microdysgenesis. Another feature that these conditions have in common is an absence of reactive gliosis; however, cortical microdysgenesis differs from schizophrenia in having more cells in layer 1 than are normally found.

These mild cortical maldevelopmental lesions are usually static. However, in some patients they are associated with the local development of relatively indolent tumours (dysembryoplastic neuroepithelial tumours). They also, of course, give rise to abnormally excitable cortex whose excessive excitatory activity may, if prolonged, produce secondary changes particularly in the hippocampus, as discussed below. It must be supposed that the presumptive maldevelopmental lesions of schizophrenia also generate abnormal cerebral function (i.e. symptoms), but in contrast to these epileptogenic lesions, this abnormal function in schizophrenia does not apparently spawn any additional structural pathology. A further distinction between these conditions and schizophrenia is that they normally present (with epilepsy) during childhood, whereas the full clinical picture of schizophrenia usually does not develop until early adulthood.

Rett's syndrome

This rare neurodevelopmental condition is an affliction that almost exclusively affects girls (reviewed in Naidu, 1997). It presents with developmental delay in the first year of life after apparently normal development in the first few months. Prenatal and perinatal brain growth are normal but there is a failure to maintain brain growth thereafter, and by 3 years of age there is severe mental retardation with loss of acquired hand use and speech, gait apraxia, seizures, and respiratory disturbances. The deterioration stabilises later in child-hood and 70 per cent survive into adulthood. MRI studies show significantly decreased cortical and caudate volume (Subramaniam *et al.*, 1997), in keeping with the 12 to 34 per cent reduced brain weight (Jellinger *et al.*, 1988). The histological data are limited but of interest. There are no gross neuronal deficiencies or migrational defects, but the size of neurons in cortex and subcortical structures is reduced and there is an increase in cell packing density (Bauman *et al.*, 1995). There is no obvious gliosis (Jellinger *et al.*, 1998). Golgi studies show reduced numbers of dendritic spines on cortical neurons (Belichenko *et al.*, 1997) and shortening of dendritic processes (Armstrong *et al.*, 1995), accompanied by reduced expression of microtubule associated protein 2 (Kaufmann *et al.*, 1995). In many respects these features bear some resemblance to those reported in schizophrenia (Chapters 2 to 4).

Autism

Autism is a syndrome apparent within the first 3 years of life, affecting language and social development, usually associated with mental retardation. It is largely genetic in origin and 80 per cent of cases are male. Like schizophrenia, some cases occur in the context of other disorders, including fragile X syndrome, metabolic diseases, and tuberous sclerosis.

The brain in autism is of normal or increased weight (Bailey *et al.*, 1998; Kemper and Bauman, 1998; Courchesne *et al.*, 1999), although the cerebellum, brainstem, hippocampal formation, and corpus callosum may all be smaller (Egaas *et al.*, 1995; Courchesne, 1997). Driven in part by these observations, histopathological studies of autism have focused on the medial temporal lobe and the cerebellum and its associated brainstem nuclei. There are two major contemporary studies to mention. Kemper and Bauman (1998) studied nine brains. The main abnormalities, present in most or all cases, were: smaller and more closely packed hippocampal and cortical neurons; reduced dendritic extent of hippocampal neurons seen with the Golgi technique (only done in two brains); a decreased number of Purkinje cells; and preserved or enlarged inferior olivary neurons. Gliosis was not a feature. Bailey *et al.* (1998) examined six cases (aged from 4 to 24 years). They also noted a marked loss of Purkinje cells. In some cases, the olivary nuclei were dysplastic with neuronal ectopias, and four individuals showed increased neuronal density or other cytoarchitectural abnor-malities in the neocortex. However, generally their findings were less striking than Kemper and Bauman (1998); they did not replicate the hippocampal alterations, but did find some variable and patchy gliosis. Clearly these hippocampal and cortical observations in autism have similarities to the changes described in schizophrenia (e.g. Zaidel *et al.*, 1997*a,b*; Chapters 2 to 4) and, given the early onset of autism, give credence to their putative developmental origin in schizophrenia (Chapter 8). Whilst the cerebellar changes have less obvious parallels, there is increasing evidence for structural and functional cerebellar involvement in schizophrenia (Andreasen *et al.*, 1996; Katsetos *et al.*, 1997; Tran *et al.*, 1998). Conversely, it is undoubtedly premature to argue that there are fundamental similarities in the neuropathology of the two disorders. Indeed, the different effects of autism and schizophrenia on brain size suggests an important distinction in either the nature or timing of the disease processes. Similarly, whilst abnormalities of dopaminergic and serotonergic activity occur in autism (Ciaranello and Ciaranello, 1995; Ernst *et al.*, 1997; Chugani *et al.*, 1999), as in schizophrenia (see Harrison, 1999), the neurochemical pathology of the two disorders cannot meaningfully be compared or contrasted.

Down's syndrome

Aside from the well-researched tendency for the Down's syndrome brain to be subject to excessive β/A4 amyloid deposition and premature development of Alzheimer's disease pathology, there are several abnormalities of the brain in Down's syndrome that are recognisable from birth (Harding and Copp, 1997). Brain weight is reduced and the brain has an abnormal shape, with a particularly steep slope to the occipital lobes and often poor development of the superior temporal gyrus. The gyral pattern may be somewhat simplified, and the brainstem and cerebellum smaller than normal. There are also non-specific microscopic abnormalities, with some irregularity in positioning of cortical neurons, but a tendency to an increased packing density and a deficiency overall in neuron numbers, particularly in the granular layers of the cortex (Ross *et al.*, 1984). Development of cortical lamination is delayed and disorganised (Golden and Hyman, 1994). As in some of the other conditions discussed here, there is a reduced dendritic arborisation and decreased numbers of dendritic spines in neonatal and infantile Down's syndrome cortical neurons (Takashima *et al.*, 1981).

In summary, these unequivocally neurodevelopmental disorders show interesting neuropathological similarities to schizophrenia, particularly with respect to the somewhat non-specific features of reduced overall brain size, increased neuronal cell packing density, reduced neuron size and dendritic arborisation, and absence of gliosis. The subdivisions of the brain that are affected overlap with, but also differ from, those affected in schizophrenia, as one might expect given their differing clinical features. In general, the similarities lend support to the view that schizophrenia is a neurodevelopmental disorder, though they clearly do not prove it.

Disorders in which schizophrenia-like symptoms may occur

Schizophrenia-like psychoses occur in many 'organic' disorders (Davison and Bagley, 1969). Consideration of the putative neuropathological explanation of the psychosis in these conditions may shed light on the neuropathology of schizophrenia in general.

Metabolic diseases

A number of metabolic diseases can be accompanied by, or even present with, a schizophrenia-like psychosis (Coker *et al.*, 1991; Hyde *et al.*, 1992). The best characterised is metachromatic leucodystrophy, but others include Kuf's disease (adult neuronal lipofuscinosis), Tay–Sach disease, Gaucher's disease, Fabry's disease, and adrenoleucodystrophy. The pathology of these diseases is quite varied, some affecting white matter predominantly, others grey matter, and some both (Lake, 1997). No pathological feature is known which separates cases with and without psychosis; rather, the psychotic features tend to develop when onset of symptoms is delayed until adolescence or early adulthood. In a review of 129 cases of metachromatic leucodystrophy, 53 per cent of cases presenting between the ages of 10 and 30 years had psychotic symptoms (Hyde *et al.*, 1992), whereas such symptoms were rare otherwise. Frequently psychotic symptoms are the first to appear and they may precede neurological deterioration by many years, waning as the disease progresses.

In considering the possible reasons for the development of psychotic features in metabolic disease, most attention has been focused on the damage to white matter, with the suggestion that this may lead to interruption in cerebral connectivity (Hyde *et al.*, 1992). Demyelination in these conditions frequently affects the frontal lobes and corpus callosum early on. In contrast, it is usual for the immediately subcortical fibres in affected lobes to be spared. The fact that psychotic features fade as the neurological disorder and neuropathological damage become more severe suggests that manifestation of psychotic symptoms requires a relatively intact brain. It is noteworthy that another long-lasting neurological disease characterised by demyelination—multiple sclerosis (MS)—is not associated with an increased risk of psychosis (Lishman, 1998). However, the character of the lesions in MS is very different from that of the leucodystrophies, the lesions being small, multiple, and often periventricular in MS, instead of widespread and diffuse as in leucodystrophies. The interruption in axonal connectivity in leucodystrophies is probably due not only to interference with conduction resulting from demyelination, but also from progressive and eventually quite substantial axonal loss as well. This axonal loss is likely to affect fibres in the corpus callosum, of interest since altered callosal fibre numbers have also been described in schizophrenia (Highley *et al.*, 1999). (See also Benes *et al.*, 1994 for discussion of myelination and its relevance for schizophrenia.)

Another neuropathological feature of possible significance in the leucodystrophies for the development of psychosis is the regenerative effort apparent in the oligodendrocyte population. These cells express increased amounts of myelin synthetic enzymes, even though, in long-standing cases, the number of oligodendrocytes is decreased (Morris *et al.*, 1994). This is particularly noticeable in deep cortex and the preserved subcortical white matter. It raises the speculative possibility that growth factors may be released to sustain this regenerative effort, a response which has secondary effects, perhaps on cortical neuronal plasticity (McAllister *et al.*, 1999), that may favour the development of psychosis.

Epilepsy

Schizophrenia-like psychosis occurs in subjects with epilepsy more frequently than would be expected by chance, with estimates in epidemiological studies ranging from 2 to 10 per cent (Sachdev, 1998). The psychosis usually begins several years after onset of seizures, and appears particularly common in temporal lobe epilepsy (also called complex partial epilepsy or psychomotor epilepsy; Slater and Beard, 1963; Mendez *et al.*, 1993; Umbricht *et al.*, 1995; Kanemoto *et al.*, 1996).

The pathology of temporal lobe epilepsy is complex and variable. In 50 to 60 per cent of cases there is a loss of hippocampal neurons and gliosis on the side of the focus; pyramidal neurons in CA1 are most vulnerable, followed by those in CA3 and CA4, with neurons in CA2 and dentate gyrus granule cells least affected (see Fig. 2.1 in Chapter 2). This pathological appearance is called mesial temporal sclerosis. Its pathogenesis remains controversial. Though clearly associated with prolonged seizures in early childhood, it is still unclear whether seizures are a cause or a consequence of the pathology (Mathern *et al.*, 1995; Swanson, 1995; Meldrum, 1997). Both processes may occur, with the initial seizures causing excitotoxic damage (perhaps in a hippocampus predisposed by a pre-existing, silent developmental malformation; Sloviter and Pedley, 1998). The excitotoxic process then provokes local secondary changes including sprouting of mossy fibres and alteration in the balance of excitatory and inhibitory influences on remaining hippocampal pyramidal neurons, rendering them hyperexcitable, setting the scene for repeated epileptic discharges.

Various neuropathological correlates of schizophrenia-like psychosis in temporal lobe epilepsy have been described. For example, the co-occurrence has been reported to be commoner when the lesion is pre- or perinatal in origin, such as a hamartoma (Roberts *et al.*, 1990). Conversely, Kanemoto *et al.* (1996) found an association with childhood febrile convulsions and mesial temporal sclerosis; others report a higher frequency of psychosis in cases with any focal lesion (e.g. cortical dysplasia, tumours) compared to those without (Taylor, 1975; Suckling *et al.*, submitted). Although schizophrenia has been linked with left-sided rather than right-sided foci (Flor-Henry, 1969; see Chapter 6) this association has not been consistently borne out (Sachdev, 1998). From a somewhat different perspective, Bruton *et al.* (1994) compared subjects who had epilepsy and psychosis, with subjects who had epilepsy but no psychosis. The former group were distinguished by larger ventricles, excess periventricular gliosis, more focal cerebral damage, and perivascular white matter softening.

It is clear from these differing reports that the pathological basis of psychosis in epilepsy is unknown, which is not surprising given the unresolved issues about the pathology of temporal lobe epilepsy itself. One fruitful avenue may be to search for the trigger to psychosis in the sequence of changes that follow the development of mesial temporal sclerosis, since seizures usually precede psychosis by several years (Slater and Beard, 1963; Sachdev, 1998), and psychosis is commoner if there is poor seizure control (Mendez *et al.*, 1993; Kanemoto *et al.*, 1996). Such associations suggest that recurrent seizures, and the pathological process(es) underlying them, promote the psychosis, perhaps via a process analagous to kindling (Wasterlain and Shirasaka, 1994).

Psychosis in neurodegenerative disorders

Huntington's disease is an autosomal dominant neurodegenerative disease producing dementia and choreiform movement disorders. Neuropathologically it is characterised by massive atrophy of the caudate nucleus and putamen with loss of GABAergic neurons, and accompanied by marked gliosis (Vonsattel and DiFiglia, 1998). In addition there is less conspicuous frontal cortical atrophy with loss of pyramidal neurons (Lowe *et al.*, 1997) and mediodorsal thalamic neurons (Heinsen *et al.*, 1999). The main neurochemical deficit is in GABA production in the basal ganglia, and cortico–striatal connectivity is thought to be reduced. Psychiatric features including psychosis are common; the psychosis is usually affective but sometimes schizophrenia-like (Hyde *et al.*, 1992; Lishman, 1998). Frontal cerebral glucose metabolism is lower in patients with psychosis than in those without (Kuwert *et al.*, 1989), but otherwise the neurochemical and neuropathological correlates of psychosis in Huntington's disease are unknown.

There is also an increased prevalence of psychosis in other dementias such as Alzheimer's disease, Pick's disease, and Lewy body dementia (Lishman, 1998). The psychosis is clinically less similar to schizophrenia than that occurring in the metabolic disorders or epilepsy; paranoid delusions are prominent, and hallucinations, when they occur, are more commonly visual than auditory, being particularly associated with Lewy body dementia. In general, the non-cognitive changes in degenerative disorders correlate with, and are probably attributable to, changes in nuclei that project to the cortex such as the raphe nuclei (serotonergic) and locus coeruleus (noradrenergic), or to pre- and postsynaptic alterations in cortical markers of these neurotransmitter systems (Esiri, 1996). Because they affect the elderly and are common, neurodegenerative disorders lend themselves readily to postmortem study, facilitating neurochemical and neuropathological analyses of their accompanying psychoses which may shed light on processes involved in schizophrenia itself.

In summary, epilepsy, metabolic diseases, and neurodegenerative disorders are all associated with an increased frequency of schizophrenia-like psychoses. They have little in common to provide clues as to the neuropathology of schizophrenia, except perhaps to demonstrate that clinically similar psychoses can arise from many distinct neuropathological processes. Though diverse, it is also striking that these diseases share the feature of damage to axonal connections, reinforcing the view that schizophrenia may also involve a disruption of brain connectivity. Moreover, the disorders described in this section are all conditions in which there are progressive neuropathological changes, and where the occurrence of psychotic symptoms characteristically varies with time (e.g. in the metabolic diseases symptoms tend to occur early and disappear later, while in epilepsy the onset of psychosis is delayed). These considerations may therefore be relevant to the question of static versus evolving brain abnormalities in schizophrenia.

Normal determinants of neuronal parameters and the effects of experimental lesions

Many of the changes described in schizophrenia are subtle changes in neuronal size, shape, or distribution (Chapters 2 and 3) and alterations in their processes—dendrites, axons, and synapses (Chapter 4). The extent to which these reflect morphological correlates of functionally important alterations depends upon understanding the factors which govern such parameters in the normal brain. In one respect this is equivalent to the need to understand normal cortical circuitry (Chapter 10) and its origins (Chapter 9) before putative abnormalities in neural connectivity in schizophrenia are discussed (Chapters 7 and 8).

It is a general principle that the size of a neuronal cell body (also called its soma or, less correctly, its perikaryon) is determined by '[1] the number, length and diameter of its processes, and [2] the number of synapses that it receives on its surface' (Jones and Cowan, 1983). The idea that the growth and size of nerve cells are 'influenced by the connexions that they make at both their transmitting and receiving ends' (Young, 1951) has been termed 'double dependence' (Young, 1951). Much of the work which gave rise to this doctrine was carried out in the peripheral nervous system; the extent to which it holds true in the central nervous system, particularly in the cerebral cortex, and the relative impact of the two factors (afferent versus efferent connections; dendrites versus axons) on neuronal size and shape merit some consideration.

The concept of shrinkage of neurons in response to loss of connections is well established, whether as retrograde degeneration following transection of the axon of the neuron, or transneuronal degeneration due either to loss of afferents to the cell (anterograde or orthograde transneuronal degeneration), or to degeneration of its target neurons (retrograde transneuronal degeneration; Cowan, 1970). The complementary response, namely increased size of neurons in relation to increases in peripheral target innervation (i.e. axonal volume), is also well documented, at least in the peripheral nervous system (Detwiler, 1933; Cavanagh, 1951; Fernand and Young, 1951; Pannese, 1963; Voyvodic, 1989; Causing *et al.*, 1997; see Young 1951, for review), confirming Levi's view (see Levi, 1916) of the existence of a close correlation between neuronal cell body size and the area of the periphery it supplies. In at least one case, the increased neuronal size in relation to increasing density of target innervation extends to hypertrophy of the cell's dendrites (Voyvodic, 1989). Similarly, there is evidence that motor neurons giving rise to successfully regenerated axons, which innervate larger motor units than is the case in the normal subject, show cellular hypertrophy (Edds, 1949; Bowe *et al.*, 1989).

Within the central nervous system, the size of Betz cells in the human motor cortex is proportional to height, i.e. the length of their axons; similarly, comparative anatomy of the medullary pyramids reveals a correlation between pyramidal axon diameter and Betz cell size (Lassek and Rasmussen, 1940). Direct evidence that increased axonal arborisation is accompanied by hypertrophy of neuronal call somata in the central nervous system is somewhat sparser. However, cases where such evidence of sprouting exists or can be inferred have been reported in a variety of species and sites, including the hippocampal formation (Goldschmidt and Steward, 1980; Fowler and Olton, 1984), cholinergic basal forebrain (Pearson *et al.*, 1984, 1985, 1986*a*, 1987*b*), red nucleus (Prendergast and Stelzner, 1976*a,b*), substantia nigra (Pearson *et al.*, 1986*b*, 1987*a*), globus pallidus (Najlerahim and Pearson, 1992), lateral geniculate nucleus (Headon *et al.*, 1982, 1985*a,b*; Hendrickson and Deneen, 1982), visual cortex (Fukuda and Hsiao, 1984), and the finch song-control nuclei (Bottjer *et al.*, 1986).

In contrast to the occurrence of anterograde transneuronal degeneration, where loss of incoming synapses leads to shrinkage of the postsynaptic neuronal soma, evidence that increased afferent innervation leads to hypertrophy of postsynaptic neuronal cell bodies is not compelling. Indeed, in the human cerebral cortex, loss of considerable numbers of afferent axons following prenatal white matter lesions is accompanied by significant neuronal hypertrophy (Marin-Padilla, 1997). The distinction has to be emphasised between increased afferent innervation in the periphery, where hypertrophy of sensory ganglion cells accompanies increased peripheral innervation density, and increased neuronal cell size following increased numbers of synapses impinging on the cell body and dendrites. The former, for which the evidence is overwhelming, is more properly hypertrophy accompanying axonal sprouting, since the peripheral afferent fibre is essentially the axon (or the greater part of the axon) of the cell undergoing enlargement. Although it is often stated that 'dendritic extent is proportional to the availability of afferent supply' (Coleman and Buell, 1985), instances of increased dendritic extent are most often associated with changes in afferent synaptic activity (e.g. after stimulation, training, or rearing in complex environments) and increase in work-related activity (Jones and Schallert, 1994), rather than demonstrable increases in afferent synaptic density (see Coleman and Buell, 1985). Activity-related neuronal hypertrophy is common in neuroendocrine cells, where 'when peptide manufacturing neurons are stimulated to increase production, they increase in size' (Hatton, 1986). It is also seen in the peripheral nervous system (Edds, 1949; Edström, 1957; Drop and Sodetz, 1971; Gabella, 1984), and odour-specific regional mitral cell hypertrophy following early exposure to specific odours has been described in the olfactory bulb (Panhuber and Laing, 1987). Within the central nervous system, many of the cases of neuronal hypertrophy cited above might be related to increased activation in addition to or instead of axonal sprouting.

In the light of such experimental work, it is probable that the major connectional influence on neuronal cell body size is the volume of the axon which the soma maintains. This is not to doubt that afferent synapses markedly influence other structural features of the neuron, such as dendritic spine number and size (Pierce and Lewin, 1994). It is perhaps reasonable to regard the somatodendritic compartment as a single entity, since they share protein synthetic capacity, whereas the axon is dependent on the cell body for proteins and most other constituents (Jones and Cowan, 1983). When considering neuronal size within the human cerebral cortex, changes in cell size and organisation reflecting changes in connectivity are hence likely to affect primarily pyramidal neurons, since these are overwhelmingly the major (if not only) cortical neuronal type giving rise to long projections (Chapter 10). Furthermore, it is clear that the majority of the volume of a pyramidal neuron is actually contained within the axonal compartment. To take an extreme example, consider a layer V pyramidal neuron in the human primary motor cortex projecting to the sacral spinal cord. Its axon can be considered as a cylinder (ignoring intracortical and intraspinal collateralisation) with a radius of say 5 μm and a length of 1 m, giving a simple axonal volume of 7.5×10^7 μm^3; human frontal cortical pyramidal neurons have around six basal dendrites, and a total basal dendritic length of 3×10^3 μm (Koenderink and Uylings, 1995); assuming a mean dendritic radius of 5 μm and considering the sum of the basal dendrites as a single simple cylinder, this gives a basal dendritic volume of 2.25×10^5 μm^3. Even if the apical dendritic tree doubles this total volume, the dendritic volume will not exceed 5×10^5 μm^3. If the soma is considered as a cone, with a radius of as much as 50 μm and a height of 100 μm, its volume would approximate to 2.5×10^5 μm^3, giving an approximate total somatodendritic volume of 7.5×10^5 μm^3, i.e. only 1 per cent of the estimated axonal volume. For other pyramidal neuron populations in the cerebral cortex the axonal volume will be proportionately less, but even if the axonal volume is reduced or the somatodendritic volume increased by an order of magnitude, the axon would still represent 90 per cent of the total neuronal volume. It is thus likely that relatively small changes in neuronal somal size reflect substantial changes in the axonal arbor which the cell maintains, especially when changes in cell body size are most commonly observed as changes in cross-sectional area, or sometimes cell diameter, rather than changes in volume.

This section has focused on cell body size and its relationship to dendritic and axonal arborisations, as an example of how the origins and significance of alterations in these parameters in schizophrenia (or any other disorder) can be informed by reference to the experimental literature. To finish with a second example, dendritic spine densities are reportedly reduced on cortical pyramidal neurons in schizophrenia (Garey et al., 1998; Glantz and Lewis, 2000), a change interpreted as being suggestive of a neurodevelopmental abnormality in pruning or plasticity. Whilst this may be correct, experimental data show that dendritic spines are dynamic structures, appearing and disappearing over hours or days in response to various influences, as well as being regulated by genetic and longer term environmental factors (Horner, 1993; Engert and Bonhoeffer, 1999; Kirov et al., 1999). Establishing the cause of a loss of dendritic spines in a postmortem study is, therefore, not straightforward.

Suggestions for future studies

Investigation of structural brain changes in schizophrenia needs a period of consolidation with the aim of achieving a greater consensus. There is also a need for better defined hypotheses (see Chapter 9) that can suggest logical approaches to the study of what are likely to be only slight differences from normal. It is indeed the presumed subtlety of these differences that almost certainly contributes to the lack of consensus about what changes there are (Chapter 13). Another is the lack of a biological marker of the disease. One important principle is that stereologically sound methods should be applied for both macroscopic and microscopic studies (Chapter 14), despite the difficulties in this context (e.g. defining boundaries within the cerebral cortex). Another problem when studying schizophrenia is that it is hard to establish brain areas that can be regarded as entirely unaffected, just as it is also hard to define a hierarchy of affected areas that differ in the extent of their abnormality. Symptomatology and functional imaging studies have focused on medial temporal (Chapter 2), prefrontal (Chapter 7), and language areas, but it is difficult to build a coherent model of the disease based on the neurodevelopment of these various cortical areas. One approach might be to compare findings in parts of the cortex according to the developmental time course that they follow. Another factor that has been insufficiently considered is gender, since some recent studies have demonstrated changes that differ between male and female schizophrenics (Highley et al., 1998, 1999). Hemisphere also requires closer attention in this field than is necessary in most neuropathological studies (Chapter 6). Comparative studies that include other disorders will help in distinguishing which features are specifically associated with schizophrenia; e.g. many of the reported alterations in schizophrenia might be non-specific correlates of neurodevelopmental anomalies, or be common to psychoses in general. Finally, all investigations reporting morphometric neuronal and synaptic abnormalities in schizophrenia should take into account the known determinants of these parameters, and further experimental study of how these parameters can be influenced will be of value.

In summary, schizophrenia has tantalising links with other neuropathological conditions. These broadly reinforce the idea that it is developmental in origin. We do not believe that schizophrenia has a specific neuropathology as described at the start of this chapter. Nevertheless we are in no doubt that there is a constellation of anatomical features characteristic of the condition. Systematic studies of the types suggested above should be capable of identifying them.

References

Akbarian S, Bunney WE, Potkin SG, Bunney WE Jr, Jones EG (1993) Altered distribution of nicotinamide-adenine dinucleotide phosphate-diaphorase cells in frontal lobe of schizophrenics implies disturbances of cortical development. *Archives of General Psychiatry* **50**, 169–177.

Akbarian S, Kim J, Potkin SG, Hetrick W, Bunney WE Jr, Jones EG (1996) Maldistribution of interstitial neurons in prefrontal white matter of the brains of schizophrenic patients. *Archives of General Psychiatry* **53**, 425–436.

Andreasen NC, O'Leary DS, Cizadio T *et al.* (1996) Schizophrenia and cognitive dysmetria: A positron emission tomography study of dysfunctional prefronto-thalamic-cerebellar circuitry. *Proceedings of the National Academy of Sciences USA* **93**, 9985–9990.

Armstrong DD (1993) The neuropathology of temporal lobe epilepsy. *Journal of Neuropathology and Experimental Neurology* **52**, 433–443.

Armstrong D, Dunn JK, Antalffy B, Trivedi R (1995) Selective dendritic alteration in the cortex of Rett syndrome. *Journal of Neuropathology and Experimental Neurology* **54**, 195–201.

Arriagada OV, Growdon JH, Hedley-Whyte TE, Hyman BT (1992). Neurofibrillary tangles but not senile plaques parallel duration and severity of Alzheimer's disease. *Neurology* **42**, 631–639.

Bailey A, Luthert P, Dean A *et al.* (1998) A clinicopathological study of autism. *Brain* **121**, 889–905.

Bauman ML, Kemper TL, Arin DM (1995) Pervasive neuroanatomic abnormalities of the brain in three cases of Rett syndrome. *Neurology* **45**, 1581–1586.

Belichenko PV, Hagberg B, Dahlstrom A (1997) Morphological study of neocortical areas in Rett syndrome. *Acta Neuropathologica* **93**, 50–61.

Benes FM, McSparren J, Bird ED, SanGiovanni JP, Vincent SL (1991) Deficits in small interneurons in prefrontal and cingulate cortices of schizophrenic and schizoaffective sufferers. *Archives of General Psychiatry* **48**, 996–1001.

Benes FM, Turtle M, Khan Y, Farol P (1994) Myelination of a key relay zone in the hippocampal formation occurs in the human brain during childhood, adolescence and adulthood. *Archives of General Psychiatry* **51**, 477–484.

Bottjer SW, Miesner EA, Arnold AP (1986) Changes in neuronal number, density and size account for increases in volume of song-control nuclei during song development in zebra finches. *Neuroscience Letters* **67**, 263–268.

Bowe CM, Hildebrand C, Kocsis JD, Waxman SG (1989). Morphological and physiological properties of neurons after long-term axonal regeneration: observations on chronic and delayed sequelae of peripheral nerve injury. *Journal of the Neurological Sciences* **91**, 259–292

Bruton CJ, Stevens JR, Frith CD (1994) Epilepsy, psychosis, and schizophrenia. Clinical and neuropathologic correlations. *Neurology* **44**, 34–42.

Causing CG, Gloster A, Aloyz R *et al.* (1997). Synaptic innervation density is regulated by neuron-derived BDNF. *Neuron* **18**, 257–267.

Cavanagh MW (1951) Quantitative effects of the peripheral innervation area on nerves and spinal ganglion cells. *Journal of Comparative Neurology* **94**, 181–219.

Chugani DC, Muzik O, Behen M *et al.* (1999) Developmental changes in brain serotonin synthesis capacity in autistic and non-autistic children. *Annals of Neurology* **45**, 287–295.

Ciaranello AL, Ciaranello RD (1995) The neurobiology of infantile autism. *Annual Review of Neuroscience* **18**, 101–128.

Coker SB (1991). The diagnosis of childhood neurodegenerative disorders presenting as dementia in adults. *Neurology* **41**, 794–798.

Coleman PD, Buell SJ (1985). Regulation of dendritic extent in developing and aging brain. In: Cotman CW, Ed. *Synaptic plasticity*. Guildford Press, New York, pp. 311–333.

Courchesne E (1997) Brain stem, cerebellar and limbic neuroanatomical abnormalities in autism. *Current Opinion in Neurobiology* **7**, 269–278.

Courchesne E, Muller RA, Saitoh O (1999) Brain weight in autism: Normal in the majority of cases, megancephalic in rare cases. *Neurology* **52**, 1057–1059.

Cowan WM (1970) Anterograde and retrograde transneuronal degeneration in the central and peripheral nervous system. In: Nauta WJH, Ebbesson SOE, Eds. *Contemporary research methods in neuroanatomy*. Springer-Verlag, Berlin, pp. 217–249.

Davison K, Bagley CR (1969). Schizophrenia-like psychosis associated with organic disorder of the central nervous system: a review of the literature. *British Journal of Psychiatry* **113** (Suppl.), 18–69.

Detwiler SR (1933). Experimental studies upon the development of the amphibian nervous system. *Biological Review* **8**, 269–310.

Drop JJ, Sodetz FJ (1971). Autoradiographic study of neurons and neuroglia in autonomic ganglia of behaviourally stressed rats. *Brain Research* **33**, 419–430.

Edds MV (1949). Experiments on partially deneurotized nerves. II. Hypertrophy of residual fibres. *Journal of Experimental Zoology* **112**, 29–47.

Edström J-E (1957). Effects of increased motor activity on the dimensions and the staining properties of the neuron soma. *Journal of Comparative Neurology* **107**, 295–304.

Egaas B, Courchesne E, Saitoh O (1995) Reduced size of corpus callosum in autism. *Archives of Neurology* **52**, 794–801.

Engert F, Bonhoeffer T (1999) Dendritic spine changes associated with hippocampal long-term synaptic plasticity. *Nature* **399**, 66–70.

Ernst M, Zametkin AJ, Matochik JA, Pascualvaca D, Cohen RM (1997). Low medial prefrontal dopaminergic activity in autistic children. *Lancet* **350**, 638.

Esiri MM (1996) The basis for behavioural disturbances in dementia. *Journal of Neurology, Neurosurgery and Psychiatry* **61**, 127–130.

Fernand VSV, Young JZ (1951). The sizes of the nerve fibres of muscle nerves. *Proceedings of the Royal Society (London) B* **139**, 38–58.

Ferrer I, Pineda M, Tallada M, Oliver B, Russi A, Oller L (1992) Abnormal local-circuit neurons in epilepsia partialis continua associated with focal cortical dysplasia. *Acta Neuropathologica* **83**, 647–652.

Flor-Henry P (1969). Psychosis and temporal lobe epilepsy: a controlled investigation. *Epilepsia* **10**, 363–395.

Fowler K, Olton DS (1984). Recovery of function following injections of kainic acid: behavioural electrophysiological and neuroanatomical correlates. *Brain Research* **321**, 21–32.

Fukuda Y, Hsiao C-F (1984). Bilateral changes in soma size of geniculate relay cells and corticogeniculate cells after neonatal monocular enucleation in rats. *Brain Research* **301**, 13–23.

Gabella G (1984) Sizes of neurons and glial cells in the intramural ganglia of the hypertrophic intestine of the guinea-pig. *Journal of Neurocytology* **13**, 73–84.

Galaburda AM, Sherman GF, Rosen GD, Aboitiz F, Geschwind N (1985) Developmental dyslexia: four consecutive patients with cortical anomalies. *Annals of Neurology* **18**, 222–233.

Garey LJ, Ong WY, Patel TS *et al.* (1998) Reduced dendritic spine density on cerebral cortical pyramidal neurons in schizophrenia. *Journal of Neurology, Neurosurgery and Psychiatry* **65**, 446–453.

Glantz L, Lewis DA (2000) Decreased dendritic spine density on prefrontal cortical pyramidal neurons in schizophrenia. *Archives of General Psychiatry* **57**, 65–73.

Golden JA, Hyman BT (1994) Development of the superior temporal neocortex is anomalous in trisomy 21. *Journal of Neuropathology and Experimental Neurology* **53**, 513–520.

Goldman-Rakic PS (1994). Working memory dysfunction in schizophrenia. *Journal of Neuropsychiatry and Clinical Neuroscience* **6**, 348–357.

Goldschmidt RB, Steward, O (1980). Time course of increase in retrograde labeling and increases in cell size of entorhinal cortex neurons sprouting in response to unilateral entorhinal lesions. *Journal of Comparative Neurology* **189**, 359–379.

Grabowski TJ, Damasio AR (1997). Definition, clinical features and neuroanatomical basis of dementia. In: Esiri MM, Morris JH, Eds. *The neuropathology of dementia*. Cambridge University Press, Cambridge, pp. 1–20.

Harding BH, Copp AJ (1997) Malformations. In: Graham DI, Lantos PL, Eds. *Greenfield's neuropathology*, 6th Edition, Volume 1. Edward Arnold, London, pp. 397–536.

Harrison PJ (1999) Neurochemical alterations in schizophrenia affecting the putative receptor targets of atypical antipsychotics. *British Journal of Psychiatry*, **174** (Suppl. 38), 12–22.

Hatton GI (1986) Plasticity in the hypothalamic magnocellular neurosecretory system. *Federation Proceedings* **45**, 2328–2333.

Headon MP, Sloper JJ, Powell TPS (1982) Initial hypertrophy of cells in undeprived laminae of the lateral geniculate nucleus of the monkey following early monocular visual deprivation. *Brain Research* **238**, 439–444.

Headon MP, Sloper JJ, Hiorns RW, Powell TPS (1985*a*) Effect of reopening an eye after a period of monocular deprivation on sizes of neurons in the primate lateral geniculate nucleus. *Brain Research* **318**, 79–83.

Headon MP, Sloper JJ, Hiorns R, Powell TPS (1985*b*) Effects of monocular closure at different ages on deprived and undeprived cells in the primate lateral geniculate nucleus. *Developmental Brain Research* **18**, 57–78.

Heinsen H, Rub U, Bauer M *et al.* (1999) Nerve cell loss in the thalamic mediodorsal nucleus in Huntington's disease. *Acta Neuropathologica* **97**, 613–622.

Hendrickson A, Deneen JT (1982). Hypertrophy of neurons in dorsal lateral geniculate nucleus following striate cortex lesions in infant monkeys. *Neuroscience Letters* **30**, 217–222.

Highley JR, Esiri MM, McDonald B *et al.* (1998) Anomalies of cerebral asymmetry in schizophrenia interact with gender and age of onset: a postmortem study. *Schizophrenia Research* **34**, 13–25.

Highley JR, Esiri MM, McDonald B *et al.* (1999) The size and fibre composition of the corpus callosum with respect to gender and schizophrenia: a post mortem study. *Brain* **122**, 99–110.

Horner CH (1993) Plasticity of the dendritic spine. *Progress in Neurobiology* **41**, 281–321.

Hyde TM, Ziegler JC, Weinberger DR (1992) Psychiatric disturbances in metachromatic leukodystrophy: insights into the neurobiology of psychosis. *Archives of Neurology* **49**, 401–406.

Jellinger K, Armstrong D, Zoghbi H, Percy A (1988) Neuropathology of Rett syndrome. *Acta Neuropathologica* **76**, 142–158.

Jones EG, Cowan W (1983) Nervous tissue. In: Jones EG, Ed. *The structural basis of neurobiology*, Elsevier, New York.

Jones TA, Schallert T (1994) Use-dependent growth of pyramidal neurons after neocortical damage. *Journal of Neuroscience* **14**, 2140–2152.

Kanemoto K, Takeuchi J, Kawasaki J, Kawai I (1996). Characteristics of temporal lobe epilepsy with mesial temporal sclerosis, with special reference to psychotic episodes. *Neurology* **47**, 1199–1203.

Katsetos CD, Hyde TM, Herman MM (1997) Neuropathology of the cerebellum in schizophrenia—an update 1996 and future directions. *Biological Psychiatry* **42**, 213–224.

Kaufmann WE, Galaburda AM (1989) Cerebrocortical microdysgenesis in neurologically normal subjects: a histopathological study. *Neurology* **39**, 238–244.

Kaufmann WE, Hohmann CF, Israel JJ (1995) Microtubule-associated protein 2 is abnormally expressed in the neocortex of Rett syndrome subjects and in a related animal model. *Annals of Neurology* **38**, 500.

Kemper TL, Bauman M (1998) Neuropathology of infantile autism. *Journal of Neuropathology and Experimental Neurology,* **57**, 645–652.

Kirov SA, Sorra KE, Harris KM (1999) Slices have more synapses than perfusion-fixed hippocampus from both young and mature rats. *Journal of Neuroscience* **19**, 2876–2886.

Koenderink MJT, Uylings HBM (1995) Postnatal maturation of layer V pyramidal neurons in the human prefrontal cortex. A quantitative Golgi analysis. *Brain Research* **678**, 233–243.

Kuwert T, Lange H, Langen K, Herzog H, Aulich A, Feinendegen L (1989) Cerebral glucose consumption measured by PET in patients with and without psychiatric symptoms of Huntington's disease. *Psychiatry Research* **29**, 361–362.

Lake BD (1997) Lyosomal and peroxisomal disorders. In: Graham DI, Lantos PL, Eds. *Greenfield's neuropathology*, 6th Edition, Volume 1. Edward Arnold, London, pp. 658–754.

Lassek AM, Rasmussen GL (1940). A comparative fiber and numerical analysis of the pyramidal tract. *Journal of Comparative Neurology* **72**, 417–428.

Levi G (1916) I fattori che determinano il volume degli elementi nervosi. *Riv pat Nerv Ment* **21**, 625–633.

Lishman WA (1998) *Organic psychiatry*, 3rd edition. Blackwell Science, Oxford.

Lowe J, Lennox G, Leigh PN (1997) Disorders of movement and system degenerations. In: Graham DI, Lantos PL, Eds. *Greenfield's neuropathology*, 6th Edition, Volume 2. Edward Arnold, London, pp. 281–366.

McAllister A, Katz LC, Lo D (1999) Neurotrophins and synaptic plasticity. *Annual Review of Neuroscience* **22**, 295–318.

Marin-Padilla M (1997) Developmental neuropathology and impact of perinatal brain damage. II: White matter lesions of the neocortex. *Journal of Neuropathology and Experimental Neurology* **56**, 219–235.

Mathern GW, Babb TL, Vickery BG, Melendez M, Pretorius JK (1995) The clinical-pathogenic mechanisms of hippocampal neuron loss and surgical outcomes in temporal lobe epilepsy. *Brain* **118**, 105–118.

Meencke HJ, Janz D (1984) Neuropathological findings in primary generalised epilepsy: a study of eight cases. *Epilepsia* **25**, 8–21.

Meldrum BS (1997) Epileptic brain damage: a consequence and a cause of seizures. *Neuropathology and Applied Neurobiology* **23**, 185–202.

Mendez MF, Grau R, Doss RC, Taylor JL (1993) Schizophrenia in epilepsy: seizure and psychosis variables. *Neurology* **43**, 1073–1077.

Morris CS, Esiri MM, Sprinkle TJ, Gregson N (1994). Oligodendrocyte reactions and cell proliferation markers in human demyelinating diseases. *Neuropathology and Applied Neurobiology* **20**, 272–281.

Nagy Zs, Esiri MM, Jobst KA *et al.* (1995) Relative roles of plaques and tangles in the dementia of Alzheimer's disease: correlations using three sets of neuropathological criteria. *Dementia* **6**, 21–31.

Nagy Zs, Jobst KA, Esiri MM *et al.* (1996). Hippocampal pathology reflects memory deficit and brain imaging measurements in Alzheimer's disease: clinicopathologic correlations using three sets of pathologic diagnostic criteria. *Dementia* **7**, 76–81.

Naidu S (1997). Rett syndrome: a disorder affecting early brain growth. *Annals of Neurology* **42**, 3–10.

Najlerahim A, Pearson RCA (1992). Changes in glutamic acid decarboxylase mRNA in the pallidum of the rat following unilateral damage of the striatum. *Experimental Neurology* **118**, 352–356.

Panhuber H, Laing DG (1987). The size of mitral cells is altered when rats are exposed to an odor from their day of birth. *Developmental Brain Research* **34**, 133–140.

Pannese E (1963). Investigations on the ultrastructural changes of the spinal ganglion neurons in the course of axon regeneration and cell hypertrophy. II. Changes during cell hypertrophy and comparison between the ultrastructure of nerve cells of the same type under different functional conditions. *Zeitschrift fur Zellforschung Mikroskopische Anatomie* **61**, 561–586.

Pearson RCA, Powell TPS (1989). The neuroanatomy of Alzheimer's disease. *Reviews in the Neurosciences* **2**, 101–121.

Pearson RCA, Sofroniew MV, Powell TPS (1984) Hypertrophy of immunohistochemically identified cholinergic neurons of the basal nucleus of Meynert following ablation of the contralateral cortex in the rat. *Brain Research* **311**, 194–198.

Pearson RCA, Sofroniew MV, Powell TPS (1985) Hypertrophy of cholinergic neurons of the rat basal nucleus following section of the corpus callosum. *Brain Research* **338**, 337–340.

Pearson RCA, Neal JW, Powell TPS (1986*a*) Hypertrophy of the cholinergic neurons in the basal nucleus of the rat following damage of the contralateral nucleus. *Brain Research* **382**, 149–152.

Pearson RCA, Neal JW, Powell TPS (1986*b*) Bilateral morphological changes in the substantia nigra of the rat following unilateral damage of the striatum. *Brain Research* **400**, 127–132.

Pearson RCA, Neal JW, Powell TPS (1987*a*) Increase in immunohistochemical staining of GABAergic axons in the superior colliculus and thalamus of the rat following damage of the ipsilateral striatum and frontal cortex. *Brain Research* **412**, 352–356.

Pearson RCA, Sofroniew MV, Powell TPS (1987*b*) The cholinergic nuclei of the basal forebrain of the rat: hypertrophy following contralateral cortical damage or section of the corpus callosum. *Brain Research* **411**, 332–340.

Pierce JP, Lewin GR (1994) An ultrastructural size principle. *Neuroscience* **58**, 441–446.

Prendergast J, Stelzner DJ (1976*a*) Increases in collateral axon growth rostral to a thoracic hemisection in neonatal and weanling rats. *Journal of Comparative Neurology* **166**, 145–162.

Prendergast J, Stelzner DJ (1976*b*) Changes in the magnocellular portion of the red nucleus following thoracic hemisection in the neonatal and adult rat. *Journal of Comparative Neurology* **166**, 163–172.

Rajkowska G, Selemon L, Goldman-Rakic PS (1998) Neuronal and glial somal size in the prefrontal cortex: a post mortem morphometric study of schizophrenia and Huntington disease. *Archives of General Psychiatry* **55**, 215–224.

Roberts GW, Done DJ, Bruton C, Crow TJ (1990) A 'mock-up' of schizophrenia: temporal lobe epilepsy and schizophrenia-like psychosis. *Biological Psychiatry*, **28**, 127–143.

Ross MH, Galaburda AM, Kemper TL (1984) Down's syndrome: is there a decreased population of neurons? *Neurology* **34**, 909–916.

Sachdev P (1998) Schizophrenia-like psychosis and epilepsy: The status of the association. *American Journal of Psychiatry* **155**, 325–336.

Selemon LD, Rajkowska G, Goldman-Rakic PS (1995) Abnormally high neuronal density in the schizophrenic cortex. A morphometric analysis of prefrontal area 9 and occipital area 17. *Archives of General Psychiatry* **52**, 805–818.

Slater E, Beard A (1963) The schizophrenia-like psychoses of epilepsy. *British Journal of Psychiatry* **109**, 95–150.

Sloviter RS, Pedley TA (1998) Subtle hippocampal malformation. Importance in febrile seizures and development of epilepsy. *Neurology* **50**, 840–849.

Subramaniam B, Naidu S, Reiss AL (1997) Neuroanatomy in Rett syndrome: Cerebral cortex and posterior fossa. *Neurology* **48**, 399–407.

Suckling J, Roberts H, Walker M, Esiri MM (2000) Temporal lobe epilepsy with and without psychosis: exploration of hippocampal pathology including that in subpopulations of neurons defined by the content of immunoreactive calcium binding proteins. *Acta Neuropathologica* (in press).

Swanson TH (1995) The pathophysiology of human mesial temporal lobe epilepsy. *Journal of Clinical Neurophysiology* **12**, 2–22.

Takashima S, Becker LE, Armstrong DL, Chan F (1981) Abnormal neuronal development in the visual cortex of the human retina and infant with Down's syndrome: a quantitative and qualitative Golgi study. *Brain Research* **225**, 1–21.

Taylor DC (1975) Factors influencing the occurrence of schizophrenia-like psychosis in patients with temporal lobe epilepsy. *Psychological Medicine* **5**, 249–254.

Tran KD, Smutzer GS, Doty RL, Arnold SE (1998) Reduced Purkinje cell size in the cerebellar vermis of elderly patients with schizophrenia. *American Journal of Psychiatry* **155**, 1288–1290.

Umbricht D, Degreef G, Barr WB, Lieberman JA, Pollack S, Schaul N (1995) Postictal and chronic psychoses in patients with temporal lobe epilepsy. *American Journal of Psychiatry* **152**, 224–231.

Vinters H, Fisher RS, Cornford ME, Mah V, Secor DL, De-Rosa MJ (1992) Morphological substrates of infantile spasms: studies based on surgically resected cerebral tissue. *Childhood Nervous System* **8**, 8–17.

Vital A, Marchal C, Loiseau H, Rougier A, Pedespan JM, Rivel J (1994) Glial and neuroglial malformative lesions associated with medically intractable epilepsy. *Acta Neuropathologica* **87**, 196–201.

Vonsattel JPG, DiFiglia M (1998) Huntington disease. *Journal of Neuropathology and Experimental Neurology* **57**, 369–384.

Voyvodic JT (1989) Peripheral target regulation of dendritic geometry in the rat superior cervical ganglion. *Journal of Neuroscience* 9, 1997–2010.

Walsh CA (1999) Genetic malformations of the human cerebral cortex. *Neuron* **23**, 19–29.

Wasterlain C, Shirasaka Y (1994) Seizures, brain damage and brain development. *Brain and Development* **16**, 279–295.

Wilcock GK, Esiri MM (1982) Plaques, tangles and dementia: a quantitative study. *Journal of the Neurological Sciences* **56**, 343–356.

Young JZ (1951) Growth and plasticity in the nervous system. *Proceedings of the Royal Society (London) B* **139**, 18–37.

Zaidel DW, Esiri MM, Harrison PJ (1997a) Size, shape and orientation of neurons in the left and right hippocampus: investigation of normal asymmetries and alterations in schizophrenia. *American Journal of Psychiatry* **154**, 812–818.

Zaidel DW, Esiri MM, Harrison PJ (1997*b*) The hippocampus in schizophrenia: lateralized increase in neuronal density and altered cytoarchitectural asymmetry. *Psychological Medicine* **27**, 703–713.

12 Animal Models of Schizophrenia

Barbara K. Lipska and Daniel R. Weinberger

Modeling schizophrenia in animals: some general considerations
Neurodevelopmental models of schizophrenia
   Models of prenatal aetiological factors
   Models of disrupted neurogenesis
   Models of early postnatal experiential factors
   Lesion models
Future approaches to modeling schizophrenia in animals

Animal models are commonly used in medical research as convenient and often the only available tools for studying pathophysiological mechanisms of disease and, most importantly, for designing new treatment and prevention strategies. However, despite numerous scientific reports and reviews, animal models of psychiatric disorders, notably schizophrenia, have gained little popularity and have proved a rather frustrating task (Stein and Wise, 1971; Borison *et al.*, 1977; Kornetsky and Markowitz, 1978; Coyle and Johnston, 1980; Kokkinidis and Anisman, 1980; McKinney and Moran, 1981; Robinson and Becker, 1986; Ellenbroek and Cools, 1990; Robbins, 1990; Feldon and Weiner, 1992; Machiyama, 1992; Rupniak and Iversen, 1993; Lillrank *et al.*, 1995; Sams-Dodd, 1996). Part of the problem with modeling schizophrenia in animals is, of course, that schizophrenia is an inherently complex, human disease. Another impediment is that schizophrenia was long regarded as a social or psychological disorder, not a brain disorder with a particular neurobiological cause. As discussed in this book, the situation is changing rapidly in light of mounting neuroimaging (Chapter 1) and postmortem (Chapters 2 to 5) evidence linking schizophrenia to neuropathological processes in the brain. Inspired by results of these studies, several groups have become proponents of the so-called 'neurodevelopmental hypothesis' of schizophrenia, which is presently popular because of its capacity to explain potential mechanisms underlying a number of aspects of schizophrenia, including pathomorphological changes in brain. The theory, discussed in detail in Chapter 8, postulates that schizophrenia is caused by a subtle defect in cerebral development that disrupts late-maturing, highly evolved neocortical functions, and which fully manifests itself years later in adult life. In addition to developmental genes, the putative causal factors for the aberrant development include a range of early environmental events such as maternal viral infection, malnutrition, alcohol exposure, and birth complications (Chapter 8).

We have recently witnessed a renewal of interest in animal models of schizophrenia based on the neurodevelopmental hypothesis. Their common feature is the use of an early developmental insult to disrupt indirectly certain brain functions in an animal's adult life. This chapter will review these newer models. Firstly, the feasibility of modeling a human psychiatric illness in a phylogenetically lower species will be considered. Secondly, the recent attempts to produce neurodevelopmental animal models of schizophrenia in rodents and primates based on various concepts about the origin and pathophysiology of the disease will be presented and their heuristic value discussed. The final section will focus on future possibilities in this field.

Modeling schizophrenia in animals: some general considerations

Investigating the mechanisms underlying a disease and designing new treatments often are benefited by animal models that mimic closely the human pathological condition. Is it then possible to model in a rodent or in a non-human primate a disease like schizophrenia whose most prominent symptoms—hallucinations, delusions, and thought disorder—can only be revealed by examining one's mental and emotional state, and whose origin is unknown? It seems obvious that certain features are human-specific and thus impossible to reproduce or detect in any other species. Conversely, other phenomena characteristic of schizophrenia, such as motor behaviors, memory impairment, and information processing deficits, may be approachable in a phylogenetically lower animal. Moreover, the effects of pharmacological interventions on some of these behaviors or on brain chemistry may show isomorphisms across species. But is it appropriate to gauge the fidelity of a model based solely on how closely it mimics the behavioral features of the disease? Models generated by genetic engineering provide examples that this may not always be the appropriate criterion. Animal models that seek to reproduce a cellular phenotype and involve targeted gene deletions or gene transfer techniques often result in behavioral phenotypes that are not isomorphic with the disease. This is because genetic mutation can have remarkably different phenotypes when placed on different genetic backgrounds (for review, see Erickson, 1996). Nevertheless, such models are faithful in terms of their cellular characteristics and can be very useful in dissecting molecular mechanisms leading to pathological changes. This approach is, of course, possible only if the disease can be linked to specific human genes. So far, it has been successfully employed in studying many neurological disorders, including Alzheimer's disease (Johnson-Wood et al., 1997), Down's syndrome (Davisson, 1995), Lesch–Nyhan syndrome (Wu and Melton, 1993), and Niemann–Pick disease (Loftus et al., 1997). The transgenic animals provide almost perfect models because they are, in a sense, 'humanized' by introduction of human genes involved in the disease or the mutated animal homologues, particularly if introduced onto the proper genetic background (Erickson, 1996; Loring et al., 1996).

Unfortunately, it is not yet possible to construct such models of schizophrenia because putative causal genetic mutations have not been identified. Even if it were possible to model such a complex disorder at the cellular level without knowledge of its cause, it would still represent at best an approximation, not the disease itself. This compromise may be acceptable—and heuristically meaningful—even if a model is only a simplified version of the condition, provides useful novel information about either pathophysiology or therapy of the disorder, or both.

An animal model may parallel a disease on three different levels; it may reproduce the inducing factor(s) (i.e. the etiopathogenic and pathophysiological processes), the phenomenology (e.g. an array of positive and negative symptoms of schizophrenia), and the responsiveness to drugs (e.g. neuroleptics of different classes) (Kornetsky and Markowitz, 1978; McKinney and Moran, 1981; Ellenbroek and Cools, 1990). Animal models have thus been subdivided into three major categories according to the aspects that they aspire to represent, i.e. models with construct, face, or predictive validity, respectively, in descending order of fidelity. It has been assumed that models with construct validity usually possess both face and predictive validity, and similarly, that face validity models fulfil also the criteria of models with predictive validity (Ellenbroek and Cools, 1990). However, transgenic animals provide important exceptions to this rule. For instance, genetic models which in many instances have perfect construct and predictive validity, do not always have face validity, as in the case of the Duchenne's muscular dystrophy *mdx* mutation mouse which is hardly symptomatic (Erickson, 1996); or the mouse model of Alzheimer's disease generated using a platelet-derived growth factor β promoter driving an amyloid precursor protein (APP) minigene possessing the V to F mutation at position 717 which overexpresses APP but does not have an isomorphic behavioral phenotype (Johnson-Wood *et al.*, 1997). Similarly, mice deficient in the gene product causing Lesch–Nyhan syndrome have no recognizable phenotype analogous to the human syndrome (Wu and Melton, 1993).

Most traditional models of schizophrenia have some predictive validity and have been used to screen responsiveness to available neuroleptics. This usually involves, however, behavioral paradigms bearing no resemblence whatsoever to schizophrenia (e.g. antagonism of apomorphine-induced emesis). Nevertheless, many of these models provide excellent correlations between the behavioral changes and the antipsychotic or parkinsonism-inducing potencies of various drugs (for review, see Costall and Naylor, 1995). The majority of other models have some degree of face validity and usually address only a single symptom or a narrow range of symptoms (e.g. stereotypy in amphetamine models).

Even a seemingly identical appearance of behaviors across species does not imply that they are indeed homologous in terms of meaning, purpose, or underlying mechanisms. As noted by McKinney and Moran (1981), 'even when there is marked parallelism between the model and the human condition, the model may be only isomorphic; that is, the cause of the condition in the animal may be quite different from the cause of the condition in the human'. Nonetheless, older models, although limited in their capacity to recreate a broader range of aspects of schizophrenia, have enhanced our understanding of the mechanisms of action and extrapyramidal side-effects of antipsychotic drugs and the mechanisms underlying certain behavioral phenomena. These traditional animal models have served this purpose well. It seems today, however, that this purpose is too narrow. Neuroleptics, even the so-called novel or atypical ones, do not cure schizophrenia. Animal models that have helped to develop and screen them are limited in exploring novel therapeutic strategies that are not based on the traditional dopamine theory. It is desirable, therefore, to develop new models that would reflect the present state of knowledge about schizophrenia and that would re-examine various other concepts of the etiology and pathophysiology of this disorder. Because the etiology of schizophrenia is unknown, the major role of contemporary models which aspire to construct validity is to test the plausibility of theories concocted from the available sets of data. The models are then used as tools to validate a particular theoretical construct about the disease; as such they need to be updated and re-examined as new clinical findings emerge, and new and more specific theories are formulated. In this respect, an important aspect of the research is a give-and-take between animal experimentation and clinical research.

Neurodevelopmental animal models of schizophrenia

As interest in schizophrenia research shifted from the dopamine hypothesis to neurodevelopmental theories, animal models followed a similar trend. The earlier animal models were based on direct pharmacological manipulations within the dopaminergic system to simulate the putative overactivity of dopamine transmission. It is not surprising then that the drugs that emerged as a result of such models all exert antidopaminergic efficacy. Novel animal models (Table 12.1) address the possibility that a disruption of dopaminergic function is but a secondary manifestation of cortical, presumably neurodevelopmental, malfunction, albeit of an as yet unknown origin (Lillrank *et al.*, 1995). Thus, these models carry the prospect of novel treatment strategies based on different mechanisms (Weinberger and Lipska, 1995).

Models of prenatal aetiological factors

Several animal models address the possibility that a particular prenatal or perinatal factor may cause schizophrenia. Based on the various epidemiological findings (Chapter 8), the concepts of gestational malnutrition, perinatal infections, and hypoxic events during birth

Table 12.1 Examples of neurodevelopmental models relevant to schizophrenia

Prenatal etiological factors
    Prenatal malnutrition
    Prenatal viral infection (influenza, Borna virus)
    Hypoxia at birth
In utero disrupted neurogenesis
    X-ray radiation
    Gestational methylazoxymethanol
Postnatal experiential factors
    Maternal deprivation
    Social isolation
Postnatal brain damage
    Hippocampal lesion
    Neocortical lesion
    Thalamic lesion

See text for references.

have been tested in rats. A common feature of these models is an experimentally induced putative cause, which results in biochemical and/or behavioral changes as the animal matures.

Gestational malnutrition

Gestational malnutrition, or more precisely, protein deprivation in rat mothers that begins prior to and continues throughout pregnancy, results in severe permanent changes in brain development (for reviews, see Morgane *et al.*, 1993; Brown *et al.*, 1996). Malnutrition affects neurogenesis, cell migration and differentation, and leads to deviations in normal brain development including disrupted formation of neural circuits and neurotransmitter systems. Consequently, it has debilitating effects on cognitive function and learning abilities. It is thus not surprising that malnutrition was proposed as a causative factor in the emergence of seemingly analogous dysfunctions in human schizophrenia. However, in contrast to schizophrenia, morphological abnormalities following severe malnutrition in rats are widespread. Behavioral consequences with regard to their similarity to schizophrenia have either not been investigated so far, or are inconsistent. For instance, deficits in prepulse inhibition of startle (PPI), a phenomenon thought to reflect abilities in information processing and shown to be disrupted in patients with schizophrenia (Braff and Geyer, 1990), emerge after puberty in prenatally malnourished rats, but only in females (Printz *et al.*, 1997). To test the plausibility of the malnutrition theory of schizophrenia, more data on behavioral phenotype associated with malnutrition and on responsiveness to neuroleptics are needed.

Viral infections

The role of viral infections in schizophrenia has been the subject of a large number of clinical studies with varying results. Similarly, the animal models that test the viral hypotheses provide either negative or confusing data. Cotter *et al.* (1995) investigated whether prenatal exposure to influenza might induce pyramidal disarray in mice analogous to that reported by Scheibel and Kovelman (1981) and Conrad *et al.* (1991) in the hippocampi of schizophrenic patients. Overall, mice offspring whose mothers were inoculated with influenza between days 9 and 16 of pregnancy failed to demonstrate any cytoarchitectural abnormalities in the hippocampus, although in a small subgroup of animals infected on day 13, some disarray was observed (Cotter *et al.*, 1995). The analysis, however, was performed in the dorsal hippocampus, whereas anterior (i.e. ventral in rodents) hippocampus has been more often implicated in schizophrenia (Jeste and Lohr, 1989; Suddath *et al.*, 1990), so potentially some of the effects could have been missed. A possibility that a viral infection at different time at gestation is critical for the defects to emerge has yet to be tested. Unfortunately, there are no other behavioral, biochemical, or pharmacological data available for this model.

Besides influenza, Borna disease virus (BDV) has been hypothesized to be involved in schizophrenia, on the basis of reports of increased frequency of BDV seropositivity (Rott *et al.*, 1985; Waltrip *et al.*, 1995; but see Horimoto *et al.*, 1997). BDV seems an attractive potential causative agent because it shows tropism for the limbic system, including hippocampus and prefrontal cortex, and because the behavioral changes following infection in rats include stereotypies and hyperactivity. Also, BDV-infected rats demonstrate dopaminergic changes, such as elevated 3,4-dihydroxyphenylacetic acid (DOPAC) levels in the prefrontal cortex, and a reduced dopamine level, dopamine uptake, D2 and D3 binding in the nucleus accumbens as well as reduced D2 binding in the striatum. Nevertheless, the parallels with schizophrenia appear far fetched. The changes cannot be easily reconciled either with findings in schizophrenia or with the BDV infection-associated behavioral abnormalities (Solbrig *et al.*, 1994, 1996*a,b*). As such, though further research using the BDV model may provide insight into the mechanisms involved in infection-induced frontal lobe dysfunction, its relevance to schizophrenia remains unclear.

Birth complications

Other possible adverse factors being considered are birth complications, including anoxia around birth. In general, obstetrical and birth complications have been linked to schizophrenia later in life, although it is not clear if they constitute a causative factor for the disease or reflect already perturbed development of the fetus. Nonetheless, studies in rats on the effects of cesarean (C-) birth suggest marked changes in the limbic dopamine system. In adulthood, animals born by C-section show decreased dopamine levels and increased dopamine turnover in the prefrontal cortex, elevated dopamine concentration and reduced dopamine turnover in the nucleus accumbens, as well as hyper-responsiveness of the dopamine system to stress (Brake *et al.*, 1997; El-Khodor and Boksa, 1997). Surprisingly, these effects are not observed (or at least, their intensity is significantly reduced), in animals that in addition to C-section were subject to periods of anoxia during or shortly after birth, although the overall physical condition of the anoxic animals seemed worse than those born by C-section alone (El-Khodor and Boksa, 1997). This would suggest that C-section constitues a greater risk factor for schizophrenia than the more dramatic birth trauma of anoxia. In humans, C-section is generally assumed to involve less stress to the fetus and has not been noted as one of the obstetrical complications linked to schizophrenia. Clearly, more studies are needed to elucidate the mechanisms underlying the C-section-related phenomena, and to establish if C-section is a risk factor for schizophrenia itself.

Taken together, although these aetiological models aspire to construct validity because they reproduce putative causes of the disease and putative pathological mechanisms, their face validity is rather limited, and their predictive validity has not been generally assessed. At present, none provides compelling evidence for the plausibility of any of the aetiological theories proposed.

Models of disrupted neurogenesis

In contrast to the etiological models described above, these models do not attempt to reproduce causative factors implicated in schizophrenia, but mimic cellular events that presumably would follow a disruption of early cortical development. A common feature is prenatal interruption of cell proliferation. Brain damage thus provoked would result in certain phenotypic changes detected as the animal matures. The examples include cortical neuronal dysgenesis modeled by gestational X-ray irradiation (Mintz *et al.*, 1997) and *in utero* exposure to a mitotic toxin, methylazoxymethanol acetate (MAM), that destroys populations of rapidly dividing neurons (Johnston *et al.*, 1988). Animals that have undergone these manipulations exhibit a variety of behavioral alterations including hyperactivity, stereotypies, cognitive impairments, and disruption of latent inhibition and PPI (Johnston *et al.*, 1988; Mintz *et al.*, 1997). Morphological changes are, however, usually more profound and wide-spread, and the behavioral impairments more severe, than observed in schizophrenia, although more circumscribed damage can be achieved by altering the embryonic age and duration of treatment (Talamini *et al.*, 1998). Predictive validity of these models has not been tested, but they clearly merit further attention.

Models of early postnatal experiential factors

These models focus on the lasting consequences of stress for brain development and for shaping adult behavioral responses. They have been variably used as models of depression, anxiety, and schizophrenia, diseases in which stress appears to play a prominent role. In rodents, early exposure to varying degrees of experiential stress such as neonatal handling, maternal separation (Liu *et al.*, 1997), and social isolation (Jones *et al.*, 1992; Geyer *et al.*, 1993; Wilkinson *et al.*, 1994) produces numerous hormonal, neurochemical, and behavioral changes. The latter include locomotor hyperactivity in a novel environment, maze learning impairments, anxiety, and deficits in PPI. Of particular interest is that some of these alterations emerge in adult life. Moreover, the effects of the adverse early life events on adult reactivity are strongly influenced by genetic factors (de Kloet *et al.*, 1996; Zaharia *et al.*, 1996). The models provide important evidence for the interaction between genetic predisposition and early life experiences and demonstrate that both are involved in shaping the adult stress response system and adult patterns of behavior, and might thus represent an interesting approach to study the neurodevelopmental theory of schizophrenia.

Ellenbroek *et al.* (1998) demonstrated that maternal deprivation (lasting 24 hours between postnatal days 6 and 9) disrupts PPI in adults but not prepubertal male and female rats; moreover, the deficits can be ameliorated with an acute dose of a typical antipsychotic, haloperidol (0.1 mg/kg), or an atypical one, quetiapine (1 mg/kg). Similarly, isolation-induced (for 8 weeks from weaning) disruption of PPI can be reversed by both typical and atypical antipsychotics (Varty and Higgins, 1995). Interestingly, the glycine/NMDA receptor antagonist L-701,324 also reverses PPI deficits in social isolates (Bristow *et al.*, 1995) suggesting that this model may be useful in identifying novel therapeutic agents for schizophrenia. It should be pointed out, however, that various other agents, not necessarily effective in treating schizophrenia, also reverse alterations in these stress models. For instance, certain antidepressants can reverse the maternal separation-induced changes (Hawks *et al.*, 1997; Ladd *et al.*, 1997), and are active in social isolates (Fulford and Marsden, 1997). In terms of their predictive value, these models may thus produce some false positives. Moreover, although face and predictive validity of these models appears to be better than of most others, their construct validity is limited.

Lesion models

Our own studies have focused on neonatal damage induced by infusion of an excitotoxin into restricted cortical regions in rats (Lipska *et al.*, 1993). This work has been followed up and extended in other laboratories (Chambers *et al.*, 1996; Flores *et al.*, 1996*a,b*; Wan *et al.*, 1996; Brake *et al.*, 1997; Stine *et al.*, 1997; Wan and Corbett, 1997), and some of our findings have been reproduced and elaborated in monkeys (Beauregard *et al.*, 1995; Beauregard and Bachevalier, 1996; Bertolino *et al.*, 1997; Saunders *et al.*, 1998). The main objective of these studies is to inflict relatively subtle damage early in life in the hippocampus, the brain area most consistently implicated in schizophrenia (Chapter 2), and thus disrupt development of the widespread cortical and subcortical circuitry in which the hippocampus participates. We speculated that this early hippocampal disruption would have behavioral consequences different from those seen after similar damage produced in adulthood, and that it would indirectly affect function of the dopamine system.

The results of our studies revealed that neonatal (on postnatal day 7, PD7) excitotoxic lesions of the rat ventral hippocampus (VH) produce a temporally specific pattern of abnormalities in a number of dopamine-related behavioral paradigms. When tested before puberty (PD35), the rats do not demonstrate abnormalities in behaviors related to dopamine function. They differ, however, from normal controls in social behaviors—the VH lesioned rats make less social contacts with unfamiliar partners and show more anxiety in this testing situation (Sams-Dodd *et al.*, 1997). At a postpubertal age (PD56), the VH lesioned animals display markedly changed behaviors thought to be primarily linked to increased mesolimbic/nigrostriatal dopamine transmission, and show enhanced sensitivity to glutamate antagonists, a reaction also noted in patients with schizophrenia (Lipska *et al.*, 1993, 1995a, 1998; Lipska and Weinberger, 1993, 1994a,b). Neonatally lesioned rats, when tested after puberty, also demonstrate deficits in PPI (Lipska *et al.* 1995b). Because PPI is usually reduced by D2 dopamine receptor activation and restored by antidopaminergic drugs, these data again suggest excessive dopaminergic activity associated with this lesion at PD56. Behavioral changes related to a hyperdopaminergic state may reproduce positive symptoms of schizophrenia in this animal model. Changes in social behaviors and working memory impairments, which are also associated with this developmental lesion (Sams-Dodd *et al.*, 1997), may correspond to the negative symptoms. Thus, this model appears to mimic some of the key neurobiological features of schizophrenia and may have predictive validity as clozapine shows some superior effects over haloperidol in blocking hyperlocomotion in the VH lesioned rats, although it does not ameliorate social deficits (Lipska and Weinberger 1994a; Sams-Dodd *et al.*, 1997). Our data also suggest that age at lesion is a critical factor determining behavioral outcome. We have recently demonstrated that the delayed emergence of abnormal behaviors related to heightened dopaminergic transmission is seen in animals lesioned on PD3 or PD7, but not on PD14 or in adulthood (Wood *et al.*, 1997). Thus, this model requires an early and time-limited defect in limbic cortical development, consistent with the putative timing of the origins of schizophrenia (Chapter 8). The model also seems to reproduce functional pathology in brain regions interconnected with the hippocampal formation and targeted by antipsychotic drugs (Chambers *et al.*, 1996; Lillrank *et al.*, 1996; Sams-Dodd *et al.*, 1997). In addition, removal of the presumably dysfunctional medial prefrontal cortex in the VH lesioned animals normalized some of the hyperactive behaviors (Lipska *et al.*, 1998). It is noteworthy that recent findings in the primate also suggest that early postnatal damage of the hippocampus alters development of the prefrontal cortex and the mechanisms whereby it regulates subcortical dopamine function (Bertolino *et al.*, 1997; Saunders *et al.*, 1998).

The effects of neonatal damage of other brain structures implicated in schizophrenia have also been studied as potential models, but the results of these studies are rather limited. For instance, thalamic excitotoxic lesions in PD7 rats were shown to result in adult emergence of apomorphine- and amphetamine-induced locomotion (Rajakumar *et al.*, 1996), but no other tests have yet been performed. Intracerebroventricular infusions of kainic acid into neonatal (PD7) rats resulted in adulthood in a reduction in neuronal populations in the dorsal hippocampus and were associated with changes in dopaminergic and glutamatergic function (Bardgett *et al.*, 1995). No other data are available on this model. Finally, neonatal (PD7) excitotoxic damage of the medial prefrontal cortex was also reported to produce delayed behavioral effects accompanied by dopamine receptor changes (Flores *et al.*, 1996*b*), although these data were not confirmed (Lipska *et al.*, 1998).

Future approaches to modeling schizophrenia in animals

Although genome-wide searches have not yielded consistently positive results, there is little doubt that schizophrenia is a genetic disorder, probably involving multiple genes. A genetic component, however, has so far rarely been addressed in animal models of the disorder. One strategy that can be employed in animal studies is identification of predisposing candidate genes by selecting rodent lines or strains for particular behavioral traits. Such candidates may then be used to identify homologous human genes involved in schizophrenia. For instance, in a search for a genetic animal model of schizophrenia, animals were bred for high susceptibility for apomorphine-induced gnawing or a high response to novelty (APO-SUS rats). These animals, in contrast to apomorphine non-responsive (APO-UNSUS) rats, demonstrated various behavioral (e.g. PPI and latent inhibition deficits), biochemical (e.g. elevated levels of tyrosine hydroxylase mRNA in the substantia nigra and D2 receptor binding in the dorsal striatum), and immunological (e.g. reduced sensitivity to rheumatoid arthritis) features implicated in schizophrenia (Ellenbroek *et al.*, 1995). Other studies suggest that Fisher 344 rats, a highly stress-responsive strain, show particular susceptibility to the behavioral effects of early hippocampal damage. Lewis rats, on the other hand, bred for low stress responsiveness, appear resistant to the motor effects of identical lesions (Lipska and Weinberger, 1995). This animal model can then be used to identify genetic factors that mediate behavioral responses to neonatal hippocampal damage, and by extension, that might predispose to schizophrenia.

More generally, these data emphasize the point that effects of a given gene are affected both by genetic background—the influence of so-called 'modifiers' (allelic variants at other loci), interacting with environmental experiences. Although experimentally challenging, such complexities are entirely appropriate for modeling schizophrenia where just such an interaction of genes and environment appears to be etiologically important. In terms of future transgenic approaches, choosing the right combination of mutation and modifier genes, as well as appropriate environmental modification of gene expression (e.g. by early experiential stress), may allow an almost perfect animal model of even so human a disease as schizophrenia to be created.

References

Bardgett, M. A., Jackson, J. L., Taylor, G. T., Csernansky, J. G. (1995) Kainic acid decreases hippocampal neuronal number and increases dopamine receptor binding in the nucleus accumbens: An animal model of schizophrenia. *Behavioral Brain Research*, **70**, 153–164.

Beauregard, M., Bachevalier, J. (1996) Neonatal insult to the hippocampal region and schizophrenia: A review and a putative animal model. *Canadian Journal of Psychiatry*, **41**, 446–456.

Beauregard M., Malkova L., Bachevalier J. (1995) Stereotypies and loss of social affiliation after early hippocampectomy in primates. *NeuroReport*, **6**, 2521–2526.

Bertolino, A., Saunders, R. C., Mattay, V. S., Bachevalier, J., Frank, J. A., Weinberger, D. R. (1997) Altered development of prefrontal neurons in rhesus monkeys with neonatal mesial temporo-limbic lesions: A proton magnetic resonance spectroscopic imaging study. *Cerebral Cortex*, **7**, 740–748.

Borison, R. L., Havdala, H. S., Diamond, B. I. (1977) Chronic phenylethylamine stereotypy in rats: a new animal model for schizophrenia? *Life Sciences*, **21**, 117–122.

Braff, D. L., Geyer, M. A. (1990) Sensorimotor gating and schizophrenia: Human and animal model studies. *Archives of General Psychiatry*, **47**, 181–188.

Brake, W., Noel, M. B., Boksa, P., Gratton, A. (1997) Influence of perinatal factors on the nucleus accumbens dopamine response to repeated stress during adulthood: An electrochemical study in rat. *Neuroscience*, **77**, 1067–1076.

Bristow, L. J., Landon, L., Saywell, K. L., Tricklebank, M. D. (1995) The glycine/NMDA receptor antagonist, L-701,324 reverses isolation-induced deficits in prepulse inhibition in the rat. *Psychopharmacology*, **118**, 230–232.

Brown, A. S., Susser, E. S., Butler, P. D., Richardson, A. R., Kaufmann, C. A., Gorman, J. M. (1996) Neurobiological plausibility of prenatal nutritional deprivation as a risk factor for schizophrenia. *Journal of Nervous and Mental Disorders,* **184**, 71–85.

Chambers, R. A., Moore, J., McEvoy, J. P., Levin, E. D. (1996) Cognitive effects of neonatal hippocampal lesions in a rat model of schizophrenia. *Neuropsychopharmacology*, **15**, 587–594.

Conrad, A. J., Abebe, T., Ron, A., Forsythe, S., Scheibel, B. (1991) Hippocampal pyramidal cell disarray in schizophrenia as a bilateral phenomenon. *Archives of General Psychiatry*, **48**, 413–417.

Costall, B., Naylor, R. J. (1995) Animal neuropharmacology and its prediction of clinical response. In: S. R. Hirsch and D. R. Weinberger, eds. *Schizophrenia*, pp. 401–424. Blackwell Science, Oxford.

Cotter, D., Takei, N., Farrell, M. *et al.* (1995) Does prenatal exposure to influenza in mice induce pyramidal cell disarray in the dorsal hippocampus? *Schizophrenia Research*, **16**, 233–241.

Coyle, J. T., Johnston, M. V. (1980) Functional hyperinnervation of cerebral cortex by noradrenergic neurons results from fetal lesions: parallels with schizophrenia. *Psychopharmacology Bulletin*, **16**, 27–29.

Davisson, M. T. (1995) A mouse model for Down syndrome exhibits learning and behaviour deficits. *Nature Genetics,* **11**, 177–184.

de Kloet, E. R., Rots, N. Y., Cools, A. R. (1996) Brain-corticosteroid hormone dialogue: slow and persistent. *Cellular and Molecular Neurobiology*, **16**, 345–356.

El-Khodor, B. F., Boksa, P. (1997) Long-term reciprocal changes in dopamine levels in prefrontal cortex versus nucleus accumbens in rats born by Cesarean section compared to vaginal birth. *Experimental Neurology,* **145**, 118–129.

Ellenbroek, B. A., Cools, A. R. (1990) Animal models with construct validity for schizophrenia. *Behavioral Pharmacology*, **1**, 469–490.

Ellenbroek, B. A., Geyer, M. A., Cools, A. R. (1995) The behavior of APO-SUS rats in animal models with construct validity for schizophrenia. *Journal of Neuroscience*, **11**, 7604–7611.

Ellenbroek, B. A., van den Kroonenberg, P. T. J. M., Cools, A. R. (1998) The effect of a stressful early life event on sensorimotor gating in adult rats. *Schizophrenia Research*, **30**, 251–260.

Erickson, R. P. (1996) Mouse models of human genetic disease: which mouse is more like a man? *Bioessays*, **18**, 993–998.

Feldon, J., Weiner, I. (1992) From animal model of an attentional deficit towards new insights into the pathophysiology of schizophrenia. *Journal of Psychiatric Research*, **26**, 345–366.

Flores, G., Barbeau, D., Quirion, R., Srivastava, L. K. (1996*a*) Decreased binding of dopamine D3 receptors in limbic subregions after neonatal bilateral lesion of rat hippocampus. *Journal of Neuroscience*, **16**, 2020–2026.

Flores, G., Wood, G. K., Liang, J.-J., Quirion, R., Srivastava, L. K. (1996*b*) Enhanced amphetamine sensitivity and increased expression of dopamine D2 receptors in postpubertal rats after neonatal excitotoxic lesions of the medial prefrontal cortex. *Journal of Neuroscience*, **16**, 7366–7375.

Fulford, A. J., Marsden, C. A. (1997) Social isolation in the rat enhances alpha-2-autoreceptor function in the hippocampus in vivo. *Neuroscience*, **77**, 57–64.

Geyer, M. A., Wilkinson, L. S., Humby, T., Robbins, T. W. (1993) Isolation rearing of rats produces a deficit in prepulse inhibition of acoustic startle similar to that in schizophrenia. *Biological Psychiatry*, **34**, 361–372.

Hawks, B. W., Plotsky, P. M., Garlow, S. J. (1997) Long term regulation of serotonin 1A and transporter by early postnatal maternal separation. *Society for Neuroscience Abstracts*, **23**, 1080.

Horimoto, T., Takahashi, H., Sakagichi, M. *et al.* (1997) A reverse-type sandwich enzyme-linked immunosorbent assay for detecting antibodies to Borna disease virus. *Journal of Clinical Microbiology*, **35**, 1661–1666.

Jeste, D. V., Lohr, J. B. (1989) Hippocampal pathologic findings in schizophrenia: a morphometric study. *Archives of General Psychiatry*, **46**, 1019–1024.

Johnson-Wood, K., Lee, M., Motter, R. *et al.* (1997) Amyloid precursor protein processing and A-beta-42 deposition in a transgenic mouse model of Alzheimer disease. *Proceedings of National Academy of Sciences, USA,* **94**, 1550–1555.

Johnston, M. V., Barks, J., Greenmyre, T., Silverstein, F. (1988) Use of toxins to disrupt neurotransmitter circuitry in the developing brain. *Progress in Brain Research*, **73**, 425–446.

Jones, G. H., Hernandez, T. D., Kendall, D. A., Marsden, C. A., Robbins, T. W. (1992) Dopaminergic and serotonergic function following isolation rearing in rats: Study of behavioral responses and postmortem and in vivo neurochemistry. *Pharmacology Biochemistry and Behavior*, **43**, 17–35.

Kokkinidis L., Anisman H (1980) Amphetamine models of paranoid schizophrenia: an overview and elaboration of animal experimentation. *Psychological Bulletin*, **88**, 551–579.

Kornetsky, C., Markowitz, R. (1978) Animal models of schizophrenia. In: M. A. Lipton, A. DiMascio, K. F. Killam, eds. *Psychopharmacology: a generation of progress*, pp. 583–593. Raven Press, New York.

Ladd, C. O., Lyss, P. J., Owens, M. J., Plotsky, P. M. (1997) Effects of mirtazapine on behavioral, hormonal, and neurochemical parameters in maternally-separated rats. *Society for Neuroscience Abstracts*, **23**, 985.

Lillrank, S. M., Lipska, B. K., Weinberger, D. R. (1995) Neurodevelopmental animal models of schizophrenia. *Clinical Neuroscience*, **3**, 98–104.

Lillrank, S. M., Lipska, B. K., Bachus, S., Wood, G. K., Weinberger, D. R. (1996) Amphetamine-induced c-fos mRNA expression is reduced in rats with neonatal ventral hippocampal lesions. *Synapse*, **23**, 182–191.

Lipska, B. K., Weinberger, D. R. (1993) Delayed effects of neonatal hippocampal damage on haloperidol-induced catalepsy and apomorphine-induced stereotypic behaviors in the rat. *Developmental Brain Research*, **75**, 13–222.

Lipska, B. K., Weinberger, DR. (1994*a*) Subchronic treatment with haloperidol or clozapine in rats with neonatal excitotoxic hippocampal damage. *Neuropsychopharmacology*, **10**, 199–205.

Lipska, B. K., Weinberger, D. R. (1994*b*) Gonadectomy does not prevent novelty- or drug-induced hyperresponsiveness in rats with neonatal excitototxic hippocampal damage. *Developmental Brain Research*, **78**, 253–258.

Lipska, B. K., Weinberger, D. R. (1995) Genetic variation in vulnerability to the behavioral effects of neonatal hippocampal damage in rats. *Proceedings of National Academy of Sciences, USA*, **92**, 8906–8910.

Lipska, B. K., Jaskiw, G. E., Weinberger, D. R. (1993) Postpubertal emergence of hyperresponsiveness to stress and to amphetamine after neonatal hippocampal damage: A potential animal model of schizophrenia. *Neuropsychopharmacology*, **9**, 67–75.

Lipska, B. K., Chrapusta, S. J., Egan, M. F., Weinberger, D. R. (1995*a*) Neonatal excitotoxic ventral hippocampal damage alters dopamine response to mild chronic stress and haloperidol treatment. *Synapse*, **20**, 125–130.

Lipska, B. K., Swerdlow, N. R., Geyer, M. A., Jaskiw, G. E., Braff, D. L., Weinberger, D. R. (1995*b*) Neonatal excitotoxic hippocampal damage in rats causes postpubertal changes in prepulse inhibition of startle and its disruption by apomorphine. *Psychopharmacology*, **122**, 35–43.

Lipska, B. K., Al-Amin, H. A., Weinberger, D. R. (1998) Excitotoxic lesions of the rat medial prefrontal cortex: effects on abnormal behaviors associated with neonatal hippocampal damage. *Neuropsychopharmacology*, **19**, 451–464

Liu, D., Diorio, J., Tannenbaum, B. *et al.* (1997) Maternal care, hippocampal glucocorti-coid receptors, and hypothalamic-pituitary-adrenal responses to stress. *Science*, **277**, 1659–1662.

Loftus, S. K., Morris, J. A., Carstea, E. D. *et al.* (1997) Murine model of Niemann–Pick C disease: mutation in a cholesterol homeostasis gene. *Science*, **277**, 232–235.

Loring J. F., Paszty, C., Rose, A. *et al.* (1996) Rational design of an animal model for Alzheimer's disease: introduction of multiple human genomic transgenes to reproduce AD pathology in a rodent. *Neurobiology of Aging*, **17**, 173–182.

Machiyama, Y. (1992) Chronic methamphetamine intoxication model of schizophrenia in animals. *Schizophrenia Bulletin*, **18**, 107–113.

McKinney, W. T., Moran, E. C. (1981) Animal models of schizophrenia. *American Journal of Psychiatry*, **138**, 478–483.

Mintz, M., Youval, G., Gigi, A., Myslobodsky, M. S. (1997) Rats exposed to prenatal gamma-radiation at day 15 of gestation exhibit enhanced perseveration in T-maze. *Society of Neuroscience Abstract*, **23**, 1365.

Morgane, P. J., Austin-LaFrance, R., Bronzino, J. *et al.* (1993) Prenatal malnutrition and development of the brain. *Neuroscience and Biobehavioral Reviews,* **17**, 91–128.

Printz, D. J., Butler, P. D., Palmer, A. A. *et al.* (1997) Effects of prenatal protein depri-vation on NMDA receptor number and prepulse inhibition of startle. *Society for Neuroscience Abstract,* **23**, 1928.

Rajakumar, N., Williamson, P. C., Stoessl, J. A., Flumerfelt, B. A. (1996) Neurodevelop-mental pathogenesis of schizophrenia. *Society for Neuroscience Abstract*, **22**, 1187.

Robbins, T. (1990) The case for frontostriatal dysfunction in schizophrenia. *Schizophrenia Bulletin* **16**, 391–402.

Robinson, T. E., Becker, J. B. (1986) Enduring changes in brain and behavior produced by chronic amphetamine administration: a review and evaluation of animal models of amphetamine psychosis. *Brain Research Reviews,* **11**, 157–198.

Rott, R., Herzog, S., Fleischer, B., Winokur, A., Amsterdam, J., Dyson, W., Koprowski, H. (1985) Detection of serum antibodies to Borna disease virus in patients with psychi-atric disorders. *Science*, **228**, 755–756.

Rupniak, N. M. J., Iversen, S. D. (1993) Cognitive impairment in schizophrenia: how exper-imental models using nonhuman primates may assist improved drug therapy for negative symptoms. *Neuropsychologia*, **31**, 1133–1146.

Sams-Dodd, F. (1996) Phencyclidine-induced stereotyped behavior and social isolation in the rat: a possible animal model of schizophrenia. *Behavioral Pharmacology*, **7**, 3–23.

Sams-Dodd, F., Lipska, B. K., Weinberger, D. R. (1997) Neonatal lesions of the rat ventral hippocampus result in hyperlocomotion and deficits in social behaviour in adulthood. *Psychopharmacology*, **132**, 303–310.

Saunders, R. C., Kolachana, B. S., Bachevalier, J., Weinberger, D. R. (1998) Neonatal lesions of the medial temporal lobe disrupt prefrontal cortical regulation of striatal dopamine. *Nature*, **393**, 169–171.

Scheibel, A. B., Kovelman, J. A. (1981) Disorientation of the hippocampal pyramidal cell and its processes in the schizophrenic patient. *Biological Psychiatry*, **16**, 101–102.

Solbrig, M. V., Koob, G. F., Fallon, J. H., Lipkin, W. I. (1994) Tardive dyskinetic syndrome in rats infected with Borna disease virus. *Neurobiology of Disease*, **1**, 111–119.

Solbrig, M. V., Koob, G. F., Joyce J. N., Lipkin, W. I. (1996*a*) A neural substrate of hyperactivity in Borna disease: changes in brain dopamine receptors. *Virology*, **222**, 332–338.

Solbrig, M. V., Koob, G. F., Fallon, J. H., Reid, S., Lipkin, W. I. (1996*b*) Prefrontal cortex dysfunction in Borna disease virus (BDV)-infected rats. *Biological Psychiatry*, **40**, 629–636.

Stein, L., Wise, C. D. (1971) Possible etiology of schizophrenia: progressive damage to the noradrenergic reward system by 6-hydroxydopamine. *Science*, **171**, 1032–1036.

Stine, C. D., Lu, W. X., Xue, C.-J., Wolf, M. E. (1997) Cortical and subcortical glutamate receptor expression and glutamate transmission in a rat model of schizophrenia. *Society for Neuroscience Abstract*, **23**, 1928.

Suddath, R. L., Christison, G. W., Torrey, E. F., Casanova, M. F., Weinberger, D. R. (1990) Anatomical abnormalities in the brains of monozygotic twins discordant for schizophrenia. *New England Journal of Medicine*, **322**, 789–794.

Talamini, L. M., Koch, T., Ter Horst, G. J., Korf, J. (1998) Methylazoxymethanol acetate-induced abnormalities in the entorhinal cortex of the rat; parallels with morphological findings in schizophrenia. *Brain Research*, **789**, 293–306.

Varty, G. B., Higgins, G. A. (1995) Examination of drug-induced and isolation-induced disruptions of prepulse inhibition as models to screen antipsychotic drugs. *Psychopharmacology* **122**, 15–26.

Waltrip, R. W. II, Buchanan, R. W., Summerfeld, A. *et al.* (1995) Borna disease virus and schizophrenia. *Psychiatry Research*, **56**, 33–44.

Wan, R.-Q., Corbett, R. (1997) Enhancement of postsynaptic sensitivity to dopaminergic agonists induced by neonatal hippocampal lesions. *Neuropsychopharmacology*, **16**, 259–268.

Wan, R.-Q., Giovanni, A., Kafka, S. H., Corbett, R. (1996) Neonatal hippocampal lesion induced hyperresponsiveness to amphetamine: behavioral and in vivo microdialysis studies. *Behavioral Brain Research*, **78**, 211–223.

Weinberger, D. R., Lipska, B. K. (1995) Cortical maldevelopment, anti-psychotic drugs, and schizophrenia: a search for common ground. *Schizophreina Research*, **16**, 87–110.

Wilkinson, L. S., Killcross, S. S., Humby, T., Hall, F. S., Geyer, M. A., Robbins, T. W. (1994) Social isolation in the rat produces developmentally specific deficits in prepulse inhibition of the acoustic startle response without disrupting latent inhibition. *Neuropsychopharmacology*, **10**, 61–72.

Wood, G. K., Lipska, B. K., Weinberger, D. R. (1997) Behavioral changes in rats with early ventral hippocampal damage vary with age at damage. *Developmental Brain Research*, **101**, 17–25.

Wu, C. L., Melton, D. W. (1993) Production of a model for Lesch–Nyhan syndrome in hypoxanthine phosphoribosyltransferase-deficient mice. *Nature Genetics*, **3**, 235–240.

Zaharia, M. D., Kulczycki, J., Shanks, N., Meaney, M. J., Anisman, H. (1996) The effects of early postnatal stimulation on Morris water-maze acqusition in adult mice: genetic and maternal factors. *Psychopharmacology*, **128**, 227–239.

13 A Sceptical View of the Neuropathology of Schizophrenia

Siew E. Chua and Peter J. McKenna

Perhaps the most appropriate place to begin a sceptical review of the neuropathology of schizophrenia is with a review of the same field carried out over 40 years ago by David (1957). He noted that there had been numerous reports of structural brain abnormality in the disorder, some by researchers as distinguished as Nissl and Alzheimer; the findings ranged from macroscopic cortical atrophy, affecting particularly the frontal lobes, to histological findings including but not limited to cell loss, shrinkage and ballooning, dwarf cells, metachromatic bodies, cellular inclusions, demyelination, and gliosis. After carefully examining the literature, David dismissed all of the alleged abnormalities with the exception of demyelination, on the grounds that they were either not well replicated or had also been documented in normal individuals. Demyelination itself he considered questionable as it could have been due to fixation artefacts.

David (1957) was also critical of two studies which claimed to find cortical atrophy, 'generally accompanied by ventricular dilatation' in schizophrenic patients examined during life using the technique of air encephalography. Here, though, his conclusions were premature. After a hiatus of 20 years the first study which applied the new technology of CT scanning to schizophrenia (Johnstone *et al.*, 1976) found evidence of lateral ventricular enlargement, and this went on to be replicated in the majority of over 50 further studies (e.g. see Lewis, 1990). Nevertheless, there were still lessons to be learnt. It quickly became clear that the degree of enlargement was small—Weinberger *et al.* (1979) found that only 17 per cent of a group of 58 chronic schizophrenic patients showed clinically detectable abnormality, and Andreasen *et al.* (1990*b*) found the difference in ventricular size between cases and controls to be scarcely greater than that between normal females and normal males. This made the CT scan findings in schizophrenia vulnerable to a methodological problem concerning choice of controls. Several of the early studies employed 'medical' controls, i.e. patients with scans reported as normal by radiologists, a practice which can lead to individuals who have lateral ventricles at the extreme upper end of the normal range being excluded. This would then tend to lower the control group mean, and in turn give rise to spuriously inflated differences from the schizophrenic group. The operation of such a systematic bias was suggested when Smith and Iacono (1986) reviewed the existing CT studies and were able to argue persuasively that the differences found were due not to larger lateral ventricles in schizophrenic patients, but rather to smaller ones in controls. In a subsequent meta-analysis of 39 studies, Van Horn and McManus (1992) concluded that the difference in lateral ventricular size between schizophrenics and controls had shown a linear decrease over the years and went on to comment, not wholly tongue-in-cheek, that if this trend continued, 'within a few years the difference … might be nullified or even reversed'.

The implications for the neuropathology of schizophrenia are clear: any abnormalities, macroscopic or microscopic, are subtle and need to be demonstrated reproducibly in well-controlled studies. This chapter considers which if any of the contemporary claims for structural brain abnormality in schizophrenia can be said to be established beyond reasonable doubt in the light of these requirements (see also Shapiro 1993; Chua and McKenna, 1995). Priority is given to recent MRI and postmortem studies which have, by and large, been carried out in full knowledge of the measures needed to expose small differences against a background of wide variations in normal brain structure.

Overall brain dimensions

Postmortem findings

The most straightforward way of measuring brain size is to weigh it. However, such an approach is not without complications since it can be influenced by cause of death and delay before fixation (see Bruton *et al.*, 1990). Further tissue shrinkage and weight change takes place after the brain is immersed in fixative. Another confounding variable is the presence of coexisting organic pathology such as infarcts and Alzheimer's changes which may obscure any small differences attributable to the disease process of schizophrenia. The only way to avoid this pitfall is to 'purify' samples by excluding brains which show evidence of recognisable pathology (Chapter 14).

Four studies of brain weight in schizophrenia have been carried out; these are shown in Table 13.1. Three found evidence of a decrease (Brown *et al.*, 1986; Pakkenberg, 1987;

Table 13.1 Postmortem studies of overall brain size in schizophrenia

Study	Sample	Matching	Purifica-tion	Findings in schizophrenia	Comment
Brown et al. (1986)	41 patients 29 controls	Age Body weight Height Fixation time	Yes	Trend to reduction in fresh brain weight Fixed brain weight reduced	Controls were patients with affective psychosis
Pakkenberg (1987)	29 patients 30 controls	Age Sex	No	Fixed brain weight reduced	No diagnostic criteria employed. 6 patients had simple schizophrenia, 1 had tertiary syphilis, 1 had history of alcoholism; 18 'demented in final years' but dementia was exclusion criteria for controls
Bruton et al. (1990)	48 patients 56 controls	Sex Aged controlled for	Yes*	Fresh brain weight NSD Fixed brain weight reduced	Brain length also significantly reduced
Heckers et al. (1991b)	23 patients 23 controls	Age Sex Postmortem delay	Yes	Fresh brain weight NSD Fixed brain weight NSD	No differences in brain volume between groups

* Results shown are those for entire sample; for results on purified sample see text. NSD, no significant difference.

Bruton *et al.*, 1990), but one (Heckers *et al.*, 1991*b*) failed to do so. These decreases were small, and surprisingly constant across the studies, ranging from 5 to 8 per cent.

Two of the studies in Table 13.1 face methodological criticisms. In the study of Brown *et al.* (1986) the patients and controls were matched for age, but there were considerable differences in sex distribution (although the direction of these should have tended to minimise any differences between the groups). More importantly, the study used patients with affective psychosis as controls. In Pakkenberg's (1987) study the patients and controls were matched for age and sex, but no formal diagnostic criteria were used. More significantly, neither of the studies purified their samples, and in Pakkenberg's (1987) study 18 of the schizophrenics were described as 'demented in final years' despite dementia being an exclusion criterion for the control group; the neuropathology of their cognitive decline is unknown (Chapters 2 and 14).

The two remaining studies were methodologically scrupulous. Bruton *et al.* (1990) matched their samples for age and sex, and found a significant (4.5 per cent) reduction in fixed brain weight; however there was no significant difference in fresh brain weight. There was also a significant reduction in the length of the brain of 4.5 per cent, which, for reasons mainly related to fixation artefacts, the authors considered to be a possibly more reliable measure than brain weight. The authors then 'purified' the brains by excluding those which had Alzheimer-type changes, cerebrovascular pathology, or focal structural abnormality. When this was done, differences in fixed brain weight and brain length of comparable magnitude remained. (ANCOVA covarying for age and sex on their raw data for 38 purified cases, yields a difference in fixed brain weight at $P = 0.055$ and a difference for brain length at $P = 0.002$). Finally, Heckers *et al.* (1991*b*) compared the brains of 23 schizophrenics meeting DSM III criteria with normal controls individually matched for age and sex; only brains which did not show cerebrovascular or severe senile changes were included. In contrast to Bruton *et al.* (1990) these authors found that neither fresh nor fixed brain weight differed between the patients and controls; nor, after correcting for shrinkage, was there any significant difference in the volume of grey or white matter.

Neuroimaging findings

Some early MRI studies (e.g. Smith *et al.*, 1986; Young *et al.*, 1991) measured the area of a single brain slice and used this as a proxy variable for brain volume. Such an approach is obviously unsatisfactory for exposing small differences. A measure of brain volume can however be obtained by multiplying the area of each of a complete series of MRI slices by the distance between slices; this volumetric technique, which with some minor mathematical refinements is known as stereology, can be highly accurate, especially with the use of current thin-slice technology (e.g. Roberts *et al.*, 1993). It is also possible to segment MR images of brain matter and CSF, and so examine the entire brain volume on a voxel-by-voxel basis without recourse to manually traced regions of interest (e.g. Wright *et al.*, 1995; Chua *et al.*, 1997). MRI studies carried out up to the end of 1998, which used volumetric analysis and employed normal volunteers as comparison subjects (matched or controlling for age and sex) are shown in Table 13.2. Brain size is also a function of head size and overall body size, and varies to a minor extent with ethnicity, intelligence, and

Table 13.2 Volumetric MRI studies of overall brain size in schizophrenia

Study	Sample	Matching	Volumetric technique	Findings in schizophrenia	Comment
Kelsoe et al. (1988)	24 patients 14 controls	Age Sex Height	Summation of 10 mm coronal slices	NSD	—
Barta et al. (1990)	15 patients 15 controls	Age Sex Ethnicity Education	Summation of 5 mm axial slices	NSD	—
Shenton et al. (1992)	15 patients 15 controls	Age Sex Head size	Summation of 3 mm axial slices Computerised brain/CSF segmentation	NSD	—
Kawasaki et al. (1993)	20 patients 10 controls	Age Sex Height	Summation of 5 mm coronal and axial slices	NSD	—
Harvey et al. (1993)	48 patients 34 controls	Age Sex, ethnicity, estimated premorbid IQ, head size controlled for	Summation of 5 mm coronal slices	Smaller	Whole cerebral volume not measured
Andreasen et al. (1994b)[1]	52 patients 90 controls	Age Sex controlled for[2] Height controlled for	Summation of 1.5 mm coronal slices Computerised brain/CSF segmentation	Smaller	7 patients had a history of drug/alcohol abuse Finding remained significant when males only (36 patients and 48 controls) considered
Bilder et al. (1994)	70 patients 51 controls	Age Sex controlled for[2] Parental SES Height controlled for	Summation of 3.1 mm coronal slices Semi-automated quantitation	NSD	First-episode patients

Table 13.2 continued

Study	Sample	Matching	Volumetric technique	Findings in schizophrenia	Comment
Gur et al.[3] (1994)	81 patients 81 controls	Age Sex	Summation of 5 mm axial slices Computerised brain/CSF segmentation	Smaller	—
Schlaepfer et al. (1994)	46 patients 60 controls	Age Sex Parental SES	Summation of 5 mm axial slices Computerised grey matter/white matter/CSF segmentation	NSD	Trend to smaller brain volume in patients
Flaum et al. (1995)	102 patients 87 controls	Age Sex and height controlled for	Summation of 5 mm coronal slices	NSD	—
Nopoulos et al. (1995)	24 patients 24 controls	Age Sex Height Parental SES	Summation of 1.5 mm slices Computerised brain/CSF separation	NSD	First-episode patients
Barta et al. (1997)	28 patients 32 controls	Age Sex Ethnicity Handedness	Summation of 1.5 mm coronal slices	NSD	—
Frangou et al.[4] (1997)	32 patients 39 controls	Age Handedness Sex controlled for	Summation of 1.5 mm coronal slices	NSD	Patients all had familial schizophrenia
Pearlson et al. (1997)	46 patients 60 controls	Age Sex Parental SES	Summation of 5 mm axial slices	NSD	—
Woodruff et al. (1997)	42 patients 43 controls	Age Sex Ethnicity Handedness Paternal SES	Summation of 5 mm coronal slices	NSD	Trend to smaller total cerebral volume in patients became insignificant when minor differences in age controlled for

Table 13.2 continued

Study	Sample	Matching	Volumetric technique	Findings in schizophrenia	Comment
Buchanan et al. 1998	18 patients 24 controls	Age Sex Ethnicity Parental SES	Summation of 1.5 mm coronal slices	NSD	—
Gur et al. (1998a)	96 patients 128 controls	Age Sex Parental education	Summation of 1 mm axial slices Semi-automated quantitation	Smaller in males	—
Cannon et al. (1998)	75 patients 56 controls	Age Sex Social class	Summation of 5 mm axial slices	Smaller GM and WM	—
Whitworth et al. (1998)	30 patients (chronic) 41 patients (first episode) 32 controls	Age Sex (all male) Height Parental education	Summation of 1 mm coronal slices Semi-automated quantitation	Smaller in chronic patients NSD for first-episode patients	Overall findings for patients versus controls not given

[1] Includes patients and controls from Andreasen et al. (1994a).
[2] Authors considered that covarying for height was sufficient to deal with lack of sex matching (see also comment).
[3] Includes patients and controls from Gur et al. (1991).
[4] Includes patients and controls from Sharma et al. (1998).
GM, grey matter; NSD, no significant difference; SES, socioeconomic status; WM, white matter.

educational achievement, and so many of the studies matched or controlled for at least some of these variables.

Only four of 20 studies found a significant reduction in overall brain volume (Harvey *et al.*, 1993; Andreasen *et al.*, 1994*b*; Gur *et al.*, 1994; Cannon *et al.*, 1998). One further study found a smaller volume in male but not female patients (Gur *et al.*, 1998a), and another found a volume reduction in chronic but not first-episode patients (Whitworth *et al.*, 1998). This low rate of positive findings is similar to that of a recent review (Lawrie and Abukmeil, 1998) which found significantly smaller brain volume in schizophrenia in only three of 16 studies. Nevertheless these authors noted that 'consistent volume reductions of about 3 per cent' were evident across the studies.

In the absence of a well-replicated finding of altered total brain volume, the debate has shifted towards considering cortical grey matter and subcortical white matter separately. Once again, however, the findings have been inconsistent: some studies (Zipursky *et al.*, 1992; Harvey *et al.*, 1993; Lim *et al.*, 1996; Lauriello *et al.*, 1997; Cannon *et al.*, 1998; Zipursky *et al.*, 1998) have found a generalised reduction in grey matter volume, but others have not (Shenton *et al.*, 1992; Bilder *et al.*, 1994; Schlaepfer *et al.*, 1994; Barta *et al.*, 1997; Sharma *et al.*, 1998).

Lateral ventricular enlargement

Neuroimaging findings

Although lateral ventricular enlargement was found in the majority of over 50 CT scan studies (e.g. see Andreasen *et al.*, 1990*b*; Lewis, 1990; Van Horn and McManus, 1992), as mentioned in the introduction, some of these studies were flawed by the use of medical controls, which could have introduced systematic bias. In fact, when Lewis (1990) reviewed 21 studies which compared schizophrenic patients with control groups made up of prospectively ascertained normal volunteers, only nine were found to show significant lateral ventricular enlargement, with a further three reporting marginal increases. Andreasen *et al.* (1990a) have also drawn attention to a further potential source of bias in the CT scan studies. The measure of ventricular size invariably used in these studies has been ventricle–brain ratio (VBR), i.e. ventricular area divided by brain area on the selected slice. This is acceptable so long as there is no significant difference in cranial or cerebral size between schizophrenic patients and controls; if there is, this would inflate the VBR for the schizophrenic patients by reducing the denominator in the VBR calculation. Perhaps most importantly, the CT scan literature has made it clear that the differences between normal and schizophrenic lateral ventricles are minor. Lateral ventricular size, like overall brain size, is influenced by factors of age, sex, ethnicity, etc., and these therefore have the potential to create 'noise' in any comparison between schizophrenic patients and normal controls. Introducing further noise is the fact that virtually all CT scan studies have used area measures, typically of the slice on which the lateral ventricles are largest; this provides at best only a very approximate guide to true lateral ventricular size and can give rise to random error arising from variation in the slice angulation.

The 'state of the art' in CT scan studies of schizophrenia is represented by two recent studies, both of which illustrate the subtlety and elusiveness of ventricular enlargement. Andreasen *et al.* (1990*b*) compared 108 patients meeting DSM III criteria for schizophrenia with 75 controls who were matched not only for age and sex, but also height, weight, and level of education. VBR was greater in the schizophrenic group than in the controls; however there was a large overlap between the two groups, with only 6 per cent of the patients being more than two standard deviations above the control group mean. The study also found that significant ventricular enlargement was only present in male schizophrenics; the distributions for female patients and controls were almost identical. Jones *et al.* (1994) made lateral ventricular area (and also volume) measures in 121 patients meeting research diagnostic criteria for schizophrenia and 67 prospectively ascertained normal volunteers matched for age but not sex, socioeconomic status (SES), or ethnicity. Using an odds ratio analysis, they found evidence for a linear trend to increased raw lateral ventricular area and volume in the schizophrenic patients. When adjustment for the corresponding intracranial area/volume was made (i.e. when VBR was calculated), this became significant. However, the controls had significantly larger intracranial volumes than the patients which could have made the finding vulnerable to the systematic error noted by Andreasen *et al.* (1990*a*). Further adjustment for sex, social class, and ethnicity—the last two of which were themselves significant determinants of intracranial volume in the controls—increased the significance of the enlargement further in the schizophrenic patients. In this study, in contrast to that of Andreasen *et al.* (1990*b*), no gender effect was found.

An obvious solution to the problems surrounding CT scan studies of the ventricular system in schizophrenia is to use MRI, for which thin-slice technology and volume estimation using stereology has become the rule, so providing a more sensitive tool for detecting small differences. Also, the systematic bias in VBR measurements alluded to by Andreasen *et al.* (1990*a*) can be avoided by comparing raw ventricular volumes or by covarying out any inter-group differences in overall brain or intracranial size. Table 13.3 shows those studies which have employed prospectively ascertained volunteer controls and which have matched their groups for age and sex, or have corrected for these. Most of the studies have also controlled for other factors including height, educational level, SES, and ethnicity. In contrast to the studies of overall brain size, a majority (14 out of 21 studies) have found significant lateral ventricular enlargement, with a further study (Buchsbaum *et al.*, 1997) finding significant enlargement on the left and another (Nopoulos *et al.*, 1995) being equivocal. Enlargement has been found both in studies which compared raw ventricular volume without correction for brain or intracranial volume (six out of eight studies), and in those which corrected for this (11 out of 14 studies). Of the negative studies, one (Jernigan *et al.*, 1991) found a trend to larger overall ventricular volume, and two others (Shenton *et al.*, 1992; Roy *et al.*, 1998) had small sample sizes; this was also true of the study that found only unilateral enlargement (Buchsbaum *et al.*, 1997). In their review, Lawrie and Abukmeil (1998) also noted the predominance of positive studies and found median values for the degree of enlargement of 32 per cent in men and 12 per cent in women.

A notable example of these studies is that of Suddath *et al.* (1990) who compared a series of 15 schizophrenic patients against arguably the best possible control group—their non-schizophrenic monozygotic twins. This study was also methodologically superior in

Table 13.3 Volumetric MRI studies of the lateral ventricles in schizophrenia

Study	Sample	Matching[1]	Volumetric technique	Findings in schizophrenia	Comment
Kelsoe et al. (1988)	24 patients 14 controls	Age Sex Height Brain/intracranial volume	Summation of 10 mm coronal slices	Raw volume larger VBR larger	—
Suddath et al. (1989)	17 patients 17 controls	Age Sex Height Not brain/intracranial volume	Summation of 10 mm coronal slices	Raw volume larger	—
Suddath et al. (1990)	15 patients 15 controls	Age Sex Not brain/intracranial volume	Summation of 5 mm coronal slices	Raw volume larger	Control group consisted of unaffected MZ co-twins
Andreasen et al. (1990a)	54 patients 47 controls	Age Sex Height Education Not brain/intracranial volume	Summation of 10 mm coronal slices	Raw volume larger VBR larger	Breakdown by sex found significant enlargement in male but not female patients
Jernigan et al. (1991)	42 patients 24 controls	Age Sex[2] Education[2] Brain/intracranial volume	Summation of 5 mm axial slices	Raw volume NSD	Trend towards larger ventricular volume in patients. 23 patients also had alcohol or other substance abuse
O'Callaghan et al. (1992)	45 patients 22 controls	Age Sex Not brain/intracranial volume	Summation of 6 mm axial slices	Raw volume larger	—

Table 13.3 continued

Study	Sample	Matching[1]	Volumetric technique	Findings in schizophrenia	Comment
Shenton et al. (1992)	15 patients 15 controls	Age Sex Height Parental SES IQ Brain/intracranial volume	Summation of 3 mm axial slices Computerised brain/CSF segmentation	Raw volume NSD	—
Zipursky et al. (1992, 1994)	22 patients 20 controls	Age Sex Height Estimated premorbid IQ Brain/intracranial volume	Summation of 5 mm axial slices Semi-automated brain/CSF segmentation	Raw volume larger VBR larger	—
Harvey et al. (1993)	48 patients 34 controls	Age Sex, ethnicity, estimated Premorbid IQ Brain/intracranial volume	Summation of 5 mm coronal slices	Raw volume NSD	—
Andreasen et al. (1994b)	52 patients 90 controls	Age Height controlled for[3] Not brain/intracranial volume	Summation of 1.5 mm coronal slices Computerised brain/CSF segmentation	Raw volume larger	7 patients had a history of drug/alcohol abuse Finding remained significant when males only ($n = $ 36 and 48) considered
Gur et al. (1994)[4]	81 patients 81 controls	Age Sex Brain/intracranial volume	Summation of 5 mm axial slices Computerised brain/CSF segmentation	Raw volume larger VBR larger	Increases more marked in female patients

Table 13.3 continued

Study	Sample	Matching[1]	Volumetric technique	Findings in schizophrenia	Comment
Flaum et al. (1995)	102 patients 87 controls	Age Sex controlled for Brain/intracranial volume	Summation of 5 mm coronal slices	Raw volume larger	—
Nopoulos et al. (1995)	24 patients 24 controls	Age Sex Height Parental SES Height used to control for brain/intracranial volume	Summation of 1.5 mm slices Automated brain/CSF separation	Raw volume ?larger (see comment)	Differences significant at $P = 0.04$ using one-tailed test
Barr et al. (1997)	32 patients 42 controls	Sex Age, height and educational level controlled for Brain/intracranial volume	Summation of 3.1 mm coronal slices	Raw volume larger	First-episode patients
Buchsbaum et al. (1997)	11 patients 23 controls	Age Sex Not brain/intracranial volume	Summation of 1.2 mm slices. Semi-automated grey matter/white matter/CSF segmentation	Raw volume larger on left	—
Woodruff et al. (1997)	42 patients 43 controls	Age Sex Ethnicity Paternal SES Not brain/intracranial volume	Summation of 5 mm coronal slices	Raw volume NSD	—
Cannon et al. (1998)	75 patients 56 controls	Age Sex Social class Brain/intracranial volume	5 mm axial slices	Raw volume larger	Patient group included 63 with schizophrenia and 12 with schizoaffective disorder

Table 13.3 continued

Study	Sample	Matching[1]	Volumetric technique	Findings in schizophrenia	Comment
Sharma et al. (1998)	29 patients 39 controls	Age Sex Height Education Parental SES Brain/intracranial volume	Summation of 1.5 mm coronal slices Semi-automated quantitation	Raw volume larger	—
Roy et al. (1998)	22 patients 15 controls	Age Sex Education Brain/intracranial volume	Summation of 5 mm coronal slices	Raw volume NSD	Temporal horns significantly larger in patients
Whitworth et al. (1998)	71 patients 32 controls	Age (all male) Parental education Brain/intracranial volume	Summation of 1 mm coronal slices Semi-automated segmentation	Raw volume larger	—
Zipursky et al. (1998)	77 patients 61 controls	Age Sex Ethnicity Parental SES Brain/intracranial volume	Summation of 3 mm axial slices	Raw volume larger	—

[1] Or, in case of brain/intracranial volume, controlled for where stated.
[2] Means for sex and education similar but not stated if NSD.
[3] Authors considered that covarying for height was sufficient to deal with lack of sex matching (see also comment).
[4] Includes patients of Gur et al. (1991).
MZ, monozygotic; NSD, no significant difference; SES, socioeconomic status; VBR, ventricle - brain ratio.

other aspects of MRI technology (see Hall *et al.*, 1994). As indicated in Table 13.3, significant lateral ventricular volume enlargement was found. In addition, inspecting the scans of each twin pair, an investigator blind to diagnosis was able to pick out the affected twin in 13 of the 15 cases. The differentiation was made on the basis of ventricular size and also sulcal widening. Since Suddath *et al.* (1990), the size of the sample has been increased to 27 pairs (Torrey *et al.*, 1994). The left lateral ventricle was found to be larger in the affected co-twin in 17 of the 27 pairs, and the right lateral ventricle was larger in 13. In three twin pairs, however, the unaffected twin had grossly (90 to 500 per cent) larger ventricles than the affected one.

Regional cerebral volumes

Much of the work here (and in subsequent sections) has been driven by contemporary biological approaches to schizophrenia, where a convergence of evidence from several sources—neurochemical, neurophysiological, and neuropsychological as well as neuroanatomical/neuropathological—has implicated the frontal and temporal lobes as likely sites of dysfunction (e.g. see Gray *et al.*, 1991; Frith, 1992; Shapiro 1993). All the quantitative work in this area is from MRI; very few postmortem studies of regional brain size in schizophrenia have been carried out.

Neuroimaging findings

The relevant studies are summarised in Table 13.4. As previously discussed, only studies which used volumetric techniques and matched for age and sex, or made some effort to control for these, are included. The vast majority examined the relevant structures by employing a 'region of interest' approach, i.e. drawing round the appropriate areas on film or digitised images. Replacing this approach with a more accurate automated method has not proved easy; one such study (Andreasen *et al.*, 1994*a*) is not included in the Table, but is described separately below.

Five of 15 studies (Breier *et al.*, 1992; Harvey *et al.*, 1993; Andreasen *et al.*, 1994*b*; Buchanan *et al.*, 1998; Gur *et al.*, 1998*b*) found a reduction in frontal lobe size, with one study being equivocal (Nopoulos *et al.*, 1995). For the temporal lobe, three out of 21 studies found a significant size reduction bilaterally (Suddath *et al.*, 1989, 1990; Marsh *et al.*, 1997; Gur *et al.*, 1998*b*), plus one with borderline significant findings (Becker *et al.*, 1996). Three studies found smaller volumes unilaterally, either on the left (Suddath *et al.*, 1990; Woodruff *et al.*, 1997) or the right (Harvey *et al.*, 1993). Finally, one study (Andreasen *et al.*, 1994*b*) found no significant temporal lobe volume reductions in a sample of 52 schizophrenics compared to 90 controls, but the 36 male patients did show significant differences compared to the 48 male controls (however, the authors were sceptical about this finding).

Andreasen *et al.* (1994*a*) developed a technique to circumvent the loss of fidelity associated with the region of interest approach. Using the same thin-slice MRI technique and a subset of the patients and controls of Andreasen *et al.* (1994*b*), they linearly transformed their data to yield 'average brains' for 39 male schizophrenics and 47 age-matched male

Table 13.4 MRI studies of frontal and temporal lobe volume in schizophrenia,

Study	Samples	Matching[1]	Volumetric technique	Frontal lobes in schizophrenia	Temporal lobes in schizophrenia	Comment
Kelsoe et al. (1988)	24 patients 14 controls	Age Sex Height Brain/intracranial volume both controlled and not controlled for	Summation of 10 mm coronal slices	NSD	NSD	—
Suddath et al. (1989)	17 patients 17 controls	Age Sex Not brain/intracranial volume	Summation of 10 mm coronal slices	NSD (prefrontal)	Smaller	Temporal lobe differences due to left-sided reduction Differences due to reduction in grey matter
Bogerts et al. (1990a)	34 patients 25 controls	Age Sex and height controlled for Not brain/intracranial volume	Summation of 3 mm coronal slices	—	NSD	Right temporal lobe smaller in males. 7 controls drawn from radiology files
Suddath et al. (1990)	15 patients 15 controls	Age Sex Ethnicity Parental SES Not brain/intracranial volume	Summation of 5 mm coronal slices	NSD	Smaller on left	Control group consisted of unaffected MZ co-twins
Breier et al. (1992)	44 patients 29 controls	Age Sex Not brain/intracranial volume	Summation of 3 mm coronal slices Computerised grey matter/white matter/CSF segmentation	Smaller	—	Differences due to reduction in white matter

Table 13.4 continued

Study	Samples	Matching[1]	Volumetric technique	Frontal lobes in schizophrenia	Temporal lobes in schizophrenia	Comment
Shenton et al. (1992)	15 patients 15 controls	Age Sex Brain/intracranial volume	Summation of 3 mm axial slices Computerised brain/CSF segmentation	—	NSD	—
Swayze et al. (1992)	55 patients 47 controls	Age Sex Height Education	Summation of 10 mm coronal slices	—	NSD	Analysis based on only 5 slices
Harvey et al. (1993)	48 patients 34 controls	Age Sex, ethnicity, estimated premorbid IQ controlled for Brain/intracranial volume	Summation of 5 mm coronal slices	Smaller	Smaller on right	Right temporal lobe difference due to reduction in grey matter
Kawasaki et al. (1993)	20 patients 10 controls	Age Sex Not brain/intracranial volume	Summation of 5 mm coronal and axial slices	NSD	NSD	—
Andreasen et al. (1994b)	52 patients 90 controls	Age Height controlled for[2] Not brain/intracranial volume	Summation of 1.5 mm coronal slices Computerised brain substance and CSF segmentation	Smaller	NSD	7 patients had a history of drug/alcohol abuse. Reduced frontal lobe volume remained significant for males only (36 patients vs 48 controls)
Bilder et al. (1994)	70 patients 51 controls	Age Sex controlled for[2] Parental SES Brain/intracranial volume[2]	Summation of 3.1 mm coronal slices Semi-automated	NSD	NSD	First-episode patients

Table 13.4 continued

Study	Samples	Matching[1]	Volumetric technique	Frontal lobes in schizophrenia	Temporal lobes in schizophrenia	Comment
Zipursky et al. (1994)	22 patients 20 controls	Age Sex Height Ethnicity Handedness Estimated premorbid IQ Brain/intracranial volume	Summation of 3 mm coronal slices	—	NSD	Reduction in temporal lobe grey matter in patients
Flaum et al. (1995)	102 patients 87 controls	Age Sex controlled for Brain/intracranial volume	Summation of 5 mm coronal slices	—	NSD	—
Nopoulos et al. (1995)	24 patients 24 controls	Age Sex Height Parental SES Brain/intracranial volume[2]	Summation of 1.5 mm slices Computerised brain/CSF separation	?Smaller (see comment)	NSD	Frontal lobes significantly smaller at $P = 0.04$ using one-tailed test
Turetsky et al. (1995)	71 patients 77 controls	Age Sex Brain/intracranial volume	Summation of 5 mm axial slices	NSD	NSD	Significant changes in frontal and temporal lobe asymmetry in patients
Vita et al. (1995)	19 patients 15 controls	Age Sex Height Handedness Brain/intracranial volume	Summation of 5 mm slices	NSD	—	—
Wible et al. (1995)	14 patients 15 controls	Age Sex IQ Parental SES Brain/intracranial volume	Summation of 1.5 mm coronal slices	NSD (prefrontal)	—	—

Table 13.4 continued

Study	Samples	Matching[1]	Volumetric technique	Frontal lobes in schizophrenia	Temporal lobes in schizophrenia	Comment
Becker et al. (1996)	20 patients 20 controls	Age Sex (all male) Brain/intracranial volume	Summation of 4 mm coronal slices	—	?	Temporal lobe nearly significantly smaller on right ($P = 0.056$)
Pearlson et al. (1997)	46 patients 60 controls	Age Sex Parental SES Brain/intracranial volume	Summation of 5 mm axial slices	—	NSD	—
Woodruff et al. (1997)	42 patients 43 controls	Age Sex Ethnicity Paternal SES Not brain/intracranial volume	Summation of 5 mm coronal slices	NSD	Smaller on left	Patients had significantly lower estimated premorbid IQ and less years of education, but these not controlled for in analysis
Marsh et al. (1997)	56 patients 52 controls	Age Sex (all male) Brain/intracranial volume	Summation of 3 mm coronal slices Semi-automated brain/ CSF segmentation	—	Smaller (grey and white matter)	Patients had smaller grey matter volume in frontal lobes Entire temporal lobes not measured
Gur et al. (1998a)	40 patients 17 controls	Age Parental education	Summation of 5 mm coronal slices, semi-automated brain/CSF segmentation	Smaller	Smaller	At 30 months follow-up, frontal lobe finding remained but temporal lobe reduced in both groups

Table 13.4 continued

Study	Samples	Matching[1]	Volumetric technique	Frontal lobes in schizophrenia	Temporal lobes in schizophrenia	Comment
Sharma et al. (1998)	29 patients 39 controls	Age Sex Height Education Parental SES Brain/intracranial volume	Summation of 1.5 mm coronal slices Semi-automated segmentation	—	NSD	Relatives, as a separate group, were also NSD
Roy et al. (1998)	22 patients 15 controls	Age Sex Education Brain/intracranial volume	Summation of 5 mm coronal slices, Semi-automated segmentation	—	NSD	—
Buchanan et al. (1998)	18 patients 24 controls	Age Sex Ethnicity Parental SES	3D volume rendering of 1.5 mm coronal slices, Semi-automated segmentation	Smaller	—	—

[1] Or, in case of brain/intracranial volume, controlled for where stated.
[2] Authors considered that covarying for height was sufficient to deal with lack of sex matching, and also to control for brain/intracranial volume.
MZ, monozygotic; NSD, no significant difference; SES, socioeconomic status.

controls. Statistical comparison was then made using a numeric image subtraction technique (statistical parametric mapping) previously developed for functional imaging (PET) studies. Volume reductions of somewhat less than one standard deviation were found in the right frontal lobe white matter and the right temporal and parietal lobe white matter. Unfortunately no significance figures were given.

Temporal lobe limbic structures

Postmortem findings

Histological interest in the temporal lobe limbic structures of hippocampus and amygdala (Chapter 2) began with a report of a disturbance of the orderly palisade-like arrangement of hippocampal pyramidal cells (Scheibel and Kovelman, 1981). Soon afterwards, in the first study to examine the hippocampus and parahippocampal gyrus macroscopically, Bogerts *et al.* (1985) found that these structures 'exhibited such a marked degeneration in half the schizophrenics that the histological sections of them could be recognized during blind evaluation'; a 22 per cent reduction in the volume of amygdala was also noted. Jakob and Beckmann (1986) also claimed to have found evidence of qualitative macroscopic abnormalities in the entorhinal cortex, which forms part of the parahippocampal gyrus.

Quantitative postmortem studies of the hippocampus, amygdala, and entorhinal cortex in schizophrenia are summarised in Table 13.5. Given the typically small numbers in these studies and the irregular shape of the structures concerned, it is unlikely that a simple area measurement could hope to provide a realistic size estimate. However, as with MRI, a volumetric measure can be derived by stereology. Only such studies are, therefore, included. It would also be desirable to include only studies using diagnostic criteria for schizophrenia. However, an exception needs to be made for the studies of Bogerts and co-workers (Bogerts *et al.*, 1985, 1990*b*; Falkai and Bogerts, 1986); these made the diagnosis of schizophrenia only according to the loose guidelines of ICD 9, but were otherwise methodologically superior and played an important role in the development of the field. Having made an exception for these studies it would be unfair to exclude the study of Jeste and Lohr (1989) in which only half of the patients met DSM III criteria due to insufficient detail in the case notes.

Three of six studies (Bogerts *et al.*, 1985, 1990*b*; Falkai and Bogerts, 1986) found a significant reduction in the volume of the hippocampus, with one further study (Jeste and Lohr, 1989) finding a trend. None of these studies employed purification, and three (Bogerts *et al.*, 1985; 1990*b*; Falkai and Bogerts, 1986) also failed to match for gender. Findings for the amygdala and parahippocampal gyrus are likewise mixed and there are too few studies to judge the replicability of findings. In general it is noteworthy that all the positive findings were in studies which failed to employ diagnostic crieria for schizophrenia.

Neuroimaging findings

These studies have several advantages over postmortem studies, not the least being that death ceases to be a rate-limiting step for recruitment, and that elderly subjects with their concomitant high rates of additional brain pathology can be avoided. Nevertheless, an

Table 13.5 Postmortem studies of volume of temporal lobe limbic structures in schizophrenia

Study	Sample	Matching	Purification	Hippocampus in schizophrenia	Amygdala in schizophrenia	Parahippocampal gyrus in schizophrenia	Comment
Bogerts et al. (1985)	13 patients 9 controls	Age PM delay	No	Smaller	Smaller	Smaller	Hippocampus and parahippocampal gyrus smaller to naked eye in half of patients
Falkai & Bogerts (1986); Falkai et al. (1988)	13 patients 11 controls	Age PM delay	No	Smaller	—	Smaller (entorhinal cortex)	—
Jeste & Lohr (1989)	13 patients 16 controls	Age Sex PM delay	No[1]	Trend to smaller volumes in each of 4 sectors	—	—	Only half sample met DSM III criteria
Bogerts et al. (1990b)	18 patients 20 controls	Age PM delay Fixation time	No	Smaller	—	—	—
Heckers et al. (1990a)	18 patients 18 controls	Age Sex PM delay Fixation time	Yes	—	—	NSD	—
Heckers et al. (1990b)	20 patients 20 controls	Age Sex PM delay Fixation time	Yes	NSD	NSD	—	—
Heckers et al. (1991b)	13 patients 13 controls	Age Sex	Yes	NSD	—	—	—

[1] Paper states only that controls showed no evidence of gross or microscopic abnormality.
NSD, no significant difference; PM, postmortem.

obstacle remains in that manual or semi-manual tracing of regions of interest is still the only means of measurement and the complexity of the structures concerned can lead to unreliability. For example, in one study (Flaum *et al.*, 1995) test–retest reliabilities for the same individual were only 0.64 for the hippocampus, and were so low for the amygdala (0.23), that the data were not analysed.

The relevant studies, once again those using volumetric techniques and matching or controlling for at least age and sex, are shown in Table 13.6. Six of the 20 studies found bilateral hippocampal volume reductions (Suddath *et al.*, 1990; Bogerts *et al.*, 1993; Flaum *et al.*, 1995; Fukazako *et al.*, 1996; Becker *et al.*, 1996; Whitworth *et al.*, 1998) and three found a left-sided reduction (Breier *et al.*, 1992; Barr *et al.*, 1997; Woodruff *et al.*, 1997). A case can be made for a left-sided volume reduction in one further study (Shenton *et al.*, 1992), as the anterior hippocampus was included in this study's measure of the amygdala (which was significantly smaller on the left). Four of nine studies found volume reductions of the amygdala. Three of four studies examining the parahippocampal gyrus found it to be significantly smaller, either bilaterally (Shenton *et al.*, 1992) or on the left (Kawasaki *et al.*, 1993; Pearlson *et al.*, 1997).

The study of Suddath *et al.* (1990) is again of interest. On comparing prefrontal and temporal grey and white matter volumes across 15 monozygotic twin pairs, the only significant difference found was a smaller volume of grey matter in the left temporal lobe in the affected co-twin ($P < 0.002$). Further analysis revealed that this was due to significant volume reductions in the left hippocampus ($P = 0.006$); there was also a significant volume reduction in the right hippocampus ($P = 0.01$). No differences were found for the amygdala. Hippocampal volume was smaller in the affected twin in 14 out of the 15 pairs on the left side, and 13 out of 15 on the right. In the extended series of 27 twin pairs, the affected co-twin had a smaller hippocampus–amygdala complex in 21 cases on the left and in 22 cases on the right (Torrey *et al.*, 1994). The authors concluded that 'reduction in the size of the hippocampus–amygdala appears to be a better predictor of which twin is affected with schizophrenia than is enlargement of the cerebral ventricles'.

Other brain structures

Planum temporale

The superior temporal gyrus, and its posterior upper surface, the planum temporale, has attracted close scrutiny in schizophrenia because of its role in normal speech and language, and the possible importance of this for psychotic symptoms like formal thought disorder and auditory hallucinations (e.g. Frith, 1992). This brain region is also of interest from the perspective of neurodevelopmental theories of schizophrenia (e.g. Chua and Murray, 1996) because it is normally asymmetrical (left larger than right) from the 30th week of gestation onwards (Chapter 6).

MRI studies which have conducted quantitative analyses of the superior temporal gyrus or planum temporale are shown in Table 13.7. Three of 13 studies (Shenton *et al.*, 1992; Zipursky *et al.*, 1994; Pearlson *et al.*, 1997) have found a size reduction of the superior temporal gyrus bilaterally or unilaterally, with two more (Menon *et al.*, 1995; Marsh *et al.*,

Table 13.6 Volumetric MRI studies of temporal lobe limbic structures in schizophrenia

Study	Sample	Matching[1]	Volumetric technique	Hippocampus in schizophrenia	Amygdala in schizophrenia	Parahippocampal gyrus in schizophrenia	Comment
Kelsoe et al. (1988)	24 patients 14 controls	Age Sex Height Brain/intracranial volume controlled and not controlled for	Summation of 10 mm coronal slices	NSD (hippocampal–amygdala complex)		—	Patients had non-significantly larger amygdala/hippocampus
Bogerts et al. (1990a)	34 patients 25 controls	Age Height and sex controlled for Not brain/intracranial volume	Summation of 3 mm coronal slices	NSD	NSD	—	Significant reduction in left hippocampal volume in male patients
Suddath et al. (1990)	15 patients 15 controls	Age Sex Not brain/intracranial volume	Summation of 5 mm coronal slices	Smaller	—	—	—
Breier et al. (1992)	44 patients 29 controls	Age Sex Parental SES Not brain/intracranial volume	Summation of 3 mm coronal slices	Smaller on left	Smaller	—	—
Hoff et al. (1992)	52 patients 30 controls	Age Sex Brain/intracranial volume	Summation of 5 mm coronal slices	NSD	NSD	—	—
Shenton et al. (1992)	15 patients 15 controls	Age Sex Brain/intracranial volume	Summation of 3 mm axial slices	?NSD (see comment)	Smaller	Smaller on left	Amygdala measure included anterior hippocampus

Table 13.6 continued

Study	Sample	Matching[1]	Volumetric technique	Hippocampus in schizophrenia	Amygdala in schizophrenia	Parahippo-campal gyrus in schizophrenia	Comment
Swayze et al. (1992)	55 patients 47 controls	Age Sex Education Height Not brain/intracranial volume	Summation of 10 mm coronal slices	NSD	—	—	—
Bogerts et al. (1993)	19 patients 18 controls	Age Sex Height and education controlled for Not brain/intracranial volume	Summation of 3 mm coronal slices	Smaller	NSD	—	Hippocampus included only posterior part; amygdala included anterior part of hippocampus
Kawasaki et al. (1993)	20 patients 10 controls	Age Sex Not brain/intracranial volume	Summation of 5 mm coronal and axial slices	NSD	NSD	Smaller on left	—
Rossi et al. (1994b)	19 patients 14 controls	Age Sex (all male) Height Education Not brain/intracranial volume	Summation of 5 mm coronal slices Semi-automated segmentation	NSD (posterior)	Smaller (included anterior hippocampus)		—
Zipursky et al. (1994)	22 patients 20 controls	Age Sex Premorbid IQ Brain/intracranial volume	Summation 3 mm coronal slices	NSD	—	—	—

Table 13.6 continued

Study	Sample	Matching[1]	Volumetric technique	Hippocampus in schizophrenia	Amygdala in schizophrenia	Parahippo-campal gyrus in schizophrenia	Comment
Flaum et al. (1995)	102 patients 87 Controls	Age Sex controlled for Brain/intracranial volume	Summation of 3 mm coronal slices	Smaller	—	—	Reliability of hippocampal measure only fair
Fukazako et al. (1996)	18 patients 18 controls	Age Sex (all male) Brain/intracranial volume both controlled for and not controlled for	Summation of 1 mm coronal slices	Smaller	—	—	—
Becker et al. (1996)	20 patients 20 controlls	Age Sex (all male) Brain/intracranial volume	Summation of 4 mm coronal slices	Smaller (posterior)	NSD (included anterior hippocampus)	—	
Barr et al. (1997)	32 patients 42 controls	Sex Age, height and eduation controlled for Brain/intracranial volume	Summation of 3.1 mm coronal slices	Smaller on left	—	—	First-episode patients
Pearlson et al. (1997)	46 patients 60 controls	Age Sex Parental SES Brain/intracranial volume	Summation of 5 mm axial slices	NSD	Smaller	Smaller	—

Table 13.6 *continued*

Study	Sample	Matching[1]	Volumetric technique	Hippocampus in schizophrenia	Amygdala in schizophrenia	Parahippocampal gyrus in schizophrenia	Comment
Woodruff et al. (1997)	42 patients 43 controls	Age Sex Ethnicity Paternal SES Not brain/intracranial volume	Summation of 5 mm coronal slices	Smaller on left	—	NSD	Patients had significantly lower estimated premorbid IQ and less years of education, but these not controlled for in analysis
Marsh et al. (1997)	56 patients 52 controls	Sex (all male) Age Brain/intracranial volume	Summation of 3 mm coronal slices, semi-automated segmentation	NSD	—	—	Entire hippocampal volume not measured
Hirayasu et al. (1998)	17 patients 18 controls	Age Handedness Parental SES Brain/intracranial Volume	Summation of 1.5 mm coronal slices Semi-automated segmentation	NSD	—	—	Patients had smaller GM volume of the left posterior amygdala–hippocampal complex
Whitworth et al. (1998)	71 patients 32 controls	Age Sex (all male) Parental education	Summation of 1 mm coronal slices Semi-automated segmentation	Smaller	—	—	—

[1] Or in case of brain/intracranial volume, controlled for where stated.

GM, grey matter; NSD, no significant difference; SES, socioeconomic status.

Table 13.7 MRI studies of the planum temporale (PT) and superior temporal gyrus (STG) in schizophrenia

Study	Sample	Matching[1]	MRI measure(s)	STG in schizophrenia	PT in schizophrenia	Altered asymmetry	Comment
Rossi et al. (1992)	20 patients 12 controls	Age Sex Handedness Educational level Not brain/intracranial volume	Area	—	Smaller on left	Yes	Patients showed larger right PT
Shenton et al. (1992)	15 patients 15 controls	Age Sex Height Parental SES IQ Brain/intracranial volume	Volume	Smaller on left	—	No	Patients but not controls showed significant STG asymmetry
DeLisi et al. (1994)	85 patients 40 controls	Age Sex SES Brain/intracranial volume	Area	NSD	NSD	No	—
Kleinschmidt et al. (1994)	26 patients 26 controls	Sex Height Handedness Not brain/intracranial volume[2]	Area	—	NSD	No	Samples not age-matched
Rossi et al. (1994a)	22 patients 23 controls	Age Sex Height Handedness Educational level Not brain/intracranial volume[2]	Area	—	NSD	No	—

Table 13.7 continued

Study	Sample	Matching[1]	MRI measure(s)	STG in schizophrenia	PT in schizophrenia	Altered asymmetry	Comment
Zipursky et al. (1994)	22 patients 20 controls	Age Sex Height Handedness Premorbid IQ Brain/intracranial volume	Volume	Smaller	—	No	—
Flaum et al. (1995)	102 patients 87 controls	Age Handedness Sex controlled for Brain/intracranial volume	Volume	Larger on right	—	No	—
Kulynych et al. (1995, 1996)	12 patients 12 controls	Age Sex Handedness Brain/intracranial volume	Area (PT) Volume (STG)	NSD	NSD	No	—
Menon et al. (1995)	20 patients 20 controls	Age Sex Ethnicity Handedness Parental SES Brain/intracranial volume	Volume	NSD (total) Smaller (GM)	—	No	—
Petty et al. (1995)	14 patients 14 controls	Age Sex Handedness Parental SES Not brain/intracranial volume[2]	Area	—	Smaller on left (+ larger on right)	Yes	Reversal of normal asymmetry in patients
Vita et al. (1995)	19 patients 15 controls	Age Sex Height Handedness Brain/intracranial volume	Volume	NSD	—	No	—

Table 13.7 *continued*

Study	Sample	Matching[1]	MRI measure(s)	STG in schizophrenia	PT in schizophrenia	Altered asymmetry	Comment
Barta et al. (1997)	28 patients 32 controls	Age Sex Handedness Brain/intracranial volume	Area and volume	—	Area smaller Volume NSD	Yes	Reversal of normal PT asymmetry
Frangou et al. (1997)	32 patients 39 controls	Age Handedness Sex controlled for Brain/intracranial volume	Volume	NSD	NSD	No	Patients all had familial schizophrenia
Jacobsen et al. (1997)	16 patients 16 controls	Age Sex Handedness Brain/intracranial volume	Area	—	NSD	No	Patients had childhood-onset schizophrenia
Pearlson et al. (1997)	46 patients 60 controls	Age Sex Parental SES Brain/intracranial volume	Volume	Smaller	—	Yes	Reversal of normal STG asymmetry
Woodruff et al. (1997)	42 patients 43 controls	Age Sex Ethnicity Parental SES Not brain/intracranial volume	Volume	NSD	—	—	Patients had significantly lower estimated premorbid IQ and less education, but these not controlled for in analysis
Hirayasu et al. (1998)	17 patients 18 controls	Age Parental SES Intracranial volume	Volume	NSD	—	Yes	Patients had smaller GM volume in left posterior STG

Table 13.7 *continued*

Study	Sample	Matching[1]	MRI measure(s)	STG in schizophrenia	PT in schizophrenia	Altered asymmetry	Comment
Marsh et al. (1997)	56 patients 52 controls	Age Sex Handedness Intracranial volume	Volume	Smaller GM volume in STG bilaterally	—	No	—
Roy et al. (1998)	22 patients 15 controls	Age Sex Education Intracranial volume	Volume	NSD	—	—	—

[1]Or, in case of brain/intracranial volume, controlled for where stated.
[2]Authors used laterality coefficient as a substitute for controlling for overall differences in brain size. GM, grey matter; NSD, no significant difference; ROI, region of interest; SES, socioeconomic status.

1997) finding a significant reduction in grey matter, but not overall volume. Only two of nine studies (Rossi *et al.*, 1992; Petty *et al.*, 1995) found a reduction in planum temporale size; this was on the left side only in both cases (accompanied in the latter study by a significant size increase on the right). Barta *et al.* (1997) had equivocal results, finding reduced area but unchanged volume. Findings of significantly altered asymmetry are likewise in a minority, being present in five of 17 studies.

Planum temporale size has been reported in one postmortem study (Falkai *et al.*, 1995). 24 schizophrenic patients were compared with 24 normal controls matched for age, sex, and postmortem delay, but not for handedness. Altered asymmetry was found based on a measure of volume, but not in terms of an area measure (see also Chapter 6).

Basal ganglia

Four postmortem studies have measured the volume of one or more basal ganglia structures (Bogerts *et al.*, 1985, 1990*b*; Pakkenberg, 1990; Heckers *et al.*, 1991*b*). A smaller internal segment of the globus pallidus was found in two of these (Bogerts *et al.*, 1985, 1990*b*), but the samples were not sex matched nor purified, and the diagnosis of schizophrenia was made according to ICD 9. A third study (Pakkenberg, 1990) failed to replicate the finding, and the fourth (Heckers *et al.*, 1991*b*) found the whole globus pallidus to be increased in size. Size reductions of the caudate nucleus and putamen were not found in any of the studies, but one (Heckers *et al.*, 1991) found increased striatal volume. A smaller nucleus accumbens was found in one study (Pakkenberg, 1990) but not in two others (Bogerts *et al.*, 1985, 1990*b*).

The few MRI studies of basal ganglia have been inconsistent. There are reports of a larger lenticular nucleus (Jernigan *et al.*, 1991) and a larger left caudate nucleus (Breier *et al.* 1992). Follow-up studies of patients with first-episode schizophrenia (Chakos *et al.*, 1994; Keshavan *et al.*, 1994) have found volume increases in the caudate nuclei of 6 to 15 per cent, which may be due to neuroleptics (Chapter 15); larger caudate nucleus volumes are also seen in subjects with major depression treated with neuroleptics compared to those untreated (Doraiswamy *et al.*, 1995). However, Gur *et al.* (1998*b*) found no difference in the basal ganglia volumes of neuroleptic-treated and neuroleptic-naive patients. Finally, two recent studies report reduced caudate nucleus volumes in first-episode cases (Keshavan *et al.*, 1998; Shihabuddin *et al.*, 1998).

Histological findings

Historically, postmortem studies have taken the form of intensive examinations of restricted cerebral regions in small numbers of cases, and have sought to demonstrate unique, qualitative abnormalities; issues of quantitation, blindness, and appropriateness of controls were not uppermost in neuropathologists' minds for most of the twentieth century. However, it has been evident from at least the time of David's (1957) review that any microscopic neuropathology in schizophrenia is not going to yield to such an approach, and will probably need to be understood as subtle differences, for example in cell numbers, density, or size. This latter approach has methodological requirements which overlap with those affecting macroscopic studies, such as rigorous diagnosis of schizophrenia and careful matching of patients and controls; however, in one area, quantitation, there are unique issues concerning the differentiation of neurons from glia, the effects of tissue shrinkage, and the use of measures of cell density versus cell number (see Chapters 2 and 14; Dwork, 1997; Heckers, 1997).

The main contemporary histological abnormalities claimed in schizophrenia include, in roughly descending order of popularity, the following: absence of gliosis; hippocampal pyramidal cell disarray; other evidence of cytoarchitectonic disorganisation, especially in the parahippocampal gyrus and frontal cortex; decreased neuron number in the frontal cortex, anterior cingulate gyrus, entorhinal cortex, and hippocampus; and finally reduced cell size in the hippocampus and some other areas. The findings with respect to gliosis are consistently negative and so will not be discussed further (Chapter 5). The other findings are summarised in Tables 13.8 and 13.9.

A widely investigated neuropathological finding in schizophrenia has been hippocampal pyramidal cell disarray, a disturbance of the palisade-like arrangement of the pyramidal cells and irregularity of their dendritic domains, first reported by Scheibel and Kovelman (1981). In the wake of this, other findings concerning hippocampal cell numbers and size followed. Table 13.8 shows that none of the findings has been consistently replicated. When only the studies using automated or semi-automated methods of measurement are considered, as advocated by Benes (1988), positive findings for pyramidal cell disarray, in particular, are evident in only one of five studies (Conrad et al., 1991).

Jakob and Beckmann (1986) reported disturbed cytoarchitecture and reduced cell numbers in the entorhinal cortex in a qualitative and essentially uncontrolled study. As can be seen from Table 13.9, these findings are also poorly replicated. It is noteworthy that an initial replication of disturbed cytoarchitecture in this area of cortex by Arnold et al. (1991) was not confirmed in a subsequent, quantitative study from the same group (Arnold et al., 1995; see Chapter 2).

The anterior cingulate cortex has been investigated by Benes and coworkers in a series of studies, each of which has had some positive findings concerning cell numbers or organisation (Chapter 3). However, it is important to note that all of these findings await replication. In addition, two of the studies (Benes et al., 1986, 1991a) tested multiple areas and few if any of the findings would have remained significant if the authors had controlled for multiple comparisons.

Histological studies of the prefrontal cortex have found decreases, increases, and no change in the number and/or density of neurons, and overall there is little to suggest consistent change. In a recent series of studies, Akbarian and coworkers (Akbarian et al. 1993a, 1996) found reductions in the density of nicotinamide adenine dinucleotide phosphate-diaphorase (NADPH-D) positive neurons in the prefrontal neocortex with greater numbers in the underlying white matter. These authors have interpreted these and somewhat similar findings in the temporal cortex (Akbarian et al., 1993b) as indicating disordered migration of embryonic neurons. These studies have attracted much interest and have significant implications for developmental theories of schizophrenia (Chapter 8). However, they have been criticised by Dwork (1997), on the grounds that in two of the studies (Akbarian et al.,

Table 13.8 Histological abnormalities in the hippocampus in schizophrenia

Study	Sample	Matching	Morphometry method	Pyramidal neuron disarray in schizophrenia	Neuronal number/density in schizophrenia	Pyramidal neuron size in schizophrenia	Comment
Kovelman & Scheibel (1984)	10 patients 8 controls	Age Sex	Manual	Increased	NSD	—	2 patients were leucotomised and 1 had epilepsy
Falkai & Bogerts (1986)	13 patients 11 controls	Age	Manual	—	Reduced	—	—
Jeste & Lohr (1989)	13 patients 16 controls	Age Sex Brain weight	Semi-automated	—	NSD	—	Only 7 patients met DSM III criteria. Patients had significantly lower cell densities compared to 16 non-leucotomised controls in 2 of 4 subfields
Christison et al. (1989)	17 leuco-tomised patients, 14 leuco-tomised controls	Age	Semi-automated	NSD	—	NSD	Only 9 patients met RDC criteria. Similar findings when compared to 18 non-leucotomised controls
Altshuler et al. (1987)	7 patients 6 controls	Age Sex	Semi-automated	NSD	—	—	No diagnostic criteria used. 2 controls had neurological disease

Table 13.8 continued

Study	Sample	Matching	Morphometry method	Pyramidal neuron disarray in schizophrenia	Neuronal number/ density in schizophrenia	Pyramidal neuron size in schizophrenia	Comment
Conrad et al. (1991)	11 patients 7 controls	Age Sex	Automated	Increased	—	—	No diagnostic criteria used; 2 patients had history of seizures, 1 leucotomised
Benes et al. (1991b)	14 patients 9 controls	Age	Manual	NSD	NSD	Smaller	—
Heckers et al. (1991a)	13 patients 13 controls	Age Sex Fixation time controlled for	Manual	—	NSD	—	—
Arnold et al. (1995)	14 patients 17 controls	Age Sex PM delay Fixation	Automated	NSD	NSD	Smaller (see comment)	Neurons smaller in 1 of 4 subregions in patients
Zaidel et al. (1997a)	14 patients 10 controls	Age PM delay Fixation time	Semi-automated	NSD	—	Smaller (see comment)	Neurons smaller in left CA1, left CA2 and right CA3
Zaidel et al. (1997b)	22 patients 17 controls	Age PM delay Fixation time	Manual	—	NSD or increased (see comment)	—	Cell density increased in right CA1 and CA3. Loss of normal asymmetrical correlations in neuronal density
Benes et al. (1998)	10 patients 11 controls	Age PM delay	Manual	—	NSD for pyramidal neurons; reduced for other neurons	—	—

NSD, no significant difference; PM, postmortem; RDC, Research Diagnostic Criteria.

Table 13.9 Other histological findings in schizophrenia

Study	Sample	Matching	Morphometry method	Neuronal number/density in schizophrenia	Neuronal disarray in schizophrenia	Other findings	Comments
Entorhinal cortex							
Falkai et al. (1988)	13 patients 11 controls	Age PM delay	Manual	Reduced	—	—	—
Arnold et al. (1995)	6 leucomised patients 16 controls	None	Qualitiative assessment only	—	Yes	Abnormal invaginations of surface	Only 4 patients met diagnostic criteria. Controls were mixed neurosurgical patients and normals
Arnold et al. (1995)	14 patients 10 controls	Age Sex PM delay Fixation time	Computerised image analysis	NSD	No	Cell size smaller in 1 of 3 layers studied	—
Akil & Lewis (1997)	10 patients 10 contols	Age Sex PM delay	Qualitative assessment only	—	No	—	—
Krimer et al. (1997)	14 patients 14 controls	Age	Manual	NSD	No	—	—
Anterior cingulate cortex							
Benes et al. (1986)	10 patients 10 controls	Age PM delay and fixation time controlled for	Manual	Lower in 1 of 6 cortical layers (layer V)	—	—	—

Table 13.9 *continued*

Study	Sample	Matching	Morphometry method	Neuronal number/density in schizophrenia	Neuronal disarray in schizophrenia	Other findings	Comments
Benes & Bird (1987)	10 patients 10 controls	Age PM delay and fixation time controlled for	Semi-automated	—	Increase in 1 of 6 layers (layer III)	—	—
Benes et al. (1991a)	18 patients 12 controls	Age PM delay and fixation time controlled for	Manual	Interneurons reduced in 5 of 6 layers (layer II–VI)	—	—	Not clear that findings would have survived Bonferroni correction
Prefrontal cortex							
Benes et al. (1986)	10 patients 10 controls	Age PM delay and fixation time controlled for	Manual	Reduced in 1 of 6 cortical layers (layer VI)	—	—	Not clear that finding would have survived Bonferroni correction
Benes & Bird (1987)	10 patients 10 controls	Age PM delay and fixation time controlled for	Semi-automated	—	NSD	—	—
Benes et al. (1991a)	18 patients 12 controls	Age PM delay and fixation time controlled for	Manual	Pyramidal cells increased in 1 of 6 cortical layers (layer V)	—	Interneurons smaller in 1 of 6 layers (layer II)	—

Table 13.9 continued

Study	Sample	Matching	Morphometry method	Neuronal number/density in schizophrenia	Neuronal disarray in schizophrenia	Other findings	Comments
Pakkenberg (1993)	8 patients 16 controls	Age PM delay	Manual	NSD	—	—	Also NSD for neuronal numbers in temporal, parietal, and occipital cortex
Akbarian et al. (1995)	10 patients 10 controls	Age Sex PM delay	Manual	NSD	—	—	—
Selemon et al. (1995)	16 patients 19 controls	Age PM delay	Semi-automated	Increased	—	—	Finding of questionable significance (MANOVA insignificant, *post hoc* testing significant)
Rajkowska et al. (1998)	9 patients 10 controls	Age PM delay Fixation time	Manual	—	—	?Smaller (trend across all layers + significantly smaller in layer III)	Subset of patients of Selemon et al. (1995)
Selemon et al. (1998)	9 patients 10 controls	Age PM delay Fixation time	Manual	Increased (layers II, III, IV and VI)	—	—	Subset of patients of Selemon et al. (1995)

NSD, no significant difference; PM, postmortem.

1993*a,b*) the authors treated several different measurements obtained on each subject as an independent variable, i.e. when 10 measurements were obtained on each of seven subjects, the sample size was treated as 70 instead of seven, so drastically affecting calculations of statistical significance.

Conclusions

Having taken as its starting point the review by David (1957), and having faithfully followed his sceptical approach, it is appropriate to continue in the same vein and ask: what would David have made of the state of the field 40 years on?

David's initial reaction might well be a slight sense of dismay that he had been dismissive of the structural neuroimaging findings in schizophrenia. While the air encephalographic studies he reviewed and a number of subsequent studies had obvious methodological shortcomings, one of their main findings, of ventricular enlargement, was prophetic. This abnormality re-emerged immediately in CT studies where, notwithstanding embarrassing revelations about selection of controls, it has always enjoyed a favourable balance of positive to negative replications. The most recent wave of MRI studies establish the reality of lateral ventricular enlargement in schizophrenia beyond any reasonable doubt (Chapter 1).

David would have found it difficult not to be impressed by the MRI studies of schizophrenia whose sophistication, careful attention to confounding factors, and in some cases large sample sizes places them, as a group, above methodological reproach. This same scientific probity, however, appears to have left few survivors among the other candidates for structural brain abnormality. The minority of positive findings for overall brain volume (four of 20 studies), volume of the frontal lobe (five or six of 15 studies), and volume of the temporal lobe (six or seven of 21 studies) point to size reductions which, if they are present at all, are at the limit of detectability. It is true, as Lawrie and Abukmeil (1998) have suggested, that 'vote counting' of studies can conceal genuine abnormalities, and that volume reductions of 3 to 5 per cent have been consistently found across the above studies. But whether there are significant size differences requires meta-analysis for an answer. A single meta-analysis of overall brain size in schizophrenia has been carried out (Ward *et al.*, 1996), and this found a significant overall effect size of -0.26 ($P < 0.0001$)—this falls into the range designated 'small' for behavioural science (Cohen, 1988). However, this meta-analysis included CT and postmortem studies as well as MRI studies, and included not just volumetric studies, but studies using area measurements of a single slice, and in one case brain length. The balance of evidence in favour of volume reductions is not much better for the hippocampus (nine to 10 out of 20 studies) or the amygdala (four out of nine studies). However, a recent meta-analysis of nearly the same set of hippocampal MRI studies (Nelson *et al.*, 1998) found consistent evidence for a volume reduction of approximately 4 per cent bilaterally, which was significant at $P < 0.001$, with a moderate effect size of 0.4.

Faced with the contemporary evidence—or lack of it—for histological abnormality in schizophrenia, David might well have felt a sense of *déjà vu*. The more important question here, however, is whether he would have been impressed by the methodological improvements to postmortem studies of schizophrenia which his review made abundantly clear were needed and whose importance has been regularly rehearsed since. Sadly, the answer to this question must be, almost certainly not. Having been rescued from their much quoted status as the graveyard of neuropathology, postmortem studies of schizophrenia continue to be dogged by an informal and even sometimes casual approach, where sample sizes of less than 10 are considered acceptable, in which matching is often dealt with cursorily, and whose authors commonly seem to regard lack of replication as no obstacle to validity. David probably would have found little to disagree with in the following quote from a recent review of the hippocampal findings by Dwork (1997): 'The postmortem studies have been widely accepted, in aggregate, as demonstrating conclusively that in schizophrenia there is *some* abnormality in the hippocampal formation. They are often cited in other articles . . . reporting clinical, radiologic, and experimental evidence of hippocampal abnormality. Unquestioning acceptance of postmortem abnormalities, however, ignores several well-designed negative studies, as well as the mutual contradictions to be found among the various positive reports.'

It has been known for a long time that the brain looks normal or relatively normal in schizophrenia and so demonstration of an underlying neuropathology was always going to present a challenge, and the field was sure to be littered with the perished fruit of others' labours. Nevertheless, despite the many false starts and red herrings, it is important not to lose sight of the fact that one important objective has been achieved: the evidence for lateral ventricular enlargement, and perhaps also reduced hippocampal size, disproves the null hypothesis that there is *no* neuropathology of schizophrenia. Other abnormalities that underlie, give rise to, or are otherwise associated with, these changes, must exist. Whatever these ultimately turn out to be, surely it will not prove to be beyond the wit of researchers to uncover them sooner or later?

Acknowledgements

S. E. C. was supported by a grant from the CRCG, the University of Hong Kong. Irving Gottesman and Paul Griffiths provided helpful comments on the manuscript. The authors thank Miss Isabel W. S. Lam for her assistance in the preparation of the manuscript.

References

Akbarian, S., Bunney, W. E., Potkin, S. G. *et al.* (1993*a*) Altered distribution of nicoti-namide-adenine dinucleotide phosphate-diaphorase cells in frontal lobe of schizophrenics implies disturbances of cortical development. *Archives of General Psychiatry* **50**, 169–177.

Akbarian, S., Viela, A., Kim, J. J. *et al.* (1993*b*) Distorted distribution of nicotinamide-adenine dinucleotide phosphate-diaphorase neurons in temporal lobe of schizophrenics implies anomalous cortical development. *Archives of General Psychiatry* **50**, 178–187.

Akbarian, S., Kim, J. J., Potkin, S. E. *et al.* (1995) Gene expression for glutamic acid decarboxlase is reduced without loss of neurons in prefrontal cortex of schizophrenics. *Archives of General Psychiatry* **52**, 258–266.

Akbarian, S., Kim, J. J., Potkin, S. E. *et al.* (1996) Maldistribution of interstitial neurons in prefrontal white matter of the brains of schizophrenic patients. *Archives of General Psychiatry* **53**, 425–436.

Akil, M., Lewis, D. A. (1997) Cytoarchitecture of the entorhinal cortex in schizophrenia. *American Journal of Psychiatry* **154**, 1010–1012.

Altshuler, L. L., Conrad, A., Kovelman, J. A. *et al.* (1987) Hippocampal pyramidal cell orientation in schizophrenia: a controlled neurohistologic study of the Yakovlev Collection. *Archives of General Psychiatry* **44**, 1094–1098.

Andreasen, N. C., Ehrhardt, J. C., Swayze, V. W. *et al.* (1990*a*) Magnetic resonance imaging of the brain in schizophrenia: the pathophysiologic significance of structural abnormalities. *Archives of General Psychiatry* **47**, 35–44.

Andreasen, N. C., Swayze, V. W., Flaum, M. *et al.* (1990*b*) Ventricular enlargement in schizophrenia evaluated with computed tomographic scanning. *Archives of General Psychiatry* **47**, 1008–1015.

Andreasen, N. C., Arndt, S., Swayze, V. *et al.* (1994*a*) Thalamic abnormalities in schizophrenia visualised through magnetic resonance imaging. *Science* **266**, 294–298.

Andreasen, N.C., Flashman, L., Flaum, M. *et al.* (1994*b*) Regional brain abnormalities in schizophrenia measured with magnetic resonance imaging. *Journal of the American Medical Association* **272**, 1763–1769.

Arnold, S. E., Franz, B. R., Gur, R. C. *et al.* (1995) Smaller neuron size in schizophrenia in hippocampal subfields that mediate cortical-hippocampal interactions. *American Journal of Psychiatry* **152**, 738–748.

Arnold, S. E., Hyman, B. T., Hoesen, G. W. V. *et al.* (1991) Some cytoarchitectural abnormalities of the entorhinal cortex in schizophrenia. *Archives of General Psychiatry* **48**, 625–632.

Barr, W. B., Ashtari, M, Bilder, R. M. *et al.* (1997) Brain morphometric comparison of first-episode schizophrenia and temporal lobe epilepsy. *British Journal of Psychiatry* **170**, 515–519.

Barta, P. E., Pearlson, G. D., Powers, R. E. *et al.* (1990) Auditory hallucinations and smaller superior temporal gyrus volume in schizophrenia. *American Journal of Psychiatry* **147**, 1457–1462.

Barta, P. E., Pearlson, G. D., Brill, L. B II *et al.* (1997) Planum temporale asymmetry reversal in schizophrenia: Replication and relationship to gray matter abnormalities. *American Journal of Psychiatry* **154**, 661–667.

Becker, T., Elmer, K., Schneider, F. *et al.* (1996) Confirmation of reduced temporal lobe limbic structure volume on magnetic resonance imaging in male patients with schizophrenia. *Psychiatry Research* **67**, 135–143.

Benes, F. M. (1988) Post-mortem structural analyses of schizophrenic brain: Study designs and the interpretation of data. *Psychiatric Developments* **6**, 213–226.

Benes, F. M., Bird, E. D. (1987) An analysis of the arrangement of neurons in the cingulate cortex of schizophrenic patients. *Archives of General Psychiatry* **44**, 608–616.

Benes, F. M., Davidson, B., Bird, E. D. (1986) Quantitative cytoarchitectural studies of the cerebral cortex of schizophrenia. *Archives of General Psychiatry* **43**, 31–35.

Benes, F. M., Kwok, E. W., Vincent, S. L. *et al.* (1998) A reduction of nonpyramidal cells in sector CA2 of schizophrenics and manic-depressives. *Biological Psychiatry* **44**, 88–97.

Benes, F. M., McSparren, J., Bird. *et al.* (1991*a*) Deficits in small interneurons in prefrontal and cingulate cortices of schizophrenic and schizoaffective patients. *Archives of General Psychiatry* **48**, 996–1001.

Benes, F. M., Sorensen, I., Bird, E. D. (1991*b*) Reduced neuronal size in posterior hippocampus of schizophrenic patients. *Schizophrenia Bulletin* **17**, 597–608.

Bilder, R. M., Wu, H., Bogerts, B. *et al.* (1994) Absence of regional hemispheric volume asymmetries in first-episode schizophrenia. *American Journal of Psychiatry* **151**, 1437–1447.

Bogerts, B., Meertz, E., Schoenfeldt-Bausch, R. (1985) Basal ganglia and limbic system pathology in schizophrenia: a morphometric study of brain volume shrinkage. *Archives of General Psychiatry* **42**, 784–791.

Bogerts, B., Ashtari, M., Degreef, G. *et al.* (1990*a*) Reduced temporal limbic structure volumes on magnetic resonance imaging in first episode schizophrenia. *Psychiatry Research: Neuroimaging* **35**, 1–13.

Bogerts, B., Falkai, P., Haupts, M. *et al.* (1990*b*) Post-mortem volume measurements of limbic system and basal ganglia structures in chronic schizophrenics. *Schizophrenia Research* **3**, 295–301.

Bogerts, B., Lieberman, J. A., Ashtari, M. *et al.* (1993) Hippocampus–amygdala volumes and psychopathology in chronic schizophrenia. *Biological Psychiatry* **33**, 236–246.

Breier, A., Buchanan, R. W., Elkashef, A. *et al.* (1992) Brain morphology and schizophrenia. *Archives of General Psychiatry* **49**, 921–926.

Brown, R., Colter, N., Corsellis , J. A. N. *et al.* (1986) Post-mortem evidence of structural brain changes in schizophrenia: differences in brain weight, temporal horn area, parahippocampal gyrus compared with affective disorder. *Archives of General Psychiatry* **43**, 36–42.

Bruton, C. J., Crow, T. J., Frith, C. D. *et al.* (1990) Schizophrenia and the brain: a prospective post-mortem study. *Psychological Medicine* **20**, 285–304.

Buchanan, R. W., Katalin, V., Barta, P. E., Pearlson, G. D. (1998) Structural evaluation of the prefrontal cortex in schizophrenia. *American Journal of Psychiatry* **155**, 1049–1055.

Buchsbaum, M..S., Stanley, Y., Hazlett, E. *et al.* (1997) Ventricular volume and asymmetry in schizotypal personality disorder and schizophrenia assessed with magnetic resonance imaging. *Schizophrenia Research* **27**, 45–53.

Cannon, T. D., van Erp, T. G., Huttunen, M. *et al.* (1998) Regional gray matter, white matter, and cerebrospinal fluid distributions in schizophrenic patients, their siblings and controls. *Archives of General Psychiatry* **55**, 1084–1091.

Chakos, M. H., Lieberman, J. A., Bilder, R. M. *et al.* (1994) Increase in caudate nuclei volumes of first-episode schizophrenic patients taking anti-psychotic drugs. *American Journal of Psychiatry* **151**, 1430–1436.

Christison, G. W., Casanova, M. F., Weinberger, D. R. *et al.* (1989) A quantitative investigation of hippocampal pyramidal cell size, shape, and variability of orientation in schiozphrenia. *Archives of General Psychiatry* **46**, 1027–1032.

Chua, S. E., McKenna, P. J. (1995) Schizophrenia—a brain disease? A critical review of structural and functional cerebral abnormality in the disorder. *British Journal of Psychiatry* **166**, 563–582.

Chua, S. E. , Murray, R. M. (1996) The neurodevelopmental theory of schizophrenia: Evidence concerning structure and neuropsychology. *Annals of Medicine* **28**, 547–555.

Chua, S. E., Wright, I. C., Poline, J. B. *et al.* (1997) Grey matter correlates of syndromes of schizophrenia. A semi-automated analysis of structural magnetic resonance images. *British Journal of Psychiatry* **170**, 406–410.

Cohen, J. (1988) *Statistical power analysis for the behavioral sciences.* Academic Press: New York.

Conrad, A. J., Abebe, T., Austin, R. *et al.* (1991) Hippocampal pyramidal cell disarray in schizophrenia as a bilateral phenomenon. *Archives of General Psychiatry* **48**, 413–417.

David, G. B. (1957) The pathological anatomy of the schizophrenias. In: D. Richter, ed. *Schizophrenia: somatic aspects.* Oxford: Pergamon, pp. 93–130.

DeLisi, L. E., Hoff, A. L., Neale, C. *et al.* (1994) Asymmetries in the superior temporal lobe in male and female first-episode schizophrenia patients: measures of the planum temporale and superior temporal gyrus by MRI. *Schizophrenia Research* **12**, 19–28.

Doraiswamy, P. M., Tupler, L. A., Krishnan, K. R. R. (1995) Neuroleptic treatment and caudate plasticity. *Lancet* **345**, 734–735.

Dwork, A. J. (1997) Postmortem studies of the hippocampal formation in schizophrenia. *Schizophrenia Bulletin* **23**, 385–402.

Falkai, P., Bogerts, B. (1986) Cell loss in the hippocampus of schizophrenics. *European Archives of Psychiatry and Neurological Sciences* **236**, 154–161.

Falkai, P., Bogerts, B., Rozumek, M. (1988) Limbic pathology in schizophrenia: the entorhinal region—a morphometric study. *Biological Psychiatry* **24**, 515–521.

Falkai, P., Bogerts, B., Schneider, T. *et al.* (1995) Disturbed planum temporale asymmetry in schizophrenia. A quantitative post-mortem study. *Schizophrenia Research* **14**, 161–176.

Flaum, M., Swayze, V. W., O'Leary, D. S. *et al.* (1995) Effects of diagnosis, laterality and gender on brain morphology in schizophrenia. *American Journal of Psychiatry* **152**, 704–714.

Frangou, S., Sharma, T., Sigmundsson, T. *et al.* (1997) The Maudsley family study IV. Normal planum temporale asymmetry in familial schizophrenia. *British Journal of Psychiatry* **170**, 328–333.

Frith, C. D. (1992) *The cognitive neuropsychology of schizophrenia.* Laurence Erlbaum Associates: Hove, UK.

Fukazako, H., Fukazako, T., Hashiguchi, T. *et al.* (1996) Reduction in hippocampal formation volume is caused mainly by its shortening in chronic schizophrenia: assessment by MRI. *Biological Psychiatry* **39**, 938–945.

Gray, J. A., Rawlins, J. N. P., Hemsley, D. R. *et al.* (1991) The neuropsychology of schizophrenia. *Behavioral and Brain Sciences* **14**, 1–84.

Gur, R. E., Mozley, P. D., Resnick, S. M. *et al.* (1991) Magnetic resonance imaging in schizophrenia. *Archives of General Psychiatry* **48**, 407–412.

Gur, R. E., Mozley, P. D., Shtasel, D. L. *et al.* (1994) Clinical subtypes of schizophrenia: differences in brain and CSF volume. *American Journal of Psychiatry* **151**, 343–350.

Gur, R. E., Cowell, P., Turetsky, B. I. *et al.* (1998*a*) A follow-up magnetic resonance imaging study of schizophrenia. *Archives of General Psychiatry* **55**, 145–152.

Gur R. E., Maany, V., Mozley, P. D. *et al.* (1998*b*) Subcortical MRI volumes in neuroleptic-naïve and treated patients with schizophrenia. *American Journal of Psychiatry* **155**, 1711–1717.

Hall, L. D., Herrod, J., Carpenter, T. A. *et al.* (1994) Magnetic resonance imaging in schizophrenia: a review of clinical and methodological issues. In: R. J. Ancill, S. Halliday, J. Higenbottam, eds. *Schizophrenia: exploring the spectrum of psychosis.* Wiley: Chicester, pp. 115–135.

Harvey, I., Ron, M. A., Du Boulay, G. *et al.* (1993) Reduction of cortical volume in schizophrenia on magnetic resonance imaging. *Psychological Medicine* **23**, 591–604.

Heckers, S. (1997) Neuropathology of schizophrenia: cortex, thalamus, basal ganglia and neurotransmitter-specific projection systems. *Schizophrenia Bulletin* **23**, 403–421.

Heckers, S., Heinsen, H., Heinsen, Y. C. *et al.* (1990*a*) Morphometry of the parahippocampal gyrus in schizophrenia. *Journal of Neural Transmission* **80**, 151–155.

Heckers, S., Heinsen, H., Heinsen, Y. C. *et al.* (1990*b*) Limbic structures and lateral ventricle in schizophrenia: a quantitative postmortem study. *Archives of General Psychiatry* **47**, 1016–1022.

Heckers S., Heinsen H., Geiger B. *et al.* (1991*a*) Hippocampal neuron number in schizophrenia. *Archives of General Psychiatry* **48**, 1002–1008.

Heckers, S., Heinsen, H., Heinsen, Y. *et al.* (1991*b*) Cortex, white matter, and basal ganglia in schizophrenia: a volumetric post-mortem study. *Biological Psychiatry* **29**, 556–566.

Hirayasu, Y., Shenton, M. E., Salisbury, D. F. *et al.* (1998) Lower left temporal lobe MRI volume in patients with first-episode schizophrenia compared with psychotic patients with first-episode affective disorder and normal subjects. *American Journal of Psychiatry* **155**, 1384–1391.

Hoff, A., Riordan, H., O'Donnell, D. *et al.* (1992) Anomalous lateral sulcus asymmetry and cognitive function in first-episode schizophrenia. *Schizophrenia Bulletin* **18**, 257–272.

Jacobsen, L. K., Giedd, J. N., Tanrikut, C. *et al.* (1997) Three dimensional cortical morphometry of the planum temporale in childhood-onset schizophrenia. *American Journal of Psychiatry* **154**, 685–687.

Jakob, H., Beckmann, H. (1986) Prenatal developmental disturbances in the limbic allocortex in schizophrenics. *Journal of Neural Transmission* **65**, 303–326.

Jernigan, T.l., Zisook, S., Heaton, R. K. *et al.* (1991) Magnetic resonance imaging abnormalites in lenticular nuclei and cerebral cortex in schizophrenia. *Archives of General Psychiatry* **48**, 881–890.

Jeste, D. V., Lohr, J. B. (1989) Hippocampal pathologic findings in schizophrenia. *Archives of General Psychiatry* **46**, 1019–1024.

Johnstone, E. C., Crow, T. J., Frith, C. D. *et al.* (1976) Cerebral ventricular size and cognitive impairment in chronic schizophrenia. *Lancet* **ii**, 924–926.

Jones, P. B., Harvey, I., Lewis, S. W. *et al.* (1994) Cerebral ventricle dimensions as risk factors for schizophrenia and affective psychosis. *Psychological Medicine* **24**, 995–1011.

Kawasaki, Y., Maeda, Y., Urata, K. *et al.* (1993) A quantitative magnetic resonance imaging study of patients with schizophrenia. *European Archives of Psychiatry and Clinical Neuroscience* **242**, 268–272.

Kelsoe, J., Cadet, J. L., Pickar, D. *et al.* (1988) Quantitative neuroanatomy in schizophrenia. *Archives of General Psychiatry* **45**, 533–541.

Keshavan, M. S., Bagwell, W. W., Munson, R. C. *et al.* (1994) Changes in caudate volume with neuroleptic medication. *Lancet* **344**, 1434.

Keshavan, M. S., Rosenberg, D., Sweeney, J. A., Pettegrew, J. W. (1998) Decreased caudate volume in neuroleptic-naïve psychotic patients. *American Journal of Psychiatry* **155**, 774–778.

Kleinschmidt, A., Falkai, P., Huang, Y. *et al.* (1994) *In vivo* morphometry of planum temporale asymmetry in first-episode schizophrenia. *Schizophrenia Research* **12**, 9–18.

Kovelman, J. A., Scheibel, A. B. (1984) A neurohistological correlate of schizophrenia. *Biological Psychiatry* **19**, 1601–1621.

Krimer, L. S., Herman, M. M., Saunders, R. C. *et al.* (1997) A qualitative and quantitative analysis of the entorhinal cortex in schizophrenia. *Cerebral Cortex* **7**, 732–739.

Kulynych, J. J., Vladar, K., Fantie, B. *et al.* (1995) Normal asymmetry of the planum temporale in patients with schizophrenia: three dimensional cortical morphometry with MRI. *British Journal of Psychiatry* **166**, 742–749.

Kulynych, J. J., Vladar, K., Jones, D. W. *et al.* (1996) Superior temporal gyrus volume in schizophrenia: A study using MRI morphometry assisted by surface rendering. *American Journal of Psychiatry* **153**, 50–56.

Lauriello, J., Hoff, A., Wieneke, M. H. *et al.* (1997) Similar extent of brain dysmorphology in severely ill women and men with schizophrenia. *American Journal of Psychiatry* **154**, 819–825.

Lawrie, S. M., Abukmeil, S. S. (1998) Brain abnormality in schizophrenia. A systematic and quantitative review of volumetric magnetic resonance imaging studies. *British Journal of Psychiatry* **172**, 110–120.

Lewis, S. W. (1990) Computerised tomography in schizophrenia 15 years on. *British Journal of Psychiatry* **157** (Suppl. 9), 16–24.

Lim, K. O., Tew, W., Kushner, M. *et al.* (1996) Cortical gray matter volume deficit in patients with first-episode schizophrenia. *American Journal of Psychiatry* **153**, 1548–1554.

Marsh, L., Harris, D., Lim, K. O. *et al.* (1997) Structural magnetic resonance imaging abnormalities in men with severe chronic schizophrenia and an early age at clinical onset. *Archives of General Psychiatry* **54**, 1104–1112.

Menon, R. R., Barta, P. E., Aylward, E. H. *et al.* (1995) Posterior superior temporal gyrus in schizophrenia: grey matter changes and clinical correlates. *Schizophrenia Research* **16**, 127–135.

Nelson, M. D., Saykin, A. J., Flashman, L. *et al.* (1998) Hippocampal volume reduction in schizophrenia as assessed by magnetic resonance imaging. A meta-analytic study. *Archives of General Psychiatry* **55**, 433–440.

Nopoulos, P. Torres, I., Flaum, M. *et al.* (1995) Brain morphology in first-episode schizophrenia. *American Journal of Psychiatry* **152**, 1721–1723.

O'Callaghan, E., Buckley, P., Redmond O. *et al.* (1992) Abnormalities of cerebral structure on magnetic resonance imaging: interpretation in relation to the neurodevelopmental
hypothesis. *Journal of the Royal Society of Medicine* **85**, 227–231.

Pakkenberg, B. (1987) Post-mortem study of chronic schizophrenic brains. *British Journal
of Psychiatry* **151**, 744–752.

Pakkenberg, B. (1990) Pronounced reduction of total neuron number in mediodorsal thalamic nucleus and nucleus accumbens in schizophrenics. *Archives of General Psychiatry*
47, 1023–1028.

Pakkenberg, B. (1993) Total nerve cell number in neocortex in chronic schizophrenics and
controls estimated using optical detectors. *Biological Psychiatry* **34**, 768–772.

Pearlson, G. D., Barta, P. E., Powers, R. E. *et al.* (1997) Medial and superior temporal
gyral volumes and cerebral asymmetry in schizophrenia versus bipolar disorder. *Biological
Psychiatry* **41**, 1–14.

Petty, R. G., Barta, P. E., Pearlson, G. D. *et al.* (1995) Reversal of asymmetry of
the planum temporale in schizophrenia. *American Journal of Psychiatry* **152**, 715–
721.

Rajkowska, G., Selemon, L. D., Goldman-Rakic, P. S. (1998) Neuronal and glial somal
size in the prefrontal cortex: a postmortem morphometric study of schizophrenia and
Huntington disease. *Archives of General Psychiatry* **55**, 215–224 .

Roberts, N., Cruz-Orive, L. M., Reid, N. M. K. *et al.* (1993) Unbiased estimation of human
body composition by the Cavalieri method using magnetic resonance imaging. *Journal
of Microscopy* **171**, 239–253.

Rossi, A., Stratta, P., Mattei, P. *et al.* (1992) Planum temporale in schizophrenia: a magnetic
resonance imaging study. *Schizophrenia Research* **7**, 19–22.

Rossi, A., Serio, A., Stratta, P. *et al.* (1994*a*) Planum temporale asymmetry and thought
disorder in schizophrenia. *Schizophrenia Research* **12**, 1–7.

Rossi, A., Stratta, P., Mancini, F. *et al.* (1994*b*) Magnetic resonance imaging findings of
amygdala–anterior hippocampus shrinkage in male patients with schizophrenia. *Psychiatry
Research* **52**, 43–53.

Roy, P. D., Zipursky, R. B., Saint-Cyr, J. A. *et al.* (1998) Temporal horn enlargement is
present in schizophrenia and bipolar disorder. *Biological Psychiatry* **44**, 418–422.

Scheibel, A. B., Kovelman, J. A. (1981) Disorientation of the hippocampal pyramidal cell
and its processes in the schizophrenic patient. *Biological Psychiatry* **16**, 101–102.

Schlaepfer, T. E., Harris, G. J., Tien, A. Y. *et al.* (1994) Decreased regional cortical gray
matter volume in schizophrenia. *American Journal of Psychiatry* **151**, 842–848.

Selemon, L. D., Rajkowska, G. and Goldman-Rakic, P. S. (1995) Abnormally high neuronal
density in the schizophrenic cortex: A morphometric analysis of prefrontal area 9 and
occipital area 17. *Archives of General Psychiatry* **52**, 805–818.

Selemon, L. D., Rajkowska, G., Goldman-Rakic, P. S. (1998) Elevated neuronal density
in prefrontal area 46 in brains from schizophrenic patients: application of a three-
dimensional, stereologic counting method. *Journal of Comparative Neurology* **392**,
402–412.

Shapiro, R. M. (1993) Regional neuropathology in schizophrenia: where are we? Where
are we going? *Schizophrenia Research* **10**, 187–239.

Sharma, T., Lancester, E., Lee, D. *et al.* (1998) Brain changes in schizophrenia: volumetric MRI study of families multiply affected with schizophrenia—the Maudsley Family Study 5. *British Journal of Psychiatry* **173**, 132–138.

Shenton, M. E., Kikinis, R., Jolesz, F. A. *et al.* (1992) Abnormalities of the left temporal lobe and thought disorder in schizophrenia. *New England Journal of Medicine* **327**, 604–612.

Shihabuddin, L., Buchsbaum, M. S., Hazlett, E. A. *et al.* (1998) Dorsal striatal size, shape and metabolic rate in never-medicated and previously medicated schizophrenics performing a verbal learning task. *Archives of General Psychiatry* **55**, 235–243.

Smith, G. N., Iacono, W. G. (1986) Lateral ventricular size in schizophrenia and choice of control group. *Lancet* **i**, 1450.

Smith, R. C., Baumgartner, R., Calderon, M. (1986) Magnetic resonance imaging studies of the brains of schizophrenic patients. *Psychiatry Research* **20**, 33–46.

Suddath, R. L., Casanova, M. F., Goldberg, T. E. *et al.* (1989) Temporal lobe pathology in schizophrenia: a quantitative magnetic resonance imaging study. *American Journal of Psychiatry* **146**, 464–472.

Suddath, R. L., Christison, G. W., Torrey, E. F. *et al.* (1990) Anatomical abnormalities in the brains of monozygotic twins discordant for schizophrenia. *New England Journal of Medicine* **322**, 789–794.

Swayze, V. W. II, Andreasen, N. C., Alliger, R. J. *et al.* (1992) Subcortical and temporal structures in affective disorder and schizophrenia: a magnetic resonance imaging study. *Biological Psychiatry* **31**, 221–240.

Torrey, E. F., Bowler, A. E., Taylor, E. H. *et al.* (1994) *Schizophrenia and manic-depressive disorder: the biological roots of mental illness as revealed by the landmark study of identical twins.* Basic Books: New York.

Turetsky, B., Cowell, P. E., Gur, R. C. *et al.* (1995) Frontal and temporal lobe volumes in schizophrenia. Relationship to symptoms and clinical subtype. *Archives of General Psychiatry* **52**, 1061–1070.

Van Horn, J. D. and McManus, I. C. (1992) Ventricular enlargement in schizophrenia: a meta-analysis of studies of the ventricle–brain ratio (VBR) *British Journal of Psychiatry* **160**, 687–697.

Vita, A., Dieci, M., Giobbio, G. M. *et al.* (1995) Language and thought disorder in schizophrenia: brain morphological correlates. *Schizophrenia Research* **15**, 243–251.

Ward, K. E., Friedman, L., Wise, A. *et al.* (1996) Meta-analysis of brain and cranial size in schizophrenia. *Schizophrenia Research* **22**, 197–213.

Weinberger, D. R., Torrey, E. F., Neophytides, A. N. *et al.* (1979) Lateral cerebral ventricular enlargement in schizophrenia. *Archives of General Psychiatry* **36**, 735–739.

Whitworth, A. B., Honeder, M., Kremser, C. *et al.* (1998) Hippocampal volume reduction in male schizophrenic patients. *Schizophrenia Research* **31**, 73–81.

Wible, C. G., Shenton, M. E., Hokama, H. *et al.* (1995) Prefrontal cortex and schizophrenia: A quantitative magnetic resonance imaging study. *Archives of General Psychiatry* **52**, 279–288.

Woodruff. P. W., Wright, I. C., Shuriquie, N. *et al.* (1997) Structural brain abnormalities in male schizophrenics reflect fronto-temporal dissociation. *Psychological Medicine* **27**, 1257–1266.

Wright, I. C., McGuire, P. K., Poline, J-B. *et al.* (1995) A voxel-based method for the statistical analysis of gray and white matter density applied to schizophrenia. *Neuroimage* **2**, 244–252.

Young, A. H., Blackwood, D. H. R., Roxburgh, H. *et al.* (1991) A magnetic resonance imaging study of schizophrenia. *British Journal of Psychiatry* **158**, 158–164.

Zaidel, D. W., Esiri, M. M. and Harrison, P. J. (1997*a*) Size, shape and orientation of neurons in the left and right hippocampus: Investigation of normal asymmetries and alterations in schizophrenia. *American Journal of Psychiatry* **154**, 812–818.

Zaidel, D. W., Esiri, M. M. and Harrison, P. J. (1997*b*) The hippocampus in schizophrenia: lateralized increase in neuronal density and altered cytoarchitectural asymmetry. *Psychological Medicine* **27**, 703–713.

Zipursky, R. B., Lim, K. O., Sullivan, E. V. *et al.* (1992) Widespread cerebral gray matter volume deficits in schizophrenia. *Archives of General Psychiatry* **49**, 195–205.

Zipursky, R. B., Marsh, L., Lim, K. *et al.* (1994) Volumetric MRI assessment of temporal lobe structures in schizophrenia. *Biological Psychiatry* **35**, 501–516.

Zipursky R. B., Lambe, E. K., Kapur, S., Mikulis, D. J. (1998) Cerebral gray matter volume deficits in first episode psychosis. *Archives of General Psychiatry* **55**, 540–546.

14 Methodological Issues

Paul J. Harrison and Joel E. Kleinman

Methodological issues in case collection and selection
    Diagnostic issues
    Brain collection
    Neuropathological purification
    Toxicology
    Tissue handling and processing
    Confounding variables
Methodological issues for studies of neurochemical pathology
    Molecular studies
    Immunological methods
    Biochemical indices
Methodological issues for morphometric studies
    Perimortem confounders
    Stereology

There are no methodological problems unique to schizophrenia neuropathology. Rather, the field must contend with the problems common to all schizophrenia research, as well as with the factors which introduce noise into postmortem brain studies and which are magnified because of the subtlety of the pathology being sought. Though the technical and statistical sophistication of research has improved dramatically over the past 20 years, limitations continue to hamper progress to an unnecessary extent, contributing to the persisting short-comings in the data discussed elsewhere in this book, especially in Chapter 13.

The conceptual and technical issues complicating all types of schizophrenia research are summarised in Table 14.1 and those affecting investigations of brain structure in Table 14.2. These general issues are not discussed further. The rest of the chapter focuses on the methodological issues specifically affecting neuropathological studies. For complementary reviews, see Benes (1988) and Casanova and Kleinman (1990). Confounding by medication is considered in Chapter 15.

Table 14.1 Methodological issues common to all schizophrenia research

Matching for demographics: Age, sex, education, social class, etc.

Validity of the diagnosis

Does the variable being measured relate to the syndrome of schizophrenia, or to a symptom ? Is it categorical or dimensional?

Is there heterogeneity?

Is the variable affected by antipsychotic drugs or other treatments?

Are subjects included in research representative?

Use of a psychiatric control group

Use of an antipsychotic-treated control group

Is the experimenter blind to diagnosis?

What is the hypothesis being tested?

Use of appropriate statistics

Table 14.2 Methodological issues affecting all structural studies of the brain in schizophrenia

Availability of enough cases, with adequate documentation

Variable, usually prolonged, duration of disease

Dealing with pathologies which may have produced a schizophrenia-like psychosis

Confounding by concurrent illnesses and medications

Hemispheric structural asymmetries

Is the neuropathology a result of schizophrenia, *E.g.* persistent symptoms, poor environment?

Selecting which brain areas to study

Adherence to stereological principles

Choice of suitable image analysis methods

Methodological issues in case collection and selection

Diagnostic issues

Finding the label 'schizophrenia' in the case notes is insufficient for research purposes, as it will include false positive diagnoses (mostly of other functional psychoses) compared to formal DSM (version IIIR or IV) or ICD 10 criteria for the disorder. Conversely, careful review of case notes of deceased patients by experienced psychiatrists does allow a reliable diagnosis of schizophrenia to be made (Keilp *et al.*, 1995; Hill *et al.*, 1996). The Diagnostic Evaluation after Death (DEAD) checklist (Zalcman and Endicott, 1983) is an attempt to operationalise such diagnoses, but it is cumbersome and has not been widely utilised.

Brain collection

The rate-limiting step in the field is the collection of adequate numbers of brains (Wagman, 1992). This problem has been worsened by two factors. Firstly, there has been a steep decline in autopsy rates in many countries, and the research value of autopsies overlooked. Secondly, in the United Kingdom in particular, the move to community care means that most subjects with schizophrenia die at home, and either do not get an autopsy or are referred to the coroner (medical examiner in American terms) which places significant legal and practical constraints on tissue collection for research purposes. Legal changes pertaining to these matters are likely in the near future, but whether their impact is beneficial or detrimental remains to be seen.

Such difficulties are not insurmountable, but they do mean that increasing efforts and collaborations are required to collect a brain series of sufficient size within a reasonable time. These efforts need to be more sustained and proactive than applies to brain banks for most neurological and neuropsychiatric disorders (Ravid and Swaab, 1993; Cairns and Lantos, 1996). A highly successful strategy has been that of the Stanley Foundation's Consortium, which by funding pathologists based in co-operative medical examiners' offices, as well as a central storage and processing facility, has collected a large number of brains from subjects with schizophrenia and affective disorder as well as healthy controls for the use of the research community (Torrey *et al.*, 2000). The protocol includes contact with relatives to provide additional diagnostic and demographic information about each case. An alternative option adopted by some research groups is to set up a prospective series in which schizophrenics are diagnostically and neuropsychologically assessed in life, and the patient's wish for their brain to be used for research recorded (Arnold *et al.*, 1995). This approach has the advantage of increasing the information available on each case, and the chances that consent to brain tissue collection will be granted by next-of-kin after death. The drawbacks are the slow rate of brain collection, the marked bias towards recruitment of elderly subjects, and the difficulty acquiring comparable, well-evaluated control subjects.

Neuropathological purification

About half the brains examined from patients with schizophrenia contain non-specific focal degenerative abnormalities, such as small infarcts or white matter changes (Riederer *et al.*, 1995). These are presumably coincidental, in that they are variable in distribution and nature, do not affect the clinical picture (Johnstone *et al.*, 1994), and in some instances are documented as having occurred long after the onset of symptoms. A related point is that ~3 to 5 per cent of cases diagnosed as schizophrenia turn out to be due to an atypical presentation of another disorder, such as temporal lobe epilepsy, syphilis, Wilson's disease, metachromatic leukodystrophy, and so on (Davison, 1983; Johnstone *et al.*, 1987). One school of thought argues that cases in both these categories should be included in neuropathological studies of schizophrenia, since there are no grounds a priori for exclusion, and these 'outliers' may provide crucial and unexpected clues—and if not will at least help establish the pathological heterogeneity of the syndrome (Heckers, 1997; Stevens, 1997). On the other hand, omission of subjects with coincidental pathologies, or those with a neurological schizophrenia-like disorder, allows 'true' schizophrenia to be examined (Bruton *et al.*, 1990; Dwork, 1997); an argument in favour of the latter strategy is that the excess of miscellaneous lesions in schizophrenia may be an artefact of how tissue is acquired: researchers can afford to pick and choose control brains, but cases with schizophrenia are scarce and hence more likely to be included even if there is a complex or incomplete medical history. These issues contributed significantly to the controversy surrounding the presence of gliosis in schizophrenia (see Chapter 5).

In practice, most if not all contemporary histological studies of schizophrenia have been carried out on brains which were neuropathologically screened, to greater or lesser degree. In our opinion this is essential, and a formal evaluation for Alzheimer's disease using the Consortium to Establish a Registry for Alzheimer Disease (CERAD) criteria (Mirra *et al.*, 1991) is desirable given the prevalence of this disorder in elderly subjects whether or not they have schizophrenia (Chapters 3 and 15). Other relatively common disorders such as vascular dementia, Lewy body disease, and Parkinson's disease should also be excluded. The extent (e.g. what areas were examined?) and nature (e.g. what stains and diagnostic criteria were used?) of the neuropathological screen should be stated in research reports.

Toxicology

Antipsychotics and other medications are not the only compounds which can potentially confound neuropathological studies of schizophrenia (Chapter 15). Use and abuse by cases and controls of legal and illegal recreational drugs, notably nicotine, alcohol, amphetamines, cocaine, and cannabis, must also be considered. Equally, some patients allegedly on medication have a negative drug screen at death presumably due to non-compliance— a form of pseudo-confounding. Drug analysis of blood, urine, or hair is therefore desirable, especially for neurochemical studies, but is not often carried out; one advantage of tissue acquisition through the medical examiner is that toxicology is routinely performed.

Tissue handling and processing

No one tissue handling and processing protocol can suit every investigator and every technique. Tough, and at times arbitrary, decisions have to be made and adhered to if a meaningful tissue collection is to result. Fundamental questions to be addressed include: is the tissue is to be fixed (and how) or frozen (and how)? Is the brain to be fixed or frozen whole, or in slices, or dissected into blocks immediately? Are 'grind and bind' methods or slide-mounted sections to be used? What is the optimal section thickness, and how should the slides be processed? What effect do all these factors have on the parameter under investigation?

Two principles apply here. Firstly, horses for courses: the tissue must be suitable for the proposed method and vice versa. Secondly, investigators should demonstrate in pilot studies what effect the handling and processing variables have on their measurements. The key variables of this kind are summarised in Table 14.3 and discussed below.

Table 14.3 Methodological issues specifically affecting schizophrenia neuropathology research

---

Premortem events (agonal state)
Hypoxia/acidosis (pH)
Pyrexia
Coma
Acute medication, e.g. opioids, antibiotics

Postmortem events
Postmortem interval (death to freezing or processing)
  Time from death to refrigeration
  Time from refrigeration to fixation or freezing
Temperature from death to refrigeration

Issues for frozen tissue
Mode and speed of freezing
Temperature of storage
Duration of storage
Partial thawing during storage

Issues for fixed tissue
Duration of fixation
Fixative composition and buffering
Embedding medium
Post fixation antigen/mRNA retrieval (e.g. microwaving, autoclaving)

Other factors
Ensuring control and case material comes from same source (to avoid systematic variation in one or more of the above factors)

Confounding variables

Having detailed information about variables of known confounding effect is the secret to minimising their influence. In this way, the groups being compared can be matched in terms of mean and range, and appropriate statistics (e.g. analysis of covariance, partial correlations) used to reduce further their potential confounding of the results. Matching should always occur for age, sex, postmortem interval, and arguably cerebral hemisphere, since these basic demographic factors affect many neuropathological and neurochemical parameters. Information about duration of fixation or freezer storage time, as appropriate, should also be collected routinely, as these factors correlate with signal for many types of analysis. Beyond these basic issues, further variables come into play according to the methods being applied.

Methodological issues for studies of neurochemical pathology

Molecular studies

One of the main developments of the past decade has been the application of molecular methods to the neuropathology of schizophrenia (Harrison, 1996). These have centred upon hybridisation measurements of mRNAs (using *in situ* hybridisation histochemistry, reverse transcriptase-polymerase chain reaction (RT-PCR) and nuclease assays) and antibody-based analyses of proteins (using immunocytochemistry, western blotting, and allied methods). In the near future, these will be complemented by gene expression arrays allowing simultaneous investigation of thousands of transcripts. The very power and sensitivity of these techniques leaves them open to confounding by many variables other than schizophrenia, and to which adequate attention has not always been paid.

For mRNA studies, the mode of death is crucial. The key determinant is pH (Harrison *et al.*, 1995; Kingsbury *et al.*, 1995; Johnston *et al.*, 1997), a marker of premortem brain acidosis which in turn reflects the mode and speed of death of the patient (Bowen *et al.*, 1976; Perry *et al.*, 1982). The influence on mRNA is probably via activation of acid ribonucleases. The pH effect is seen whether the technique is *in situ* hybridisation (e.g. Porter *et al.*, 1997) or RT-PCR (Eastwood *et al.*, 1997a; Johnston *et al.*, 1997)—or, presumably, any other form of mRNA analysis. pH is simple to measure, stable for a prolonged period after death and after freezer storage, and is similar throughout the brain (and CSF) of an individual (Hardy *et al.*, 1985; Alafuzoff and Winblad, 1993). A pH of ~6.8 is seen after a very rapid death, whereas prolonged agonal states can produce a pH of <6.0. Parenthetically, suicide victims tend to have a high pH (Harrison *et al.*, 1995), presumably because they die rapidly (e.g. due to hanging, jumping, exsanguination) more often than do those dying of natural causes; hence some findings interpreted as being related to suicide may just be a reflection of mode and speed of death.

The pH influence is of a magnitude such that pH screening and omission of brains with a low pH (e.g. pH <6.1) is a sensible strategy. (Even having done so, effects of pH are still observed; Eastwood and Harrison, 2000). Conversely, without pH, quantitative mRNA studies are unreliable, since it cannot be assumed that controls and schizophrenics die in the same fashion; indeed cases collected in Oxford have had a significantly lower pH than that of controls, perhaps because we have been less likely to reject a schizophrenic brain than a control brain if the medical history is complicated. Other premortem factors such as coma and pyrexia, which are not independent of pH, can also affect preservation of mRNAs (Harrison *et al.*, 1991; Morrison-Bogorad *et al.*, 1995). Complicating the issue, different mRNAs are differentially sensitive to premortem events, which should thus be examined and ideally controlled for statistically for each new transcript investigated (Harrison *et al.*, 1995); it also means that normalisation of one mRNA to another does not entirely overcome the problem of interbrain differences in RNA content.

In contrast to the above sensitivities, postmortem interval is unexpectedly unimportant for studies, with most mRNAs being stable for 48 h and often more (Barton *et al.*, 1993), though there are individual exceptions reported.

Immunological methods

Some proteins are influenced by perimortem events. For example, immunological detection of glutamate receptors is affected by pH (Eastwood *et al.*, 1997b), and that of some cytoskeletal proteins is decreased by postmortem interval and probably by hypoxia (Schwab *et al.*, 1994; Geddes *et al.*, 1995). However, in general, proteins are more robust than mRNAs to these factors. Instead, a major problem for protein studies is the effect of formalin, which jeopardises immunochemical methods for many proteins in proportion to fixation time (e.g. Eastwood *et al.*, 1994). All such studies should include documentation of fixation protocols and include this variable in the statistical analysis. The deleterious effect of fixation can often be largely overcome by microwaving and other antigen-retrieval techniques, but it is essential to demonstrate that such methods are valid for quantitative analyses.

Biochemical indices

Activities of brain enzymes and synaptosomal preparations are susceptible to both pre- and postmortem variables (Perry and Perry, 1983; Hardy *et al.*, 1985; Dodd *et al.*, 1988; Palmer *et al.*, 1988). For example, glutamic acid decarboxylase activity is lower in those with prolonged agonal states or who die after coma (Bowen *et al.*, 1976; Butterworth *et al.*, 1983; Harrison *et al.*, 1991), a vulnerability which likely explains the earlier reported decrease in schizophrenia (Bird *et al.*, 1977).

Levels of transmitters and metabolites are labile after death (e.g. Spokes, 1979; Kontur *et al.*, 1994) and can be affected by agonal state (Perry *et al.*, 1982).

Measurement of binding site densities (B_{max}) and affinities (K_d) are relatively resistant, but by no means immune, to perimortem factors. For example, [^{3}H]MK-801 binding is higher in those dying rapidly (Piggott *et al.*, 1992), increasing postmortem interval is associated with lower muscarinic M1 receptor binding but higher benzodiazepine receptor binding (Whitehouse *et al.*, 1984), and [^{3}H]glutamate binding decreases with freezer storage (Kornhuber *et al.*, 1988). Many receptor binding sites show declines with age (e.g. Burnet *et al.*, 1994; Dean *et al.*, 1997), whilst some increase (Burnet and Harrison, 2000).

Methodological issues for morphometric studies

Perimortem confounders

Morphometric indices such as cell density, size, and shape may also be affected by perimortem factors (Table 14.4). In particular they are influenced by the composition and duration of time in fixative and the mode of embedding, all of which have effects on tissue and neuronal shrinkage and thereby upon morphometric parameters (Kretschmann *et al.*, 1982; Haug, 1986; Quester and Schröder, 1997). pH can even influence cell size (P.J.H. unpublished observations 1999), presumably via swelling secondary to acidosis. Overall the perimortem effects on morphometry are likely to be comparable in magnitude as the differences between schizophrenics and controls reported in most studies, so it is essential that they are evaluated and controlled for.

Stereology

As well as having to attend to these kinds of variables, morphometric studies now have to contend with serious criticisms of the methods themselves and the way they have been

Table 14.4 Relative sensitivity of different neuropathological variables to perimortem factors

Parameter or method	Sensitivity to			
	Agonal state	PMI	Fixation	Freezer storage
Neurotransmitters	++	+++	n/a	++
Enzyme activity	++	++	n/a	+
mRNA	+++	+	n/a[1]	+ or ++[2]
Immunochemistry	+	+	+++	+
Radioligand binding	+	+	n/a	++
Neuronal morphometry	+	+	+++	n/a
Electron microscopy	++?	+++	+++	n/a

+, low; ++, moderate; +++, high sensitivity; ?, few data; n/a, not applicable. Ratings are approximations.
Individual molecules within each group may behave differently.
[1]Good mRNA signal possible if fixed tissue is autoclaved (Oliver et al., 1997; Eastwood and Harrison, 1999) or microwaved (Lucassen et al, 1995).
[2]If there is partial thawing during storage. Anecdotal observations also suggest greater mRNA vulnerability on slide-mounted sections (even if post fixed) than in tissue blocks.
PMI, postmortem interval.

applied over the years (Mayhew and Gundersen, 1996). These concern two main areas: how the tissue is sampled, and how the parameters are measured. The vogue is now for stereological methods since these eliminate most of the potential for error and bias which are either inherent in, or more problematic with, the older techniques. Excellent reviews of the principles and practice of stereological neuropathology are provided by West (1993) and Howard and Reed (1998); see also discussion in Chapters 2 and 3.

The application of stereology to schizophrenia is exemplified by the pioneering work of Pakkenberg (1990) and Heckers et al. (1991) and, in a welcome move, is now being widely adopted in the field. However, it would be wrong to dismiss all non-stereological studies; indeed they have produced much valuable morphometric data and continue to do so (Guillery and Herrup, 1997). Moreover, stereology has its own conceptual and technical limitations. For example, a 'hardline' stereologist requires that any structure from which measurements are to be made (e.g. the superior temporal gyrus) must be unambiguously definable and available in its entirety to be sampled from. It is often difficult to satisfy these criteria in postmortem brains, and it is fortunate that more pragmatic but stereologically valid approaches are being adopted (e.g. Gomez-Isla et al., 1997). A second relevant issue is that stereologists dismiss density as a measure (number of particles per unit volume) because it is heavily influenced by tissue shrinkage and is readily misinterpretable, especially if the reference volume is unknown (Oorschot, 1994). Certainly, an elevated neuronal density may simply reflect the same number of neurons in smaller volume, whilst a decreased neuronal number will not affect neuronal density if volume is reduced in parallel. Nevertheless, we view density measurements as remaining valuable and reliable (assuming appropriate methodology and cautious interpretation). Firstly, neuronal density informs about the cytoarchitecture of an area, including the status of the neuropil with its dendrites, synapses, and so on, which is likely to be functionally important independent of the absolute number of neurons (Chapters 4 and 11). Secondly, for many molecular and immunological methods it is impractical or impossible to avoid some form of relative quantitation, usually with density-based units; this does not intrinsically reduce the value of the data. The essential points, as always, are that (a) techniques are clearly described and suitable for the question being asked; and (b) interpretation is appropriate to the method and results.

References

Alafuzoff I, Winblad B (1993) How to run a brain bank: potentials and pitfalls in the use of human post-mortem brain material in research. *Journal of Neural Transmission,* Suppl. 39, 235–243.

Arnold SE, Gur RE, Shapiro RM *et al.* (1995) Prospective clinicopathologic studies of schizophrenia: Accrual and assessment of patients. *American Journal of Psychiatry,* **152**, 731–737.

Barton AJL, Pearson RCA, Najlerahim A, Harrison PJ (1993) Pre- and postmortem influences on brain RNA. *Journal of Neurochemistry,* **61**, 1–11.

Benes FM (1988) Post mortem structural analyses of schizophrenic brain: study designs and the interpretation of data. *Psychiatric Developments,* **3**, 213–226.

Bird ED, Barnes J, Iversen LL, Spokes EG, Mackay AVP, Shepherd M (1977) Increased brain dopamine and reduced glutamic acid decarboxylase and choline acetyltransferase activity in schizophrenia and related disorders. *Lancet,* **ii**, 1157–1159.

Bowen DM, Goodhardt MJ, Strong AJ *et al.* (1976) Biochemical indices of brain structure, function and 'hypoxia' in cortex from baboons with middle cerebral artery occlusion. *Brain Research,* **117**, 503–507.

Burnet PWJ, Eastwood SL, Harrison PJ (1994) Detection and quantitation of 5-HT$_{1A}$ and 5-HT$_{2A}$ receptor mRNAs in human hippocampus using a reverse transcriptase-polymerase chain reaction (RT-PCR) technique and their correlation with binding site densities and age. *Neuroscience Letters,* **178**, 85–89.

Burnet PWJ, Harrison PJ (2000) Substance P (NK1) receptors in the cingulate cortex in unipolar and bipolar mood disorder and schizophrenia. *Biological Psychiatry* **47**, 80–83.

Butterworth J, Yates CM, Simpson J (1983) Phosphate-activated glutaminase in relation to Huntington's disease and agonal state. *Journal of Neurochemistry,* **41**, 440–447.

Cairns NJ, Lantos PL (1996) Brain tissue banks in psychiatric and neurological research. *Journal of Clinical Pathology,* **49**, 870–873.

Casanova MF, Kleinman JE (1990) The neuropathology of schizophrenia: a critical assessment of research methodologies. *Biological Psychiatry,* **27**, 353–362.

Davison K (1983) Schizophrenia-like psychoses associated with organic cerebral disorders: a review. *Psychiatric Developments,* **1**, 1–33.

Dean B, Pavey G, Opeskin K (1997) [^{3}H]raclopride binding to brain tissue from subjects with schizophrenia: Methodological aspects. *Neuropharmacology,* **36**, 779–786.

Dodd PR, Hambley JW, Cowburn RF, Hardy JA (1988) A comparison of methodologies for the study of functional transmitter neurochemistry in human brain. *Journal of Neurochemistry,* **50**, 1333–1345.

Dwork AJ (1997) Postmortem studies of the hippocampal formation in schizophrenia. *Schizophrenia Bulletin,* **23**, 385–402.

Eastwood SL, Harrison PJ (1999) Detection and quantitation of synaptophysin mRNA in the hippocampus in schizophrenia using autoclaved formalin-fixed paraffin wax-embedded sections. *Neuroscience,* **93**, 99–106.

Eastwood SL, Harrison PJ (2000) Hippocampal synaptic pathology in schizophrenia, bipolar disorder and major depression: a study of complexin mRNAs. *Molecular Psychiatry* (in press).

Eastwood SL, Burnet PWJ, McDonald B, Clinton J, Harrison PJ (1994) Synaptophysin gene expression in human brain: A quantitative *in situ* hybridization and immunocytochemical study. *Neuroscience,* **59**, 881–892.

Eastwood SL, Burnet PWJ, Harrison PJ (1997*a*) GluR2 glutamate receptor subunit flip and flop isoforms are decreased in the hippocampal formation in schizophrenia: A reverse transcriptase-polymerase chain reaction (RT- PCR) study. *Molecular Brain Research,* **44**, 92–98.

Eastwood SL, Kerwin RW, Harrison PJ (1997*b*) Immunoautoradiographic evidence for a loss of α-amino-3-hydroxy- 5-methyl-4-isoxazole propionate-preferring non-*N*-methyl-D-aspartate glutamate receptors within the medial temporal lobe in schizophrenia. *Biological Psychiatry,* **41**, 636–643.

Geddes JW, Bondada V, Tekirian TL, Pang Z , Siman RG (1995) Perikaryal accumulation and proteolysis of neurofilament proteins in the post-mortem rat brain. *Neurobiology of Aging,* **16**, 651–660.

Gomez-Isla T, Hollister R, West H *et al.* (1997) Neuronal loss correlates with but exceeds neurofibrillary tangles in Alzheimer's disease. *Annals of Neurology,* **41**, 17–24.

Guillery RW, Herrup K (1997) Quantification without pontification: choosing a method for counting objects in sectioned tissues. *Journal of Comparative Neurology,* **386**, 2–7.

Hardy JA, Wester P, Winblad B, Gexelius C, Bring G, Eriksson A (1985) The patients dying after long terminal phase have acidotic brains; implications for biochemical measurements on autopsy tissue. *Journal of Neural Transmission,* **61**, 253–264.

Harrison PJ (1996) Advances in post mortem molecular neurochemistry and neuropathology: Examples from schizophrenia research. *British Medical Bulletin,* **52**, 527–538.

Harrison PJ, Procter AW, Barton AJL *et al.* (1991) Terminal coma affects messenger RNA detection in post mortem human temporal cortex. *Molecular Brain Research,* **9**, 161–164.

Harrison PJ, Heath PR, Eastwood SL, Burnet PWJ, McDonald B, Pearson RCA (1995) The relative importance of premortem acidosis and postmortem interval for human brain gene expression studies: Selective mRNA vulnerability and comparison with their encoded proteins. *Neuroscience Letters,* **200**, 151–154.

Haug H (1986) History of neuromorphometry. *Journal of Neuroscience Methods,* **18**, 1–17.

Heckers S (1997) Neuropathology of schizophrenia: Cortex, thalamus, basal ganglia, and neurotransmitter-specific projection systems. *Schizophrenia Bulletin,* **23**, 403–421.

Heckers S, Heinsen H, Geiger B, Beckmann H (1991) Hippocampal neuron number in schizophrenia: A stereological study. *Archives of General Psychiatry,* **48**, 1002–1008.

Hill C, Keks N, Roberts S *et al.* (1996) Problem of diagnosis in postmortem brain studies of schizophrenia. *American Journal of Psychiatry,* **153**, 533–537.

Howard CV, Reed MG (1998) *Unbiased stereology. Three-dimensional measurement in microscopy.* Bios Scientific Press, Oxford.

Johnston NL, Cerevnak J, Shore AD, Torrey EF, Yolken RH (1997) Multivariate analysis of RNA levels from postmortem human brains as measured by three different methods of RT-PCR. *Journal of Neuroscience Methods,* **77**, 83–92.

Johnstone EC, McMillan JF, Crow TJ (1987) The occurrence of organic disease of possible or probable aetiological significance in a population of 268 cases of first episode schizophrenia. *Psychological Medicine,* **17**, 371–379.

Johnstone EC, Bruton CJ, Crow TJ, Frith CD, Owens DGC (1994) Clinical correlates of postmortem brain changes in schizophrenia: Decreased brain weight and length correlate with indices of early impairment. *Journal of Neurology, Neurosurgery and Psychiatry,* **57**, 474–479.

Keilp JG, Waniek C, Goodman RG *et al.* (1995) Reliability of post-mortem chart diagnoses of schizophrenia and dementia. *Schizophrenia Research,* **17**, 221–228.

Kingsbury AE, Foster OJ, Nisbet AP *et al.* (1995) Tissue pH as an indicator of mRNA preservation in human post- mortem brain. *Molecular Brain Research,* **28**, 311–318.

Kontur PJ, Al-Tikriti M, Innis RB, Roth RH (1994) Postmortem stability of monoamines, their metabolites, and receptor binding in rat brain regions. *Journal of Neurochemistry,* **62**, 282–290.

Kornhuber J, Retz W, Riederer P, Heinsen H, Fritze J (1988) Effect of antemortem and postmortem factors on [^{3}H]glutamate binding in the human brain. *Neuroscience Letters,* **93**, 312–317.

Kretschmann H-J, Tafesse U, Herrmann A (1982) Different volume changes of cerebral cortex and white matter during histological procedures. *Microscopica Acta* **86**, 13–24.

Lucassen PJ, Goudsmit E, Pool CW *et al.* (1995) *In situ* hybridization for vasopressin mRNA in the human supraoptic and paraventricular nucleus: Quantitative aspects of formalin-fixed paraffin-embedded tissue sections as compared to cryostat sections. *Journal of Neuroscience Methods,* **57**, 221–230.

Mayhew TM, Gundersen HJG (1996) 'If you assume, you can make an ass out of u and me': A decade of the disector for stereological counting of particles in 3D space. *Journal of Anatomy,* **188**, 1–15.

Mirra SS, Heyman A, McKeel D *et al.* (1991) The Consortium to Establish a Registry for Alzheimer's Disease (CERAD) Part II. Standardization of the neuropathologic assessment of Alzheimer's disease. *Neurology,* **41**, 479–486.

Morrison-Bogorad M, Zimmerman AL, Pardue S (1995) Heat-shock 70 messenger RNA levels in human brain: Correlation with agonal fever. *Journal of Neurochemistry,* **64**, 235–246.

Oliver KR, Wainwright A, Heavens RP, Sirinathsinghji DJS (1997) Retrieval of cellular mRNA in paraffin-embedded human brain using hydrated autoclaving. *Journal of Neuroscience Methods,* **77**, 169–174.

Oorschot, D.E. (1994) Are you using neuronal densities, synaptic densities or neurochemical densities as your definitive data? There is a better way to go. *Progress in Neurobiology,* **44**, 233–247.

Pakkenberg B (1990) Pronounced reduction of total neuron number in mediodorsal thalamic nucleus and nucleus accumbens in schizophrenics. *Archives of General Psychiatry,* **47**, 1023–1028.

Palmer AM, Lowe SL, Francis PT, Bowen DM (1988) Are post-mortem biochemical studies of human brain worthwhile? *Biochemical Society Transactions,* **16**, 472–475.

Perry EK, Perry RH (1983) Human brain neurochemistry: some postmortem problems. *Life Sciences,* **33**, 1733–1743.

Perry EK, Perry HP, Tomlinson BE (1982) The influence of agonal status on some neurochemical activities of postmortem human brain tissue. *Neuroscience Letters,* **29**, 303–307.

Piggott MA, Perry EK, Sahgal A, Perry RH (1992) Examination of parameters influencing [^{3}H]MK-801 binding in postmortem human cortex. *Journal of Neurochemistry,* **58**, 1001–1008.

Porter RHP, Eastwood SL, Harrison PJ (1997) Distribution of kainate receptor subunit mRNAs in human hippocampus, neocortex and cerebellum, and bilateral reduction of hippocampal GluR6 and KA2 transcripts in schizophrenia. *Brain Research,* **751**, 217–231.

Quester R, Schröder R (1997) The shrinkage of the human brain stem during formalin fixation and embedding in paraffin. *Journal of Neuroscience Methods,* **75**, 81–89.

Ravid R, Swaab DF (1993) The Netherlands brain bank—a clinico-pathological link in aging and dementia research. *Journal of Neural Transmission,* Suppl. 39, 143–153.

Riederer P, Gsell W, Calza L *et al.* (1995) Consensus on minimal criteria of clinical and neuropathological diagnosis of schizophrenia and affective disorders for post mortem research—Report from the European Dementia and Schizophrenia Network (BIOMED I). *Journal of Neural Transmission,* **102**, 255–264.

Schwab C, Bondada V, Sparks DL, Cahan LD, Geddes JW (1994) Postmortem changes in the levels and localization of microtubule-associated proteins (tau, MAP2 and MAP1B) in the rat and human hippocampus. *Hippocampus,* **4**, 210–225.

Spokes EGS (1979) An analysis of factors influencing measurements of dopamine, noradrenaline, glutamate decarboxylase and choline acetylase in human post-mortem brain tissue. *Brain,* **102**, 333–346.

Stevens JR (1997) Anatomy of schizophrenia revisited. *Schizophrenia Bulletin,* **23**, 373–383.

Torrey EF, Webster M, Knable M, Johnston N, Yolken RH (2000) The Stanley Foundation Brain Collection and neuropathology consortium. *Schizophrenia Research* (in press).

Wagman AMI (1992) Report of a workshop on issues in brain tissue acquisition. *Schizophrenia Bulletin,* **18**, 149–153.

West MJ (1993) New stereological methods for counting neurons. *Neurobiology of Aging,* **14**, 275–285.

Whitehouse PJ, Lynch D, Kuher MJ (1984) Effects of postmortem delay and temperature on neurotransmitter receptor binding in a rat model of the human autopsy process. *Journal of Neurochemistry,* **43**, 553–559.

Zalcman S, Endicott J (1983) *Diagnostic Evaluation after Death.* Developed for NIMH Neurosciences Research Branch, Department of Research Assessment and Training, New York State Psychiatric Institute.

15 Neuropathological Consequences of Schizophrenia Treatments

Paul J. Harrison

Neuropathological effects of antipsychotic drugs
  Animal studies
  Human studies
Neuropathological effects of other treatments
  Electroconvulsive therapy (ECT)
  Lithium
  Historical treatments
Neuropathological effects of substance misuse
Conclusions

The confounding effects of antipsychotic medication on neurochemical studies of schizophrenia are well known (Harrison, 1999a). Their influence on brain structure, though less well documented, has become apparent from imaging studies indicating that antipsychotics produce striatal enlargement in patients (Chakos et al., 1994; Keshavan et al., 1994; Doraiswamy et al., 1995; see Chapter 1) and in rats (Chakos et al., 1998). Of particular relevance here, the drugs also produce neuronal morphometric and synaptic changes which may overlap with and hence confound the cytoarchitectural alterations reported in schizophrenia. This chapter reviews the histological effects of antipsychotics. Brief mention is also made of neuropathological implications of other schizophrenia treatments, and of substances which are commonly abused by people with (or without) schizophrenia.

Neuropathological effects of antipsychotic drugs

Nearly all patients in contemporary neuropathological studies of schizophrenia have received antipsychotics, precluding comparisons of untreated with treated subgroups of patients. Indeed, drug-naive but unequivocally diagnosed cases are so rare that one would worry about their representativeness. Archival brain material from the pre-antipsychotic era (such as the Yakovlev collection) can be valuable, but suffers from limitations of diagnostic information and mode of processing which hampers many techniques. Given these factors, there are several alternative research strategies by which the neuropathological consequences of antipsychotic drugs can be investigated and distinguished from those attributable to schizophrenia. Each has advantages and disadvantages.

1. Comparison of patients on medication at death with those who had been drug free for a significant period. Drawbacks include the assumption that medication effects on brain structure are reversible within the chosen time frame, and that the two groups are otherwise clinically and pathophysiologically comparable.

2. Calculation of life-time medication exposure, usually converted to chlorpromazine dose equivalents, and then correlation of total exposure with the parameter in question. This approach assumes a cumulative relationship between the variables, and usually a linear one in which treatment many decades ago is given equal weight to that received just before death.

3. Use of an antipsychotic-treated control group, normally comprised of a mixture of cases of dementia with psychosis, delusional disorder, and bipolar disorder. Although such a group goes some way towards controlling for drug effects, their medication histories rarely approach the duration and amount received by schizophrenic subjects. Moreover, inclusion of cases with degenerative disorders adds its own neuropathological complications, whilst inclusion of other paranoid or affective psychoses is confounded by possible shared pathological features with schizophrenia.

4. Neuropathological investigation targeted specifically at the brains of antipsychotic-treated subjects regardless of diagnosis.

5. Studies of animals administered antipsychotic drugs. This approach has many methodological attractions, but is subject to the reservations inherent when extrapolating results between species.

Many of the studies of schizophrenia discussed in this book have used one of the first three approaches listed above to exclude confounding effects of antipsychotic medication. As a rule, these have not shown a demonstrable contribution of medication to the findings in schizophrenia (see Madsen *et al.*, 1998 for a possible MRI exception), and they are not discussed further here. Rather, the focus is on studies in the latter two categories which have greater power specifically to investigate the neuropathology of antipsychotic administration.

Animal studies

Experimental studies of the neuropathological effects of antipsychotic drugs have concentrated on the structure and numerical density of synapses and, to a lesser degree, of neurons. Three caveats apply generally to the data to be reviewed (with the exception of Selemon *et al.*, 1999). Firstly, all experiments have been done in rodents, which metabolise antipsychotics differently to humans, and might respond neuropathologically in different ways. Secondly, non-stereological methods have been used throughout, and the data are therefore subject to limitations and biases (see Chapter 14); on the other hand, making a virtue out of necessity, few of the equivalent studies in schizophrenia to which these findings are being related have been stereological either. Thirdly, most studies have used haloperidol, and differential or drug-specific effects of other antipsychotics cannot be excluded.

Effects on synapses

Changes in synaptic structure and circuitry induced by antipsychotics have been examined in some detail. The majority of the studies have used electron microscopy (EM), though more recently molecular markers of synapses have been applied. The two methods each have advantages and disadvantages (see Chapter 4): EM allows direct visualisation and measurements of the structure of interest, but is time-consuming, limited to small areas of tissue, and comparable measurements in human brain are problematic because of post-mortem artefacts. The newer approaches are molecularly specific, make large-scale analyses feasible, and can be adapted more readily to human brain; on the other hand, they are only proxies and the precise underlying anatomical change has to be inferred. Table 15.1 summarises the EM studies of antipsychotic treatment. Most of the studies have assessed the proportion of morphologically defined synaptic subtypes in treated compared to untreated animals. Several overlapping categorisations of synapses have been used, each with approximate functional correlates as follows.

1. The subcellular location of the synapses (e.g. axodendritic versus axospinous versus axosomatic). Axospinous synapses (synapses between axon terminals and dendritic spines) are essentially all excitatory, whereas axosomatic ones (i.e. synapses apposed to the neuronal cell body) are inhibitory, and axodendritic synapses (i.e. synapses onto dendritic shafts) are a mixture.

2. The appearance of the pre- and postsynaptic terminal regions. Synapses similar ('symmetrical') in this respect are inhibitory, whereas 'asymmetrical' ones are considered excitatory.

3. The presence of postsynaptic specialisations, notably a perforated postsynaptic density (PPD). A PPD is believed to denote a newly formed synapse, and hence an increase in PPD-containing synapses is a marker of synaptic plasticity.

4. Synaptic components have also been assessed in terms of their size. Increased size is presumed to reflect increased 'demand' or activity across the synapse, in this respect providing another indicator of synaptic plasticity. (For review of the classification and functional correlates of synaptic morphology, see Peters and Palay, 1986; Genisman et al., 1989; Calverley and Jones, 1990; Pierce and Lewin, 1994.)

Together the data provide good evidence that chronic antipsychotic treatment induces synaptic plasticity and, *pari passu*, alters the synaptic ultrastructure (Table 15.1). Both pre- and postsynaptic elements are affected. The changes are most marked in the dorsolateral striatum, with less extensive evidence for alterations in the prefrontal cortex. Other reasonably clear findings are that most (Meshul and Casey, 1989; Roberts et al., 1995) but not all (Roberts et al., 1995; Kelley et al., 1997) changes reverse within weeks of stopping the drugs, and that clozapine has different effects from haloperidol (Vincent et al., 1991; Meshul et al., 1992).

Table 15.1 Antipsychotic drug effects on synapses: ultrastructural studies

Reference	Drug, dose, and duration	Parameters measured	Significant changes in drug-treated animals
1	Haloperidol 3mg/kg/d i.m. for 16 w	Substantia nigra: number and area of axon terminals, dendrites and spines; number of synaptic vesicles	Increased axon terminals per dendrite. No other changes
2	Haloperidol 3mg/kg/d i.m. for 16 w[a]	As above, in striatum	Increase in size of axon terminals. No changes in other parameters
3	Haloperidol 3 mg/kg/d i.m. for 16 w[a]	As above, in layer VI of medial prefrontal cortex	Loss of dendritic spines and associated asymmetrical synapses; increase in other axon terminals. No other changes
4	Chlorpromazine 20 mg/kg/d p.o. for 15 m	Striatum: number, size, and shape of vesicles in axopinous synapses	Small increase in vesicular size. Number and shaped unchanged
5	Haloperidol 5 mg/kg/d i.m. for 13 d killed 8 d or 36 d later	Number and area of dopaminergic terminal boutons in striatum	Decreased number of terminal boutons and vesicles at both time points
6	Haloperidol 0.1 mg/kg/d i.m. for 3 w	Prefrontal cortex lamina VI: density of axodendritic and axospinous synapses; number, area, and mitochondrial content of axon terminals; number and density of vesicles	Increased axodendritic but decreased axospinous synapses. Axodendritic synapses: reduced axon terminal area and fewer mitochondria; postsynaptic densities longer. Axospinous synapses: minor changes
7	Haloperidol 0.5 mg/kg/d i.m. for 2 w killed 1 d or 2 w later	Caudate and nucleus accumbens: number of synapses and those with PPD; area of axon terminals	Reversible increase in synapses with PPD in caudate nucleus. No other changes
8	Haloperidol 1 mg/kg/d i.m. for 3 w	Caudate and hippocampus (CA1): parameters as in ref. 6	Caudate: increased axodendritic and axospinous synapses. Axospinous synapses have larger axon terminals with more mitochondria; larger size of postsynaptic density. Axodendritic synapses: smaller axon terminals with less mitochondria. No other changes, nor any in hippocampus

Table 15.1 continued

Reference	Drug, dose, and duration	Parameters measured	Significant changes in drug-treated animals
9	Haloperidol 1.3 mg/kg/d or clozapine 27 mg/kg/d p.o. for 12 m	Layer VI of prefrontal corex: size of dendrites, spines, and axon teminals; vesicle density; symmetric and asymmetric synapses	Haloperidol: reduced calibre of dendrites. Both groups: relative increase of symmetric axodendritic synapses. Clozapine: increase of the (small) number of symmetric axospinous synapses. No changes in vesicle density or size of axon terminals
10	Haloperidol 0.5 mg/kg/d or clozapine 35mg/kg/d i.m. for 2 w	Caudate, nucleus accumbens and layer VI of prefrontal cortex: number of synapses and those with PPD	Caudate nucleus: increased number of synapses with PPD after haloperidol. No changes with clozapine or in other areas
11	Haloperidol or raclopride, 7 mg/kg/w i.m. for 7 m	Caudate: number of synapses with PPD	Increased number of PPD synapses after both drugs
12	Haloperidol 1.5 mg/kg/d p.o. for 6 m killed 1 d or 4 w later	Striatum: synaptic density, mitochondrial size, area, and number	Decreased density of asymmetric axospinous synapses Symmetric and axodendritic synapses unaffected. Increased mitochondrial size and decreased number. All changes reversed 4 w later, except loss of mitochondria
13	Haloperidol 1.5 mg/kg/d p.o. for 6 m killed 1 d or 4 w later[c]	Striatum: dendritic spine size and density	Spine size unaffected. Spine density decreased and remained decreased 4 w later

d; days; w; weeks; m; months; i.m.; intramuscular injection; p.o.; orally; PPD; perforated post-synaptic densities.
Reference: 1: Benes et al. (1983); 2: Benes et al. (1985a); 3: Benes et al. (1985b); 4: Takeichi (1985); 5: Ihara et al; (1986); 6: Klintzova et al. (1989); 7: Meshul and Casey (1989); 8: Uranova et al. (1991); 9: Vincent et al. (1991); 10: Meshul et al. (1992); 11: See et al. (1992); 12: Roberts et al. (1995); 13: Kelley et al. (1997).
[a]Apparently the same animals as used in reference 1, and in references 5–7 of Table 15.3.
[b]Treated rats divided into those with and without dyskinesia. Latter group had greater synapse loss (especially of symmetrical type) and more marked mitochondrial changes.
[c]The same animals as in reference 12.

A more speculative interpretation of the studies in Table 15.1 is that antipsychotic treatment increases the proportion of symmetric and axodendritic synapses in the striatum relative to asymmetric and axospinous ones (Benes et al., 1985b; Klintzova et al., 1989; Vincent et al., 1991; Roberts et al., 1995; Meshul et al., 1996; cf. See et al., 1992). Given the excitatory nature of most asymmetric and axospinous synapses (see above), this pattern implies that antipsychotics alter the numerical balance in favour of inhibitory synapses. However, there is also evidence that asymmetric synaptic terminals are enlarged and are those which have increased PPDs, implying that transmission is enhanced across excitatory synapses (Benes et al., 1985a; Meshul and Casey, 1989; See et al., 1992; Meshul et al., 1994, 1996). Overall, therefore, evaluation of the net functional effects of antipsychotics upon the circuitry of the striatum (and cortex; Vincent et al., 1991) must take into account both an altered ratio of synaptic types and probable changes in the properties of constituent synapses.

These inconclusive observations emphasise that, though the existence of antipsychotic-induced ultrastructural effects is clearly established, the overall pattern and underlying mechanisms are not. This is partly due to the methodological differences between the studies and partly the incomplete data which, for example, preclude statements about the effects of doses and durations of treatment. Equally, the functional and pathophysiological consequences of the synaptic alterations are still a matter of conjecture, though it seems reasonable to postulate that changes in the striatal circuitry contribute to the extrapyramidal side-effects of antipsychotics (Roberts et al., 1995).

The results of the molecular and immunocytochemical studies of synapses (Table 15.2) are largely in keeping with the EM data. In particular, changes in the expression of presynaptic proteins support the occurrence of synaptic plasticity which differentially affects synaptic populations in striatum and frontal cortex. Also, the use of immunolabelling with glutamate in corticostriate terminals (Meshul et al., 1996) and of GABA in frontal cortex synapses (Vincent et al., 1994) provides some clarification of the neurochemical identity of the affected synapses.

Effects on neurons

Table 15.3 summarises the relatively few studies which have examined neuronal parameters in animals treated with antipsychotics. Few significant abnormalities have been demonstrated. Neither dopamine neurons in the substantia nigra (Gerlach, 1975; Benes et al., 1983) nor cortical neurons (Selemon et al., 1999) appear to be altered by the drugs. There is some evidence for a decreased density of striatal neurons (Pakkenberg et al., 1973; Nielson and Lyon, 1978; Jeste et al., 1992), but this is not always observed (Fog et al., 1976; Benes et al., 1985a; Jeste et al., 1998) and in any event is of uncertain interest as it probably just reflects striatal enlargement (Chakos et al., 1998) rather than any change in total neuron number. One study also reported an increased somal size of striatal neurons (Benes et al., 1985a). The possibility that any striatal neuropathological effects are greater for large neurons (Jeste et al., 1992) is of interest given that the same (cholinergic) cell population has been commented on in human studies (see below, also Miller and Chouinard, 1993; Holt et al., 1999) and exhibits increased synaptophysin expression suggestive of synaptic sprouting after haloperidol treatment (Eastwood et al., 1994, 1997).

The study of prefrontal cortex by Selemon et al. (1999) is doubly noteworthy, being the first morphometric study in the field to have been stereological, and carried out in primates.

Table 15.2 Antipsychotic drug effects on synapses: molecular and immunochemical studies

Reference	Drug, dose, and duration	Parameters measured	Significant changes in drug-treated animals
1	Haloperidol decanoate 10.5 mg/kg/ 3 w or 19 w	GABA-positive terminals on pyramidal neurons in medial prefrontal cortex	Increased size (or GABA content) of terminals; unchanged number
2	Haloperidol 2 mg/kg/d i.m. for 2 w	Synaptophysin and its mRNA in dorsolateral striatum and frontal cortex	mRNA increased in both areas. Same trend for protein
3	Haloperidol 2 mg/kg/d i.m. for 2w[a]	Synaptophysin mRNA in hippocampus	No differences
4	Haloperidol 1 mg/kg/d or clozapine 20 mg/kg/d i.m. for 10 d	Secretogranin II and chromogranin mRNAs in dorsolateral striatum[b]	Increase in both mRNAs, haloperidol more so than clozapine
5	Haloperidol 0.5 mg/kg/d or clozapine 30 mg/kg/d i.m. for 4 w	Glutamate-positive asymmetric striatal synapses, with or without PPD	Both drugs increased glutamate labelling. Only haloperidol did so at perforated synapses
6	Haloperidol decanoate 14 mg/kg i.m. one injection, killed 2 w later	Size and shape of met[5]-enkephalin-positive boutons in dorsal striatum	Boutons enlarged and elongated
7	Haloperidol decanoate 21 mg/kg/3 w i.m. for 16 w	Synaptophysin, its mRNA, and GAP-43 mRNA in dorsolateral striatum, frontal cortex, and hippocampus	Synatophysin results as in references 2 and 3. No change in GAP-43 mRNA in any area
8	Haloperidol 1 mg/kg/d i.m. for 3 w killed 4 d later	Synaptophysin in striatal homogenates	Increased
9	Haloperidol decanoate 25 mg/kg/ i.m. one injection, killed 4 w later	Synaptobrevin II, synaptotagmin I and IV, syntaxin IA, SNAP-25, Rab 3a, and synaptophysin mRNAs in striatum, frontal cortex, and midbrain	Synaptobrevin, synaptotagmins, syntaxin 1A, and rab-3a mRNAs decreased in n.accumbens. No other changes
10	Haloperidol 1 mg/kg/d, chlorpromazine 15 mg/kg/d, clozapine 25 mg/kg/d, risperidone 0.5 mg/kg/d, olanzapine 5 mg/kg/d i.m. for 2 w	Synaptophysin mRNA in dorsolateral striatum, frontal cortex, and hippocampus	Increased in striatum by chlorpromazine, with trend for haloperidol

d; days; w; weeks; m, months; i.m.; intramuscular injection; mRNA, messenger RNA; PPD, perforated postsynaptic density.
Reference: 1: Vincent et al. (1994); 2: Eastwood et al. (1994); 3: Eastwood et al. (1995); 4: Kroesen et al. (1995); 5: Meshul et al. (1996); 6: Mijnster et al. (1996); 7: Eastwood et al. (1997); 8: Marin and Tolosa (1997); 9: Nakahara et al. (1998); 10: Eastwood et al. (2000).
[a]Same animals as in reference 2.
[b]Other nuclei also measured.

Table 15.3 Antipsychotic drug effects on neurons

Reference	Drug, dose, and duration	Parameters measured	Significant changes in drug-treated animals
1	Perphenazine enanthate, 3.4 mg/kg/2 w i.m. for 12 m	Neuronal density in cortex and striatum	20% reduction in striatum; no change in cortex[a]
2	Group 1: as above[b]. Group 2: 40 mg/kg/2 w i.m. for 6 m	Neuronal density in substantia nigra (pars compacta and reticulata)	No changes[a]
3	Perphenazine enanthate, 40 mg/kg/2 w i.m. for 6 m[c]	Neuronal density in cortex and striatum	No changes
4	Flupenthixo decanoate, 4 mg/kg/w i.m. for 36 w; killed 14–18 w later	Neuronal density in striatum	10% cell loss in ventrolateral compared to dorsomedial striatum
5	Haloperidol 3 mg/kg/d i.m. for 16 w	Neuronal density and size in substantia nigra pars compacta	No changes
6	Haloperidol 3 mg/kg/d i.m. for 16 w[d]	Neuronal density and size in striatum	13% increase in neuronal size; density unchanged
7	Haloperidol 3 mg/kg/d i.m. for 16 w[d]	Neuronal density and size in medial prefrontal cortex	No changes
8	Fluphenazine decanoate 5 mg/kg/2 w i.m. for 4, 8. or 12 m	Neuronal density in striatum	Decreased density of large neurons after 8 m. No other changes
9	Haloperidol 1.6 mg/kg/d p.o. for 14 m, killed 2 w later	Neuronal density in striatum	No changes
10	Haloperidol 0.2 mg/kg/d, cholorpromazine 2.8 mg/kg/d, pimozide 0.2 mg/kg/d, clozapine 5.2 mg/kg/d, olanzapine 0.35 mg/kg/d or risperidone 0.2 mg/kg/d, p.o. for 6 m (n = 2 in each group)	Neuronal and glial density in dorsolateral prefrontal cortex (area 46); cortical and laminar thickness	Neuronal density unchanged. Glial density increased ~30% in laminae I and IV. Layer V enlarged. No drug-specific effects, except apparent neurotoxicity after risperidone

d, days; w, weeks; m, months; i.m., intramuscular injection. All studies carried out in rats except reference 10 (primates).
Reference: 1: Pakkenberg et al. (1973); 2: Gerlach (1975); 3: Fog et al. (1976); 4: Nielsen and Lyon (1978); 5: Benes et al. (1985a); 7: Benes et al. (1985b); 8: Jeste et al. (1992); 9: Gariano et al. (1990); 10: Selemon et al. 1999.
[a]Comment also made on morphology and arrangement of neurons and glia; no differences in treated animals were observed.
[b]The same animals as were used in reference 1.
[c]Same animals as used in reference 2.
[d]Apparently the same animals as used in reference 5.

No differences in neuronal density were found following chronic administration of antipsychotics (see Table 15.3 for details). In contrast, glial density was increased in layers I and IV, which the authors suggest may have been a response to altered glutamatergic connectivity and which, if also occurring in patients given these drugs, might contribute beneficially to the therapeutic response. The neurotoxicity reported in the two risperidone-treated animals (one showed hypoxic-ischaemic damage, one had marked loss of neurons) is difficult to interpret given the small sample size and because the pharmacokinetics and metabolism of the drug in rhesus monkeys is unknown and might be idiosyncratic.

Human studies

The major study of the neuropathological effects of antipsychotics is that by Jellinger (1977); it also includes a summary of previous case reports and series. Jellinger investigated 28 patients treated with antipsychotics, most of whom had a diagnosis of schizophrenia. Fourteen had had significant dyskinesia. The 28 cases were compared with a series of unmedicated schizophrenics, and a series of neurologically normal, age-matched controls. Treated subjects with and without dyskinesia were also compared. Thus, an attempt was made to control for the confounding variables of age, presence of underlying psychosis, and occurrence of dyskinesia. Unfortunately, the data are not presented clearly, and the analyses are not truly quantitative. Even so, several findings are worth mentioning.

The changes were observed in the caudate nucleus, especially the rostral part. The commonest findings were swollen large neurons, glial satellitosis, and sometimes a more generalised gliosis. This pattern of alterations was considered to reflect chronic partial denervation. Small neurons were unaffected. These striatal alterations were found in 13 out of 28 (46 per cent) of the antipsychotic-treated group compared to 4 per cent of the untreated schizophrenics and 2 per cent of the controls. Antipsychotic-treated cases with dyskinesia had a slightly greater incidence of pathology than those without (57 versus 37.5 per cent). The occurrence of pathological changes did not relate to diagnosis or age. No consistent pathological effects of antipsychotics on neurons or glia were found elsewhere in the brain, although the extent of the search is not stated. EM studies of the striatum were performed in two of the dyskinetic patients, and enlarged axons were found together with increased numbers of mitochondria and abnormal organelles.

The lack of clear neuropathological abnormalities outside the caudate nucleus is in contrast to the other large series, which comprised 28 patients dying with dyskinesia, 21 of whom had been treated long term with antipsychotics (Christensen *et al.*, 1970). (The paper does not allow the latter subgroup to be separated for analysis). In the dyskinetic group, a higher incidence of gliosis (89 per cent) and neuronal degeneration (89 per cent) in the substantia nigra and brainstem was reported than in controls (25 and 14 per cent, respectively). However, the control group was poorly matched, and in the light of other negative studies (see Jellinger, 1977), the robustness and interpretation of these changes is uncertain.

Neither of the two series mentioned here is strictly comparable with the quantitative and molecular data emerging from contemporary neuropathological studies of schizophrenia.

As such, it is difficult to interpret the results of Jellinger (1977) and Christensen *et al.* (1970), and their findings must be considered together with the results of the alternative approaches to the issue of medication effects. Nevertheless, it is noteworthy that the human findings are congruent in two respects to those in animals. Firstly, that the changes are greatest in the caudate nucleus (cf. refs 1, 4, 6, 8 in Table 15.1, refs 2, 4, 5, 7, 8, 9–11 in Table 15.2; refs 2, 4–8 in Table 15.3). Secondly, the human EM data, albeit from only two patients, are consistent with the axon terminal and mitochondrial alterations seen in treated animals (refs 2, 5, 8, 12 in Table 15.2; see also Kung and Roberts, 1999).

Do antipsychotics promote Alzheimer's disease?

The suggestion that antipsychotic drugs might promote the neuropathological features of Alzheimer's disease arises for two reasons. Firstly, it has sometimes been said that patients with schizophrenia are at increased risk of Alzheimer's disease (See Harrison, 1999*b* for origins of this belief; also Chapter 2). Secondly, Wisniewski *et al.* (1994) reported that the incidence of neurofibrillary tangles was higher in schizophrenics who had been treated with antipsychotics (and who died between 1954 and 1990) than those who died before 1952 and therefore had not received the drugs (74 versus 36 per cent). They also found hippocampal neuronal density to be decreased by ~25 per cent in the medicated group.

In fact, there is no good evidence that Alzheimer's disease is commoner in schizophrenia, even in those with cognitive impairment and despite the fact that the majority of patients in these studies were treated with antipsychotics (Harrison, 1997). This negative conclusion was confirmed in a meta-analysis which found an overall odds ratio of 0.86 for the prevalence of Alzheimer's disease in schizophrenia (Baldessarini *et al.*, 1997) and by recent large and better controlled series (Arnold *et al.*, 1998; Purohit *et al.*, 1998; Jellinger and Gabriel, 1999). Interpretation of the Wisniewski *et al.* (1994) findings is difficult anyway given the doubtful comparability of the two cohorts (e.g. with regard to diagnostic criteria, effect of differing storage times) and the analysis used (Baldessarini *et al.*, 1997). Parenthetically, *in vitro* data show that phenothiazines may protect against the aggregation of tau (Wischik *et al.*, 1996) and the formation (Higaki *et al.*, 1997) and neurotoxicity (Ueda *et al.*, 1997) of β-amyloid—suggesting that antipsychotics should, if anything, be protective against Alzheimer-type neuropathology.

Which neuropathological findings in schizophrenia are likely to be confounded by antipsychotic treatment?

Consideration of the data reviewed above suggests that some neuropathological studies in schizophrenia may well be affected by antipsychotic treatment, but many will not. All studies in the striatum are vulnerable, given the range of reported effects on synapses, neurons, and perhaps glia (Tables 15.1 to 15.3), although recent data suggest a different pattern of striatal synaptic pathology due to schizophrenia than that due to antipsychotics (see Roberts *et al.*, 1996; Uranova *et al.*, 1996; Kung *et al.*, 1998; Kung and Roberts, 1999). Synaptic studies in the frontal cortex, at least in lamina VI, must also be interpreted cautiously in the light of the ultrastructural and synaptic protein findings in antipsychotic-treated animals. Similarly, the data of Selemon *et al.* (1999) imply that antipsychotics may contribute to the apparent excess of gliosis in schizophrenia reported in some studies (see Chapter 5). Conversely, there is little or no evidence that antipsychotics produce neuropathological effects in the hippocampus (Tables 15.1 to 15.3), nor affect cortical neurons (Table 15.3), and hence are unlikely to be major confounders of the cytoarchitectural findings therein.

Neuropathological effects of other treatments

Electroconvulsive therapy (ECT)

A comprehensive review concluded that ECT produces no demonstrable structural effects (Devenand *et al.*, 1994). Whilst reassuring, there are caveats. The presence of subtle changes in neuronal and synaptic structural parameters following ECT akin to those reported in schizophrenia has not been investigated; in rats, where such studies have been done, alterations in synaptic proteins (Jorgensen and Bolwig, 1979), up-regulation of the glial marker glial fibrillary acidic protein (GFAP; Orzi *et al.*, 1990; Steward, 1994), and of the dendritic microtubule associated protein MAP-2 (Pei *et al.*, 1998), and perhaps hippocampal neurotoxicity (Enns *et al.*, 1996) have been reported. Though the clinical relevance of these experiments is questionable since a higher stimulus intensity and frequency has generally been used and only short-term effects measured (see Devenand *et al.*, 1994), it would be prudent to bear the data in mind if a subject had received ECT in the weeks prior to death.

Lithium

Case reports (Schneider and Mirra, 1994) and studies in monkeys (Akai *et al.*, 1977) show that fatal lithium toxicity is associated with a variety of neuropathological findings in keeping with acute neurotoxicity. Whether therapeutic levels of lithium produce any neuropathological effects is much less clear since there have been no studies of humans or monkeys treated long term with lithium. It has even been argued that lithium may be neuroprotective (Manji *et al.*, 1999). The only empirical neuropathological data are in rodents. In one study, lithium administered for 30 weeks at serum levels of 0.5 to 0.8 mmol/l (with or without concurrent haloperidol at 1 mg/kg/day) did not affect cortical neuron number, density, or size (Licht *et al.*, 1994). However, another group have reported that rats treated with lithium (0.6 to 1.2 mmol/l) for 4 weeks have a 35 per cent elevation of hippocampal and caudate GFAP (Rocha and Rodnight, 1994) and exhibit hippocampal astrocytosis (Rocha *et al.*, 1998).

There are no neuropathological studies of other mood stabilisers or antidepressants.

Historical treatments

Some subjects included in postmortem studies are elderly patients who received insulin coma therapy or leucotomy. Though the impact of these interventions is likely to be less than that of antipsychotics if only because fewer subjects have received them, they are still potential neuropathological confounders (Roizin, 1972; Pakkenberg, 1989).

Neuropathological effects of substance misuse

The population prevalence of known and occult substance misuse, and its probable higher level amongst people with schizophrenia, means that the possibility that alcohol and illicit drugs might have relevant neuropathological effects should not be overlooked. For example, methamphetamine produces neuronal loss in substantia nigra (Sonsalla *et al.*, 1996) and alters striatal (Ihara *et al.*, 1986) and cortical (Dawirs *et al.*, 1993) synaptic terminals. Opioids decrease neuronal size in the ventral tegmentum (Sklair-Tavron *et al.*, 1996) and reduce the density of dendritic spines (Robinson and Kolb, 1999). In chronic alcohol misuse, localised alterations in neuronal soma size, dendritic arborisation, and cell density, as well as cortical gliosis, have been described (Harper and Kril, 1990; Ibanez *et al.*, 1995; Arango *et al.*, 1996); neuronal number may also be decreased in some areas (Kril *et al.*, 1997) but this was not apparent in the cortex as a whole (Jensen and Pakkenberg, 1993) nor in hippocampus (Harding *et al.*, 1997). Instead, decreased hippocampal glial number has been reported in a stereological study of alcoholics (Korbo, 1999).

Conclusions

The best documented histological effects of antipsychotic drugs are in the striatum, where neuronal and synaptic structure have been shown to be affected in rats, with circumstantial evidence for a comparable process in humans. There is also reasonable evidence for a subtle synaptic reorganisation in deep laminae of the frontal cortex, and possible effects on glial density in more superficial laminae. Caution should therefore be exercised when interpreting equivalent neuropathological findings in these areas in schizophrenia; this applies not only to ultrastructural and morphometric analyses, but also to measurements of gene products used as proxies (Chapter 4). There is no indication that antipsychotic treatment produces neuronal or synaptic changes in hippocampus, wherein many of the recent positive findings in schizophrenia have been reported (Chapter 2). Neither is there any good evidence to support the assertion that antipsychotics promote neurofibrillary pathology.

The potential neuropathological influence of antipsychotics *vis-à-vis* schizophrenia must continue to be taken into account, especially as new techniques are introduced, novel parameters measured, and different brain areas studied. As patients treated with atypical antipsychotics begin to be included in postmortem series, the structural consequences of these agents will need consideration. A combination of the approaches listed at the start of the chapter will ensure that the neuropathological effects of antipsychotics and other interventions can be disentangled from those of schizophrenia itself.

References

Akai, K., Roizin, L. and Liu, J. C. (1977) Ultrastructural findings of the central nervous system in lithium neurotoxicology. In: Roizin, L., Shiraki, H. and Grcevic, N. (eds). *Neurotoxicology.* New York, Raven, pp. 185–203.

Arango, V., Underwood, M. D., Pauler, D. K., Kass, R. E. and Mann, J. J. (1996) Differential age-related loss of pigmented locus coeruleus neurons in suicides, alcoholics, and alcoholic suicides. *Alcohol: Clinical and Experimental Research, 20*, 1141–1147.

Arnold, S. E., Trojanowski, J. Q., Gur, R. E., Blackwell, P., Han, L.-Y. and Choi, C. (1998) Absence of neurodegeneration and neural injury in the cerebral cortex in a sample of elderly patients with schizophrenia. *Archives of General Psychiatry, 55*, 225–232.

Baldessarini, R. J., Hegarty, J. D., Bird, E. D. and Benes F. M. (1997) Meta-analysis of postmortem studies of Alzheimer's disease-like neuropathology in schizophrenia. *American Journal of Psychiatry, 154*, 861–863.

Benes, F. M., Paskevich, P. A. and Domesick, V. B. (1983) Haloperidol-induced plasticity of axon terminals in rat substantia nigra. *Science, 221*, 969–971.

Benes, F. M., Paskevich, P. A., Davidson, J. and Domesick, V. B. (1985*a*) The effects of haloperidol on synaptic patterns in the rat striatum. *Brain Research, 329*, 265–274.

Benes, F. M., Paskevich, P. A., Davidson, J. and Domesick, V. B. (1985*b*) Synaptic re-arrangements in medial prefrontal cortex of haloperidol-treated rats. *Brain Research, 348*, 15–20.

Calverley, R. K. S. and Jones, D. G. (1990) Contributions of dendritic spines and perforated synapses to synaptic plasticity. *Brain Research Reviews, 15*, 215–249.

Chakos, M. H., Lieberman, J. A., Bilder, R. M. *et al.* (1994) Increase in caudate nucleus volumes of first-episode schizophrenic patients taking antipsychotic drugs. *American Journal of Psychiatry, 151*, 1430–1436.

Chakos, M. H., Shirakawa, O., Lieberman, J., Lee, H., Bilder, R. and Tamminga, C. A. (1998) Striatal enlargement in rats chronically treated with neuroleptics. *Biological Psychiatry, 44*, 675–684.

Christensen, E., Moller, J. E. and Faurbye, A. (1970) Neuropathological investigation of 28 brains from patients with dyskinesia. *Acta Psychiatrica Scandinavica, 46*, 14–23.

Dawirs, R. R., Teuchert-Noodt, G. and Molthagen, M. (1993) Indication of methamphetamine-induced reactive synaptogenesis in the prefrontal cortex of gerbils (*Meriones unguiculatus*). *European Journal of Pharmacology, 241*, 89–97.

Devenand, D. P., Dwork, A. J., Hutchinson, E. R., Bolwig, T. G. and Sackeim, H. A. (1994) Does ECT alter brain structure? *American Journal of Psychiatry, 151*, 957–970.

Doraiswamy, P. M., Tupler, L. A. and Krishnan, K. R. R. (1995) Neuroleptic treatment and caudate plasticity. *Lancet, 345*, 734–735.

Eastwood, S. L., Burnet, P. W. J. and Harrison, P. J. (1994) Striatal synaptophysin expression and haloperidol-induced synaptic plasticity. *Neuroreport, 5*, 677–680.

Eastwood, S. L., Burnet, P. W. J. and Harrison, P. J. (1995) Altered synaptophysin expression as a marker of synaptic pathology in schizophrenia. *Neuroscience, 66*, 309–319.

Eastwood, S. L., Heffernan, J. and Harrison, P. J. (1997) Chronic haloperidol treatment differentially affects the expression of synaptic and neuronal plasticity-associated genes. *Molecular Psychiatry, 2*, 322–329.

Eastwood, S. L., Burnet, P. W. J. and Harrison, P. J. (2000) Expression of complexin I and II mRNAs and their regulation by antipsychotic drugs in the rat forebrain. *Synapse 36*, 167–177.

Enns, M., Peeling, J. and Sutherland G. R. (1996) Hippocampal neurons are damaged by caffeine-augmented electroshock seizures. *Biological Psychiatry,* **40**, 642–647.

Fog, R., Pakkenberg, H., Juul, P., Jorgensen, O. S. and Andersen, J. (1976) High dose treatment of rats with perphenazine enanthate. *Psychopharmacology,* **50**, 305–307.

Gariano, R. F., Young, S. J., Jeste, D. V., Segal, D. S. and Groves, P. M. (1990) Effects of long-term administration of haloperidol on electrophysiologic properties of rat mesencephalic neurons. *Journal of Pharmacology and Experimental Therapeutics,* **255**, 108–113.

Genisman, Y., Morrell, F. and DeToledo-Morrell, L. (1989) Perforated synapses on double-headed dendritic spines. A possible structural substrate of synaptic plasticity. *Brain Research,* **480**, 326–329.

Gerlach, J. (1975) Long-term effect of perphenazine on the substantia nigra in rats. *Psychopharmacology,* **45**, 51–54.

Harding, A. J., Wong, A., Svoboda, M., Kril, J. J. and Halliday, G. M. (1997) Chronic alcohol consumption does not cause hippocampal neuron loss in humans. *Hippocampus,* **7**, 78–87.

Harper, C. G. and Kril, J. J. (1990) Neuropathology of alcoholism. *Alcohol Alcoholism,* **25**, 207–216.

Harrison, P. J. (1997) Schizophrenia and its dementia. In: Esiri M. M. and Morris J. H. (eds). *The neuropathology of dementia.* Cambridge, Cambridge University Press, pp. 385–397.

Harrison, P. J. (1999*a*) Neurochemical alterations in schizophrenia affecting the putative receptor targets of atypical antipsychotics: Focus on dopamine (D_1, D_3, D_4) and 5-HT_{2A} receptors. *British Journal of Psychiatry,* **174** (Suppl. 38), 12–22.

Harrison, P. J. (1999*b*) The neuropathology of schizophrenia. A critical review of the data and their interpretation. *Brain,* **122**, 593–624.

Higaki, J., Murphy, G. M. Jr and Cordell, B. (1997) Inhibition of β-amyloid formation by haloperidol: a possible mechanism for reduced frequency of Alzheimer's disease pathology in schizophrenia. *Journal of Neurochemistry,* **68**, 333–336.

Holt, D. J., Herman, M. M., Hyde, T. M. *et al.* (1999) Evidence for a deficit in cholinergic interneurons in the striatum in schizophrenia. *Neuroscience,* **94**, 21–31.

Ibanez, J., Herrero, M. T., Insausti, R. *et al.* (1995) Chronic alcoholism decreases neuronal nuclear size in the human entorhinal cortex. *Neuroscience Letters,* **183**, 71–74.

Ihara, Y., Sato, M., Otsuki, S., Kaiya, H. and Namba, M. (1986) Morphological changes in rat striatal boutons after chronic methamphetamine and haloperidol treatment. *Neuroscience Research,* **3**, 403–410.

Jellinger, K. (1977) Neuropathologic findings after neuroleptic long-term therapy. In: Roizin, L., Shiraki, H. and Grcevic, N. (eds) *Neurotoxicology.* New York, Raven Press, pp. 25–42.

Jellinger, K. and Gabriel, E. (1999) No increased incidence of Alzheimer's disease in elderly schizophrenics. *Acta Neurpathologica,* **97**, 165–169.

Jensen, G. B. and Pakkenberg, B. (1993) Do alcoholics drink their neurons away? *Lancet,* **342**, 1201–1204.

Jeste, D. V., Lohr, J. B. and Manley, M. (1992) Study of neuropathologic changes in the striatum following 4, 8 and 12 months of treatment with fluphenazine in rats. *Psychopharmacology (Berlin)* **106**, 154–160.

Jeste, D. V., Lohr, J. B., Eastham, J. M. *et al.* (1998) Adverse neurobiological effects of long-term use of neuroleptics: human and animal studies. *Journal of Psychiatric Research,* **32**, 201–214.

Jorgensen, O. and Bolwig, T. G. (1979) Synaptic proteins after electroconvulsive stimulation. *Science,* **205**, 705–707.

Kelley, J. J., Gao, X. M., Tamminga, C. A. and Roberts, R. C. (1997) The effect of chronic haloperidol treatment on dendritic spines in the rat striatum. *Experimental Neurology,* **146**, 471–478.

Keshavan, M. S., Bagwell, W. W., Haas, G. L., Sweeney, J. A., Schooler, N. R. and Pettegrew, J. W. (1994) Changes in caudate volume with neuroleptic treatment. *Lancet,* **344**, 1434.

Klintzova, A. J., Haselhorst, U., Uranova, N. A., Schenk, H. and Istomin, V. V. (1989) The effects of haloperidol on synaptic plasticity in rat's medial prefrontal cortex. *Journal für Hirnforschung,* **30**, 51–57.

Korbo, L. (1999) Glial cell loss in the hippocampus of alcoholics. *Alcohol: Clinical and Experimental Research,* **23**, 164–168.

Kril, J. J., Halliday, G. M., Svoboda, M. D. and Cartwright, H. (1997) The cerebral cortex is damaged in chronic alcoholics. *Neuroscience,* **79**, 983–998.

Kroesen, S., Marksteiner, J., Mahata, S. K. *et al.* (1995) Effects of haloperidol, clozapine and citalopram on messenger RNA levels of chromogranins A and B and secretogranin II in various regions of rat brain. *Neuroscience,* **69**, 881–891.

Kung, L. and Roberts, R. C. (1999) Mitochondrial pathology in human schizophrenic striatum: a postmortem ultrastructural study. *Synapse,* **31**, 67–75.

Kung, L., Conley, R., Chute, D. J., Smialek, J. and Roberts, R. C. (1998) Synaptic changes in the striatum of schizophrenic cases: A controlled postmortem ultrastructural study. *Synapse,* **28**, 125–139.

Licht, R. W., Larsen J. O., Smith, D. and Brændgaard, H. (1994) Effect of chronic lithium treatment with or without haloperidol on number and sizes of neurons in rat neocortex. *Psychopharmacology,* **115**, 371–374.

Madsen, A. L., Keiding, N., Karle, A., Esbjerg, S. and Hemmingsen, R. (1998) Neuroleptics in progressive structural brain abnormalities in psychiatric illness. *Lancet,* **352**, 784–785.

Manji, H. K., Moore, G. J. and Chen, G. (1999) Lithium at 50: Have the neuroprotective effects of this unique cation been overlooked? *Biological Psychiatry,* **46**, 929–940.

Marin, C. and Tolosa, E. (1997) Striatal synaptophysin levels are not indicative of dopaminergic supersensitivity. *Neuropharmacology,* **36**, 1115–1117.

Meshul, C. K. and Casey, D. E. (1989) Regional, reversible ultrastructural changes in rat brain with chronic neuroleptic treatment. *Brain Research,* **489**, 338–346.

Meshul, C. K., Janowsky, A., Casey, D. E., Stallbaumer, R. K. and Taylor, B. (1992) Coadministration of haloperidol and SCH-23390 prevents the increase in 'perforated' synapses due to either drug alone. *Neuropsychopharmacology,* **7**, 285–293.

Meshul, C. K., Stallbaumer, R. K., Taylor, B. and Janowsky, A. (1994) Haloperidol-induced morphological changes in striatum are associated with glutamate synapses. *Brain Research,* **648**, 181–195.

Meshul, C. K., Bunker, G. L., Mason, J. N., Allen, C. and Janowsky, A. (1996) Effects of subchronic clozapine and haloperidol on striatal glutamatergic synapses. *Journal of Neurochemistry,* **67**, 1965–1973.

Mijnster, M. J., Ingham, C. A., Meredith, G. E., Doctor, G. J. and Arbuthnott, G. W. (1996) Morphological changes in met^5-enkephalin-immunoreactive synaptic boutons in the rat neostriatum after haloperidol decanoate treatment. *European Journal of Neuroscience,* **8**, 716–726.

Miller, R. and Chouinard, G. (1993) Loss of striatal cholinergic neurons as a basis for tardive and L-dopa-induced dyskinesias, neuroleptic supersensitivity psychosis and refractory schizophrenia. *Biological Psychiatry*, **34**, 713–738.

Nakahara, T., Nakamura, K., Tsutsumi, T. *et al.* (1998) Effect of chronic haloperidol treatment on synaptic protein mRNAs in the rat brain. *Molecular Brain Research,* **61**, 238–242.

Nielsen, C. B. and Lyon, M. (1978) Evidence for cell loss in corpus striatum after long-term treatment with a neuroleptic drug (flupenthixol) in rats. *Psychopharmacology,* **59**, 85–89.

Orzi, F., Zoli, M., Passarelli, F., Ferraguti, F., Fieschi, C. and Agnati, L. F. (1990) Repeated electroconvulsive shock increases glial fibrillary acidic protein, ornithine decarboxylase, somatostatin and cholecystokinin immunoreactivities in the hippocampal formation of the rat. *Brain Research Reviews*, **533**, 223–231.

Pakkenberg, B. (1989) What happens in the leucotomised brain? A post-mortem morphological study of brains from schizophrenic patients. *Journal of Neurology, Neurosurgery, and Psychiatry,* **52**, 156–161.

Pakkenberg, H., Fog, R. and Nilakantan, B. (1973) The long-term effect of perphenazine enanthate on the rat brain. Some metabolic and anatomical observations. *Psychopharmacologia (Berlin),* **29**, 329–336.

Pei, Q., Burnet, P. W. J. and Zetterström, T. S. C. (1998) Changes in mRNA abundance of microtubule-associated proteins in the rat brain following electroconvulsive shock. *Neuroreport*, **9**, 391–394.

Peters, A. and Palay, S. L. (1986) The morphology of synapses. *Journal of Neurocytology,* **25**, 687–700.

Pierce, J. P. and Lewin, G. R. (1994) An ultrastructural size principle. *Neuroscience,* **58**, 441–446.

Purohit, D. P., Perl, D. P., Haroutunian, V., Powchik, P., Davidson, M. and Davis, K. L. (1998) Alzheimer disease and related neurodegenerative diseases in elderly patients with schizophrenia. *Archives of General Psychiatry,* **55**, 205–211.

Roberts, R. C., Gaither, L. A., Gao, X. M., Kashyap, S. M. and Tamminga, C. A. (1995) Ultrastructural correlates of haloperidol-induced oral dyskinesias in rat striatum. *Synapse,* **20**, 234–243.

Roberts, R. C., Conley, R., Kung, L., Peretti, F. J. and Chute, D. J. (1996) Reduced striatal spine size in schizophenia: a postmortem ultrastructural study. *Neuroreport,* **7**, 1214–1218.

Robinson, T. E. and Kolb, B. (1999) Morphine alters the structure of neurons in the nucleus accumbens and neocortex of rats. *Synapse,* **33**, 160–162.

Rocha, E. and Rodnight, R. (1994) Chronic administration of lithium chloride increases immunodetectable glial fibrillary acidic protein in the rat hippocampus. *Journal of Neurochemistry,* **63**, 1582–1584.

Rocha, A. Chaval, M., Santos, P. and Rodnight, R. (1998) Lithium treatment causes gliosis and modifies the morphology of hippocampal astrocytes in rats. *Neuroreport,* **9**, 3971–3974.

Roizin, L. (1972) Histopathologic observations in schizophrenia (including effects of somatic and biochemical therapies). In: Minckler, J. (ed.).*Pathology of the nervous system*, Volume 3. New York, McGraw Hill, pp. 2670–2677.

Schneider, J. A. and Mirra, S. S. (1994) Neuropathologic correlates of persistent neurologic deficit in lithium intoxication. *Annals of Neurology,* **36**, 928–931.

See, R. E., Chapman, M. A. and Meshul, C. K. (1992) Comparison of chronic intermittent haloperidol and raclopride effects on striatal dopamine release and synaptic ultrastructure in rats. *Synapse,* **12**, 147–154.

Selemon, L. D., Lidow, M. S. and Goldman-Rakic, P. S. (1999) Increased volume and glial density in primate prefrontal cortex associated with chronic antipsychotic drug exposure. *Biological Psychiatry,* **46**, 161–172.

Sklair-Tavron, S., Shi, W., Lane, S., Harris, H. W., Bunney, B. S. and Nestler, E. J. (1996) Chronic morphine induces visible changes in the morphology of mesolimbic dopamine neurons. *Proceedings of the National Academy of Sciences USA,* **93**, 11202–11207.

Sonsalla, P. K., Jochnowitz, N. D., Zeevalk, G. D., Oostveen, J. A. and Hall, E. D. (1996) Treatment of mice with methamphetamine produces cell loss in the substantia nigra. *Brain Research,* **738**, 172–175.

Steward, O. (1994) Electroconvulsive seizures upregulate astroglial gene expression selectively in the dentate gyrus. *Molecular Brain Research*, **25**, 217–224.

Takeichi, M. (1985) Electron microscopic morphometric studies on synaptic vesicles of long-term CPZ-administered rat striatum. *Folia Psychiatrica Neurologica Japonica*, **39**, 185–192.

Ueda, K., Tayami, T., Asakura, K. and Kawasaki, K. (1997) Chlorpromazine reduces toxicity and Ca^{2+} uptake induced by amyloid (protein (25–35) *in vitro. Brain Research,* **748**, 184–188.

Uranova, N. A., Orlovskaya, D. D., Apel, K., Klintsova, A. J., Haselhurst, U. and Schenk, H. (1991) Morphometric study of synaptic patterns in the rat caudate nucleus and hippocampus under haloperidol treatment. *Synapse*, **7**, 253–259.

Uranova, N. A., Casanova, M. F., DeVaughn, N. M., Orlovskawa, D. D. and Denisov, D. V. (1996) Ultrastructural alterations of synaptic contacts and astrocytes in postmortem caudate nucleus of schizophrenic patients. *Schizophrenia Research,* **22**, 81–83.

Vincent, S. L., McSparren, J., Wang, R. and Benes, F. M. (1991) Evidence for ultrastructural changes in cortical axo-dendritic synapses following longterm treatment with haloperidol or clozapine. *Neuropsychopharmacology*, **5**, 147–155.

Vincent, S. L., Adamec, E., Sorensen, I. and Benes, F. M. (1994) The effects of chronic haloperidol administration on GABA-immunoreactive axon terminals in rat medial prefrontal cortex. *Synapse*, **17**, 26–35.

Wisniewski, H. M., Constantinidis, J., Wegiel, J., Bobinski, M. and Tarnawski, M. (1994) Neurofibrillary pathology in brains of elderly schizophrenics treated with neuroleptics. *Alzheimer's Disease and Associated Disorders,* **8**, 211–227.

Wischik, C. M., Edwards, P. C., Lai, R. Y. K., Roth, M. and Harrington, C. R. (1996) Selective inhibition of Alzheimer disease-like tau aggregation by phenothiazines. *Proceedings of the National Academy of Sciences of the USA,* **93**, 11213–11218.

Index

Numbers in **bold** indicate the pages particularly relevant to the entry